ESTROGEN AND BREAST CANCER

W.R. Miller

ICRF Medical Oncology Unit
University Department of Clinical Oncology
Western General Hospital
Edinburgh, Scotland

MEDICAL
INTELLIGENCE
UNIT

ESTROGEN AND BREAST CANCER

W.R. Miller

ICRF Medical Oncology Unit
University Department of Clinical Oncology
Western General Hospital
Edinburgh, Scotland

CHAPMAN & HALL
ITP An International Thomson Publishing Company

New York • Albany • Bonn • Boston • Cincinnati • Detroit • London • Madrid • Melbourne •
Mexico City • Pacific Grove • Paris • San Francisco • Singapore • Tokyo • Toronto • Washington

R.G. LANDES COMPANY
AUSTIN

Medical Intelligence Unit
Estrogen and Breast Cancer

R.G. Landes Company
Austin, Texas, U.S.A.

Please address all inquiries to the Publishers:
R.G. Landes Company, 909 Pine Street, Georgetown, Texas, U.S.A. 78626
Phone: 512/ 863 7762; FAX: 512/ 863 0081

North American distributor:
Chapman & Hall, 115 Fifth Avenue, New York, New York, U.S.A. 10003

International distributor (except North America):
Springer-Verlag GmbH & Co. KG, Tiergartenstrasse 17, D-69121 Heidelberg, Germany

U.S. and Canada ISBN: 0-412-10371-0
International ISBN: 3-540-60777-3

While the authors, editors and publisher believe that drug selection and dosage and the specifications and usage of equipment and devices, as set forth in this book, are in accord with current recommendations and practice at the time of publication, they make no warranty, expressed or implied, with respect to material described in this book. In view of the ongoing research, equipment development, changes in governmental regulations and the rapid accumulation of information relating to the biomedical sciences, the reader is urged to carefully review and evaluate the information provided herein.

Library of Congress Cataloging-in-Publication Data

Miller, W.R., 1944-
    Estrogen and breast cancer / W.R. Miller
      p. cm. — (Medical intelligence unit)
    Includes bibliographical references and index.
    ISBN 0-412-10371-0 (hardcover)
    1. Breast Cancer—risk factors. 2. Estrogen—adverse effects. 3. Estrogen—physiological effects. I. Title. II. Series.
      [DNLM: 1. Breast Neoplasms—etiology. 2. Intestinal Mucosa—cytology.
      3. Breast Neoplasms—pathology. 4. Estrogens—physiology. 5. Breast—physiology.
      WP 870 1996]
RC280.B8M55 1996
616.99'449071—dc20
DNLM/DLC
for Library of Congress
                                           95-49772
                                              CIP

PUBLISHER'S NOTE

R.G. Landes Company publishes six book series: *Medical Intelligence Unit, Molecular Biology Intelligence Unit, Neuroscience Intelligence Unit, Tissue Engineering Intelligence Unit, Environmental Intelligence Unit* and *Biotechnology Intelligence Unit.* The authors of our books are acknowledged leaders in their fields and the topics are unique. Almost without exception, no other similar books exist on these topics.

Our goal is to publish books in important and rapidly changing areas of bioscience for sophisticated researchers and clinicians. To achieve this goal, we have accelerated our publishing program to conform to the fast pace in which information grows in bioscience. Most of our books are published within 90 to 120 days of receipt of the manuscript. We would like to thank our readers for their continuing interest and welcome any comments or suggestions they may have for future books.

Deborah Muir Molsberry
Publications Director
R.G. Landes Company

Dedication

To my late father, Bob Miller, for his encouragement to complete this monograph.

CONTENTS

1. **Introduction** 1
   Estrogens 1
   Breast Cancer 12

2. **Estrogens and the Normal Breast** 25
   Estrogens and Breast Development at Puberty 25
   The Mature Resting Breast 27
   Estrogen and Breast Involution at Menopause 29
   Summary 32

3. **Estrogens and the Risk of Breast Cancer** 35
   Epidemiological Evidence 35
   Clinico-Pathological Evidence 43
   Endocrinological Evidence 44
   Metabolic Evidence 50
   Molecular Evidence 51
   Estrogens as Initiators 52
   Estrogens as Co-Initiators/Promoters 52
   Conclusions 53

4. **Estrogen and Tumor Behavior** 63
   Epidemiological Evidence 63
   Clinico-Pathological Evidence 65
   Endocrinological Evidence 66
   Metabolic Data 68
   Molecular Evidence 68
   Conclusions 69

5. **Sources of Estrogen and Sites of Biosynthesis** 75
   Exogenous Sources of Estrogens 76
   Glandular Synthesis of Estrogen 78
   Adrenal Cortex 81
   Extraglandular Synthesis 81
   Summary 88

6. **Levels and Patterns of Estrogen Within the Breast,
   Its Fluids and Tissues** 95
   Introduction 95
   Milk 95
   Nipple Aspirates 96
   Breast Cyst Fluids 98
   Breast Tissues 102
   General Findings 102
   Specific Details 103

Mechanism of Accumulation 106
Summary 107

7. Mechanism of Estrogen Action 111
Estrogen Receptors.. 111
Nucleic Acid Synthesis 113
Secretion of Polypeptide Growth Factors 113
Production of Proteolytic Enzymes 116
Oncogenes 117
Summary 118

8. Estrogens and Endocrine Therapy for Breast Cancer 125
Historical Background 125
Ovarian Ablation 126
Adrenal and Pituitary Ablation.. 127
LHRH Agonist Analogues 128
Additive Therapy with Estrogens 132
Antiestrogens 132
Aromatase Inhibitors.. 137
Novel Methods of Estrogen Deprivation 142
Future Perspectives 143

9. Prediction of Estrogen Sensitivity/Dependence 151
Estrogen Receptors.. 151
Relationship Between Estrogen Receptors and Response
    to Endocrine Therapy for Advanced Breast Cancer 153
Estrogen Receptors and Prognosis
    in Patients with Early Breast Cancer 155
Progesterone Receptors 158
pS2 160
Estrogen Inducible Genes 160
HSP27 (Heat Shock Protein 27,000) 161
Type I Tyrosine Kinase Receptors 162
Summary 162

10. Estrogen Independence 171
Primary Resistance 171
Acquired Resistance 171
Resistance Associated with Individual Types of Estrogen
    Deprivation 179
Association with Other Features of Aggressive Behavior 186
Summary 187

11. Future Perspectives 197

Estrogen and the Normal Breast 198

Estrogens and Risk of Breast Cancer 198

Estrogens and Tumor Behavior 199

Sources of Estrogen 199

Levels and Patterns of Estrogen in the Breast 200

Mechanism of Estrogen Action 200

Estrogen Deprivation Therapy 200

Prediction of Estrogen Sensitivity/Dependencies 201

Resistance to Endocrine Therapy 201

Summary 202

Index 205

ACKNOWLEDGMENT

I wish to recognize the support of colleagues in the Edinburgh Breast Unit and thank Mark Miller for the more illustrative figures. Lastly, gratitude is extended to my secretary, Norma White, without whose patience and endeavor this monograph would not have appeared in print.

This book is about (i) the involvement of estrogenic hormones in the development of the normal breast and (ii) the evidence that both exogenous and endogenous estrogens influence carcinogenesis within the breast and the behavior of established cancers. Consideration will be given to sources of estrogen, sites of biosynthesis and patterns of endogenous estrogens within the breast, its fluids and tissues. The mechanism by which estrogens are synthesized and exert their action within breast cancers will be described. It will be illustrated how a greater knowledge of the biology behind such processes as derived from studies of model systems and clinical material, has lead to the development of novel therapies for patients with breast cancer and preventative measures for women at high risk to the disease. The current status of estrogen deprivation therapy in the treatment of breast cancer will be assessed, together with the markers of estrogen action and sensitivity, which may help define patients most likely to respond to endocrine therapy and lead to the discovery of why most cancers subsequently escape from such maneuvers.

CHAPTER 1

INTRODUCTION

ESTROGENS

INTRODUCTION

Estrogens are classically regarded as female sex hormones, capable, as the name suggests, of inducing estrus. However, while estrogens do have a major role in the control of reproductive function and development of secondary sex characteristics in women, they have an impact far beyond this and may also influence the development and/or function of tissues, such as skin, bone, liver and the reticulo-endothelial system. Since these in turn have profound effects on a host of other organs, there are few tissues which are not affected by estrogens. Thus, the effects of estrogens are extraordinarily widespread and they should not be regarded as exclusively female, since estrogens are also produced by males.

STRUCTURE

As is shown in Figure 1.1, the most important naturally occurring estrogens are C18 steroids. All have an aromatic A ring which is phenolic in unconjugated estrogens. Estradiol-17β is the most potent natural estrogen but estrone and its sulfate predominate in the circulation especially after the menopause and in men; estriol and its glucuronide are produced in large amounts during pregnancy by the fetal-placental unit.

SYNTHESIS

The general pathway of biosynthesis of estradiol from cholesterol is depicted in Figure 1.2. This comprises a series of degradative steps whereby cholesterol, a C27 sterol is successively converted by (i) partial removal of the side chain of the D ring into C21 steroids (progestogens and corticoids), (ii) completion of removal of the D ring side chain to C19 steroids (androgens) and finally (iii) removal of the methyl group between the A and B ring into the C18 steroids (estrogens). The mechanism by which these transformations are achieved have in common hydroxylation by mixed function oxidases, but each

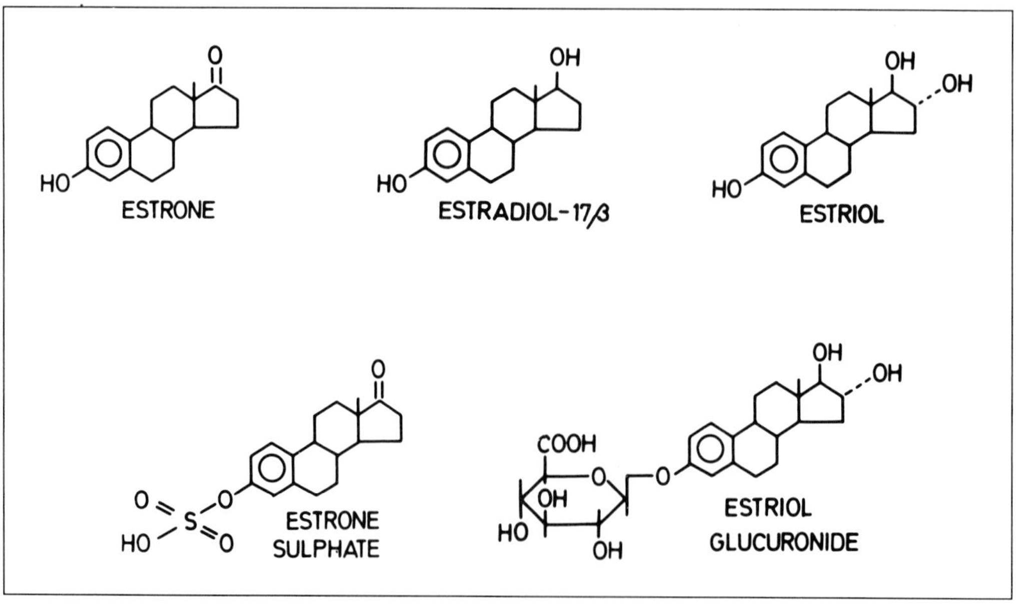

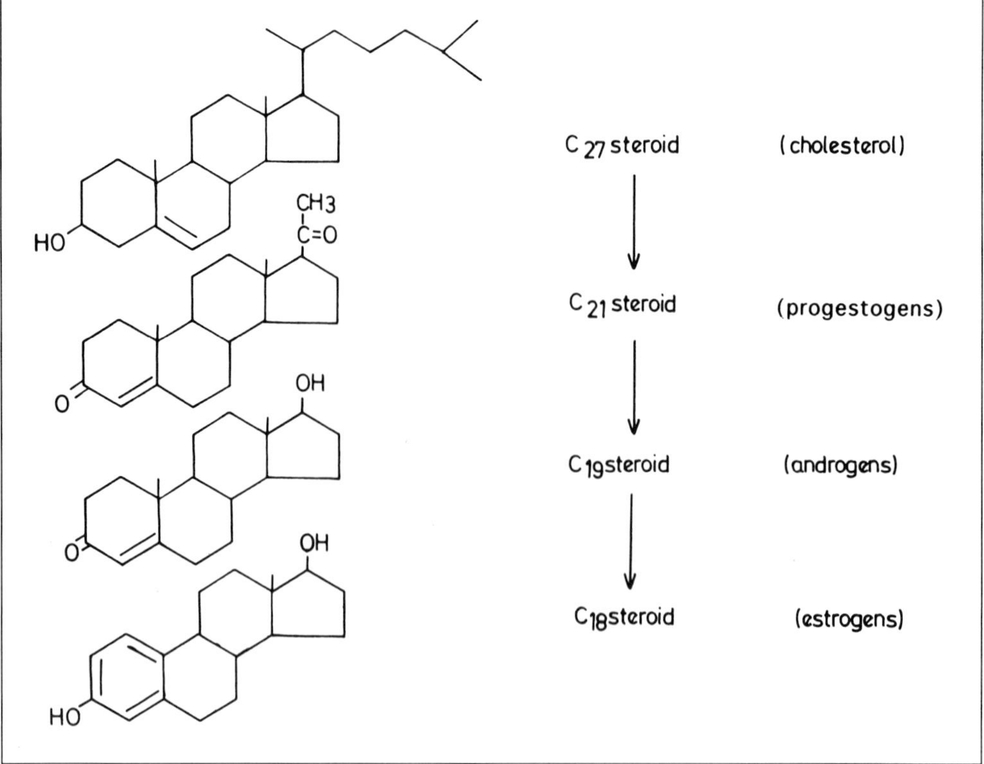

Fig. 1.1. The structure of common estrogens.

Fig. 1.2. Pathway of estrogen biosynthesis.

step is catalyzed by a different enzyme. The first step of cholesterol side-chain cleavage is rate-limiting but the last step in the sequence is unique to estrogen biosynthesis and is potentially most interesting. Thus, the removal of the methyl group between the A and B rings involves three hydroxylations, all of which utilize molecular oxygen and the reduced co-factor, NADPH. Generation of the latter involves a NADP reductase and a transfer of electrons to a specific cytochrome p450. Because the steroid A ring becomes aromatic during the removal of the methyl group, the enzyme is known as aromatase and the specific cytochrome p450, cyto p450 AROM. The aromatase reaction may utilize several androgen substrates for estrogen production; the examples shown in Figure 1.3 are the conversion of Δ4-androstenedione to estrone and testosterone to estradiol. Both transformations are thought to be catalyzed by the same enzyme molecule; indeed there seems to be a single human gene for aromatase, its product being responsible for all estrogen synthesis irrespective of androgen substrate or site of synthesis. In many tissues, androstenedione seems to be the preferred substrate for aromatization and under these conditions, full estrogenic activity

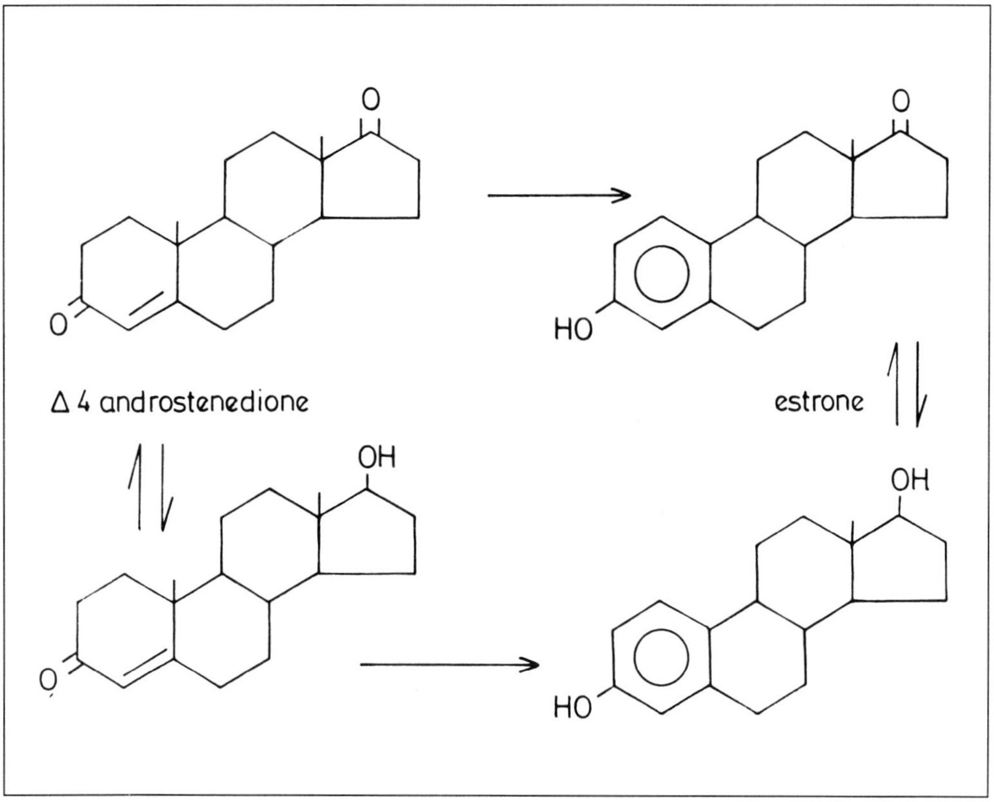

Fig. 1.3. Aromatization of androgens (Δ4-androstenedione and testosterone) to estrogens (estrone and estradiol).

requires the resulting estrone to be converted into estradiol by the enzyme, estrogen 17β dehydrogenase. However, as will be discussed later, the central role of aromatase in estrogen biosynthesis has led to development of specific inhibitors for the enzyme.

SITE OF SYNTHESIS

The major sources of estrogens are shown in Table 1.1. Thus it can be seen that in premenopausal women the ovary appears to be the primary site of estrogen biosynthesis and it has been calculated that it is responsible for between 100 and 500 μg estrogen/day depending upon the stage in the menstrual cycle. Nevertheless, during the follicular phase of the menstrual cycle, non-ovarian sources can account for about 50% of estrone. Peripheral synthesis of estrogen also assumes particular importance in women after the menopause when ovarian biosynthesis virtually ceases. However, the postmenopausal ovary may still produce substantial amounts of androgen which can be used as substrate for synthesis of estrogen at peripheral sites. These sites include fat, skin, muscle, liver and breast cancers. The adrenal cortex may also synthesize small amounts of estrogen but, like the postmenopausal ovary, its major contribution appears to be production of androgen precursor.

PRODUCTION AND LEVELS

Premenopausal Women

The complex neural and endocrine factors which regulate ovarian estrogen secretion throughout the menstrual cycle develop gradually over a number of years prior to the onset of puberty. Random fluctuations in circulating estradiol are seen early in puberty and, in mid-puberty occasional rhythmic fluctuations occur, marking the appearance of cyclical hormonal patterns. Longitudinal studies reveal a progressive rise in concentration of circulating gonadotrophins and estradiol in girls between the ages of 8 and 18 years.[1] Plasma estradiol concentrations correlate with sexual development.

The cyclical nature of hormones in the normal premenopausal woman is depicted in Figure 1.4. Following ovulation, the relatively high concentration of plasma follicle stimulating hormone (FSH) promotes the

Table 1.1. Sources of estrogen in women

Subject Status	Source	Amount (μg/day)
Premenopausal	ovary	100-500
Pregnant	fetal placental unit	35,000
Postmenopausal	peripheral tissues	15

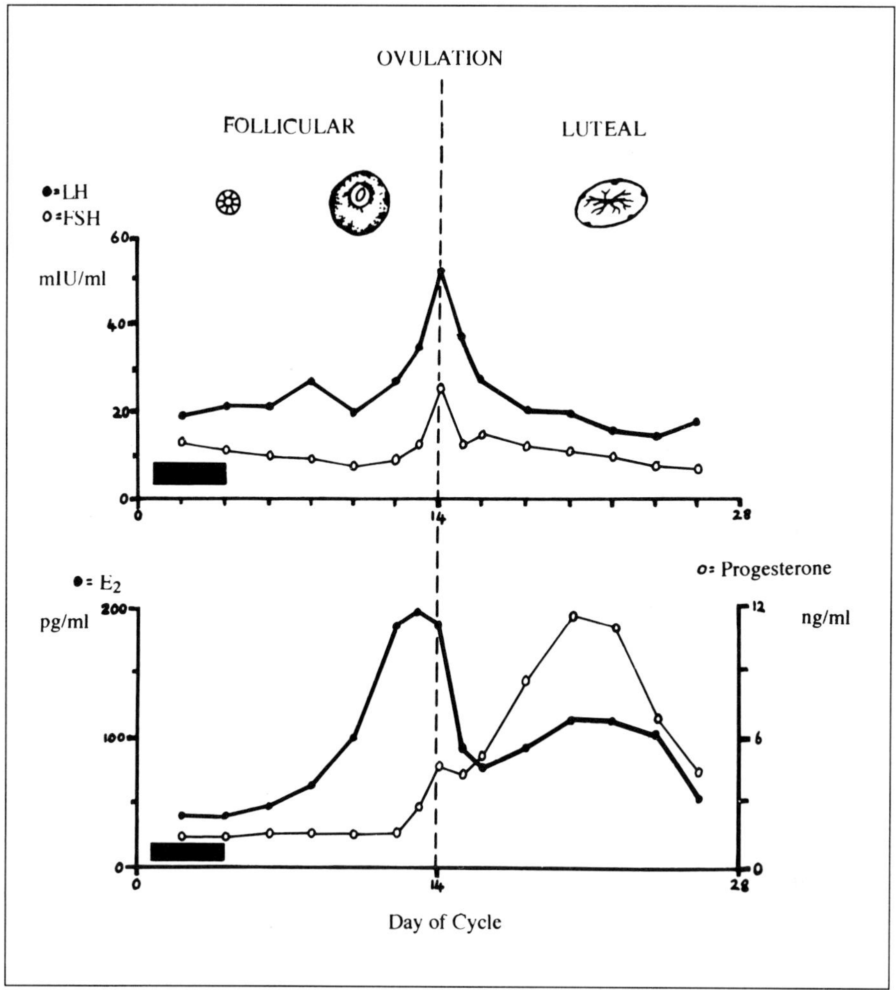

Fig. 1.4. Circulating hormone levels during the menstrual cycle of premenopausal women.

development of a new ovarian follicle. The thecal cells of the developing follicle produce estrogen and midway through the follicular phase of the menstrual cycle plasma levels of estradiol increase. This rise subsequently triggers the rapid mid-cycle release of gonadotrophins, particularly luteinizing hormone (LH) which results in ovulation. Estrogen levels fall immediately after ovulation but rise again in the luteal phase of the menstrual cycle as a consequence of synthesis by the corpus luteum. Towards the end of the luteal phase estrogen levels decline and a new cycle begins.

While the cyclical patterns of estrogens in premenopausal women are solely the consequence of ovarian activity, levels in the circulation are the sum of direct ovarian secretion of estradiol and estrone, plus peripheral conversion of C19 precursors such as androstenedione into estrogens. Since androstenedione is secreted in milligram amounts, even a small peripheral conversion can result in a significant contribution to estrogens which exist and function in microgram amounts. For example, because the production of androstenedione is about 3 mg/day, and the peripheral conversion of androstenedione to estrone is 1%, this route could account for 30 µg or 20-30% of the estrone produced per day.

The plasma levels and production rates of estrone and estradiol in menstruating females are shown in Table 1.2. The cyclical patterns of estrone and estradiol in plasma are basically similar (a tendency for lower levels in the follicular phase and raised concentrations mid-cycle) but peak levels of estradiol always exceed those of estrone. As might be expected from circulating levels of estrogen, production is lowest during the follicular phase increasing 2- to 6-fold during the luteal phase of the menstrual cycle. Highest production rates are observed at the time of ovulation. There is also evidence that estradiol is secreted episodically throughout the day.[2]

Estrone sulfate is the most abundant plasma estrogen being present at 5- to 10-fold the concentration of estradiol and 10- to 15-fold that of estrone. It displays the same marked cyclical pattern as the unconjugated estrogens.

Postmenopausal Women

At the end of reproductive life, menstrual cycles become irregular and estrogen levels can fluctuate in a haphazard fashion. However, in truly postmenopausal women, circulating estrogen are low (Table 1.2)

Table 1.2. Levels and production rates of estrogens in women

	Production Rate (µg/24 h)	Levels (ng/100 ml)
Estradiol		
Premenopausal		
Follicular	65	5.0
Midcycle	400	30.0
Luteal	250	17.5
Postmenopausal	15	1.7
Estrone		
Premenopausal		
Follicular	70	5.0
Midcycle	250	17.0
Luteal	180	11.3
Postmenopausal	60	6.5

and show no cyclical variation. Compared with premenopausal women, production of estradiol is greatly reduced while the production rate of estrone remains similar to that in the follicular phase of the menstrual cycle (Table 1.2). This is because after the menopause the ovaries produce little estrogen and plasma estradiol levels after ovariectomy are similar to those after the menopause. In contrast, estrone continues to be formed by extraglandular conversion of androstenedione, mainly in fat and muscle. Although these tissues display only low levels of estrogen synthesis, their large mass within the body means that potentially they can produce micrograms of estrogen per day. In vivo perfusion techniques suggest that muscle accounts for up to 30% and adipose tissue up to 15% of peripheral aromatization of androgens to estrogens.[3] Thus positive correlations have been found between body weight indices and plasma estrogen levels in postmenopausal women.[4,5] Factors which control peripheral production of estrogen are largely undefined.

CIRCULATION

Estradiol circulates in blood mainly in the unconjugated state while, in contrast, estrone is mostly present as its sulfate. The latter seems to result from metabolism rather than direct secretion.[6] Estrogens in blood are, however, almost totally bound to plasma proteins (mainly albumin and sex hormone-binding globulin) and only a small fraction (1-3%) is present in an unbound state. Nevertheless it seems to be the unbound estrogen which is biologically active and which is available to enter cells by passive diffusion. Estradiol most strongly associates with sex hormone-binding globulin to which it binds with relatively high affinity (K_A 10^{-8}M); about an equal proportion binds to albumin but this is of a lower affinity (K_A 10^{-4}M). Both unconjugated and sulfated estrone are largely bound to albumin with the binding of estrone sulfate being particularly extensive and of a higher affinity than the unconjugated steroid.

Clearance rates for estradiol are lower than those for estrone reflecting their different affinities for sex hormone-binding globulin and albumin. Estrone sulfate has a clearance rate only 10% of that for unconjugated estrone, probably because of its more extensive binding to albumin and its small metabolic fraction.

METABOLISM

The metabolism of estrogens largely involves the inter-conversion of estradiol, estrone and their conjugates and hydroxylation at various points in the steroid ring. Major routes of metabolism are shown in Figure 1.5. Estrone sulfate is an important circulatory estrogen and is a principal source of other metabolites. Deconjugation leads to estrone which can be transformed into a series of other metabolites. Estrone and estradiol are readily inter-converted by an estrogen 17β dehydrogenase. Hydroxylation at 2, 4 and 16 are major metabolic routes and can lead to the formation of catechol estrogens. The 2- and 4-hydroxy-estrogens have a strong structural similarity with the neurotransmitters, adrenaline and non-adrenaline and it is thus interesting that catechol estrogens may have a key endocrine function in the brain.[7]

The rate at which estrogens are metabolized depends on the sex and body weight of an individual. For example, body weight increases 16α-hydroxylation but decreases 2-hydroxylation.[8] In addition, abnormal functioning of the liver (which is the principal organ metabolizing estrogens) and thyroid can profoundly influence metabolism.[9]

EXCRETION

Like other steroids, estrogens are excreted via the kidneys almost entirely as conjugates (glucuronides and sulfates) and approximately 65% of an administered dose appears in the urine. Some estrogen is excreted into the bile, again mainly as conjugates. Biliary estrogens are in turn secreted into the intestine and are either passed as feces (about 10% of the daily production of estrogen) or re-absorbed to re-enter the blood in an entero-hepatic circulation.

DISTRIBUTION AND UPTAKE INTO TISSUES

Estrogens have been found in many body fluids (blood, urine, bile, sweat) and tissues (placenta, ovary, uterus, testis, adrenal cortex). Following administration of radioactively labelled estradiol to women, distinct patterns of uptake into different tissues can be discerned. One group of tissues, exemplified by muscle, shows rapid uptake of radioactivity (within minutes) but equally levels fall quickly. In the other group,

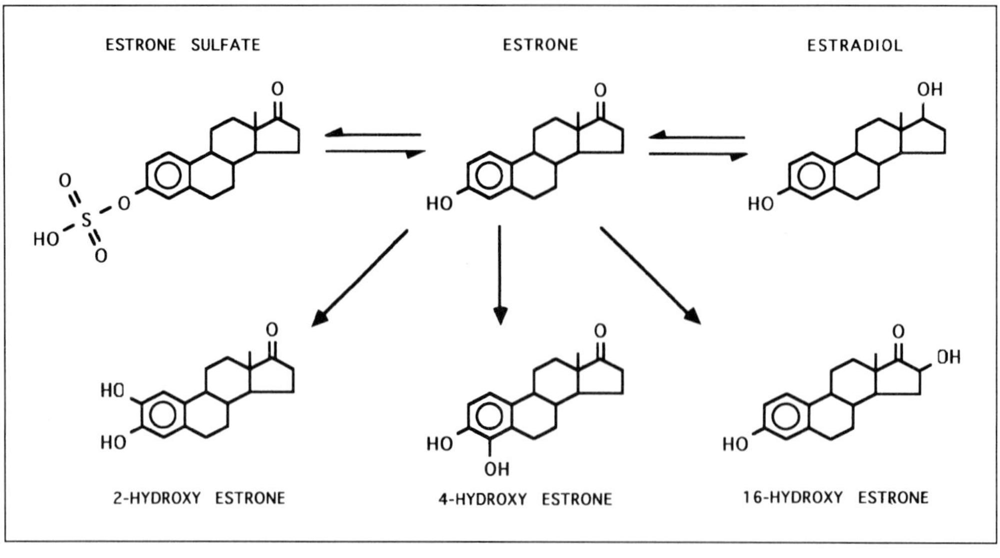

ESTRONE SULFATE   ESTRONE   ESTRADIOL

2-HYDROXY ESTRONE   4-HYDROXY ESTRONE   16-HYDROXY ESTRONE

Fig. 1.5. Major routes of estrogen metabolism.

exemplified by the uterus, uptake is also rapid but estradiol accumulates at levels beyond those in plasma and is retained over a prolonged period (hours). Thus, in endometrium, concentrations of estrone and estradiol are significantly higher than those in plasma in both the proliferative and secretory phase of the cycle. However, it is also interesting to note that whereas levels of estradiol fall in the secretory phase, those of estrone remain constant.[10] Corresponding data for breast tissues and fluids are the subject of chapter 6.

ACTIONS

The actions of estrogens are extraordinarily diverse (Table 1.3). Effects are particularly marked on the ovary, uterus, vagina, pituitary and breast (see Fig. 1.6) but influences on the development and/or function of skin, bone, liver, connective tissue and the reticulo-endothelial system are equally important. Secondary actions on many other tissues leaves virtually no organ unaffected by estrogen. The biochemical actions of estrogen are equally diverse. In target tissues estrogens may increase nucleotide incorporation into DNA, net DNA synthesis, cell number, synthesis of specific proteins, membrane trafficking, mobilization and deposition of lipids. The hepatic synthesis of several important proteins such as thyroxine-binding globulin, corticosteroid-binding globulin, sex hormone-binding globulin, and angiotensinogen appear to be controlled by estrogen. Furthermore, as will be discussed in more detail later, estrogens are able to induce the synthesis and secretion of peptide growth factors which, in turn, have autocrine and paracrine influences including proliferative responses.

MECHANISM OF ACTION

Most effects of estrogen in target organs appear to be mediated through an intracellular receptor which binds estradiol with high affinity ($Kd_{-}10^{10}M^{-1}$). The estrogen receptor appears to be similar in most

---

Table 1.3. Action of estrogen

Increased mitogenic potential	–	Nucleoside incorporation into DNA Thymidine labeling index Net DNA synthesis Cell division
Induced enzyme activity	–	Enzymes concerned with DNA synthesis e.g., thymidine kinase
Induced proteins	–	Progesterone receptor Plasminogen activator Cathepsin D CBG, SHBG, angiotensinogen

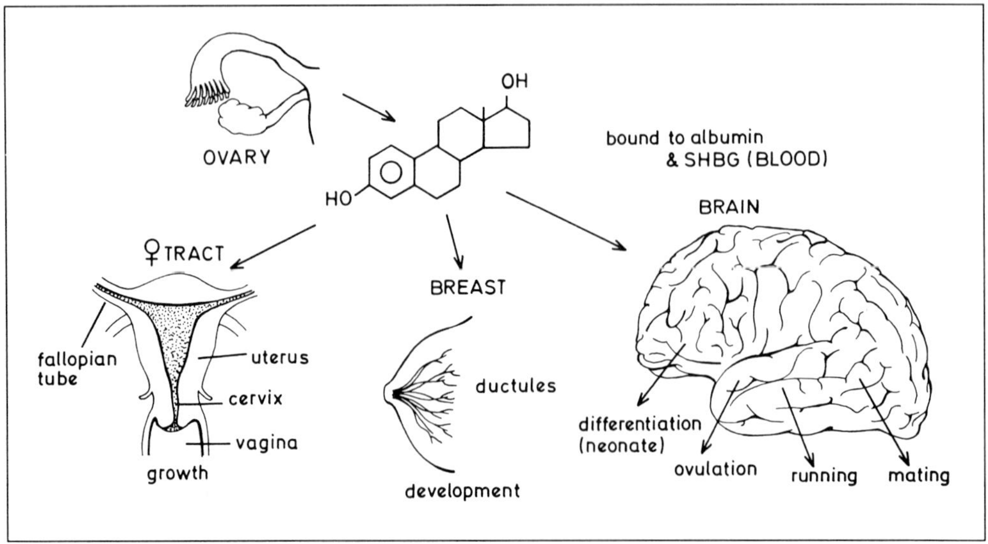

Fig. 1.6. Major target organs of estrogen action.

mammalian target organs and is a protein of about 66,000 kD in molecular weight. Although there has been controversy about the intracellular location of the estrogen receptor, it appears now that the protein primarily resides in the cell nucleus where it acts as a transcription factor. In addition to binding estradiol with high affinity, the molecule also has binding sites which attach to nuclear DNA. Both the binding sites for estrogen and particularly that for the DNA domain, have extensive homology with other receptors including those for androgen, progestogen, corticoids, Vitamin D, thyroid hormones[12] and the ErbA oncogene protein.[13] The binding of estrogen to its receptors causes a conformational change (so-called activation) and then a stabilizing dimerization which allows the complex to bind to chromatin at specific acceptor sites involving non-histone proteins. As a result transcription of DNA occurs and specific estrogen-induced species of mRNA and protein appear.

ESTROGENIC SUBSTANCES

While the classical estrogens are all C18 phenolic steroids, it is also evident that other compounds are capable of having biological effects normally associated with estrogens. Thus C19 steroids of the Δ5 series such as Δ5 androstenediol, dehydro-epiandrosterone and its sulfate (which are all secreted in large amounts by the adrenal cortex) will bind to the estrogen receptor and in certain circumstances will behave as estrogens.[14]

Phytoestrogens are a group of diphenolic compounds of plant origin which comprise two major classes (lignans and isoflavones).[15] The compounds are structurally modified by intestinal bacteria into substances which have estrogenic activity.[16] These include enterolactone, enterodiol, equol, daidzein and genistein (Fig. 1.7) all of which are capable of binding to the estrogen receptor and eliciting estrogenic responses (or anti-estrogenic effects in circumstances in which antagonism of endogenous estrogens occurs).[17]

There are also environmental contaminants of diverse chemical structures which may mimic estrogens. These include nonylphenols derived from surfactants added to detergents, pesticides and toiletries.[18]

SYNTHETIC ESTROGENS

Although estrogens may be given to women either as components of oral contraceptives or to treat menopausal symptoms, natural estrogens are rarely used because of their poor absorption properties and their susceptibility to hepatic metabolism. Synthetic compounds which avoid these characteristics and can be given orally include diethylstilbestrol, ethinyl estradiol and mestranol (Fig. 1.7).

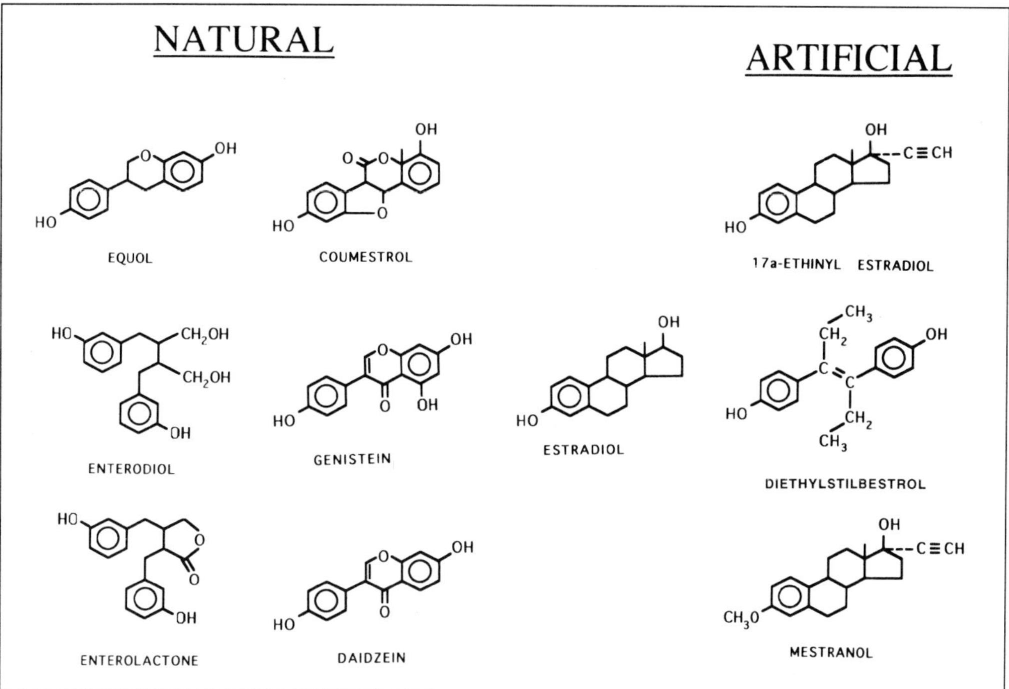

Fig. 1.7. Structure of natural and synthetic compounds with estrogenic activity.

BREAST CANCER

THE PROBLEM

Each year in the USA over 34,000 women die of breast cancer. This is a staggering figure. *The Washington Post* published the thought-provoking comparison that during the ten-year period of the Vietnam war there were 57,000 military casualties while 330,000 women died from breast cancer in the troops' homeland.[19] In the USA, one woman dies from breast cancer every 13 minutes. The statistics in the United Kingdom are no better. Each year 24,000 new cases of breast cancer are diagnosed and 15,000 die from the disease. In the United Kingdom, any individual woman has a life-time risk of 1 in 12 of developing the disease and there are at present 150,000 living women who have been treated for breast cancer. Although being overtaken by lung cancer, breast cancer is the most common female malignancy in developed countries and the most common cause of death among women in the 35 to 55 age group. There have been concerns that incidence is increasing (see Fig. 1.8),[19] although recent epidemiological evidence suggests that in the youngest cohorts of women this may not be so.[20] Nevertheless, it has been estimated that in 1975 over half a million breast cancers were diagnosed worldwide and projected figures suggest that these numbers will increase such that by the year 2000 over a million breast cancers will be detected every year. Breast cancer is thus a huge problem.

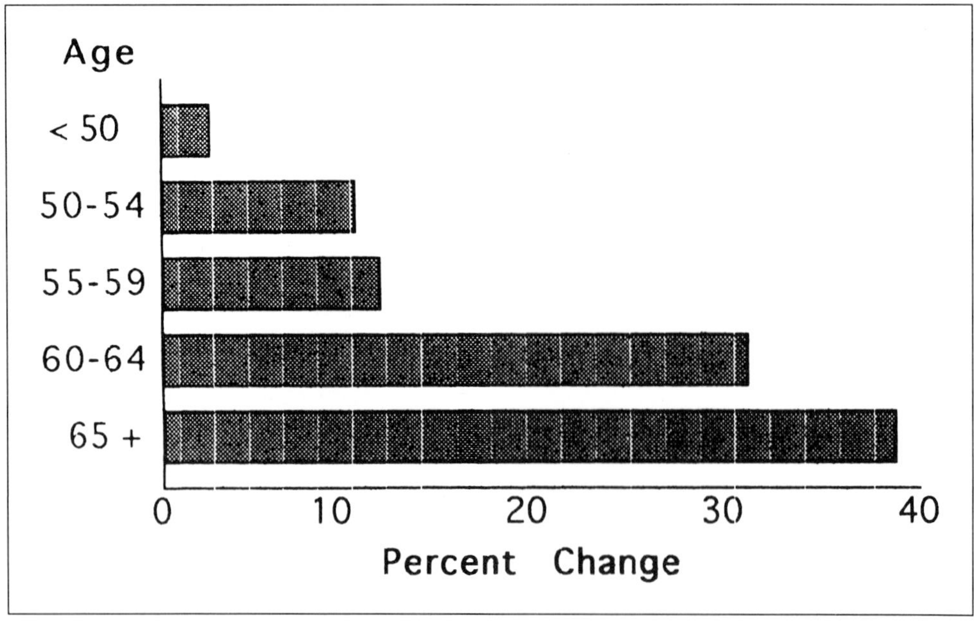

Fig. 1.8. Changes in breast cancer incidence in US females between 1973 and 1989 (age adjusted rates).

RISK FACTORS

The single greatest identified risk factor for breast cancer is to be female. Men do develop breast cancer but the incidence is 100-fold less than that in women. However, there are other factors which have a substantial impact on risk (Table 1.4).

Age

The risk of breast cancer increases with age.[21] The condition is rare before the age of 25 but increases up to the time of the menopause. There is a slight downward trend during the menopausal years but then incidence rises again with advancing years, although at a reduced rate. This age-incidence curve differs from most non-hormone dependent adult cancers which rise continuously and increasingly rapidly with age.

Geographical Variation

There are striking variations in the incidence of breast cancer in different geographical areas.[22] The most marked difference in incidence of breast cancer is between the high rate in the USA and Western Europe and the extremely low rates in South East Asia. Thus, the overall incidence of breast cancer is 5-fold higher in the USA than in Japan. Between these extremes, there are cohorts of countries with intermediate degrees of incidence (Fig. 1.9). The general impression is that the more developed or "Westernized" a country is, the higher the risk of breast cancer. Furthermore, areas within certain individual countries may differ in risk by as much as 2-fold and this again tends to relate to the degree of industrialization.[23] Studies of populations

Table 1.4. Risk factors for breast cancer

Factor	High Risk	Low Risk	Relative Excess
Gender	Female	Male	100 x
Age	Elderly	Young	> 10 x
Geography	USA/UK	Japan	5 x
Age at menarche	< 12 years	> 13 years	2 x
Age at menopause	> 50 years	< 35 years	3 x
Parity	Parous	Nulliparous	1.5 x
Age at first term birth	> 41 years	< 20 years	2 x
Body Weight	Highest percentile	Lowest percentile (postmenopausal)	1.2 x
Height	Highest percentile	Lowest percentile	1.3 x
Benign breast disease	Any benign condition	None	1.5 x
	atypical hyperplasia	None	4.0 x
Ionizing radiation	Atomic Bomb (100 rad)	no exposure	3 x
Family History	Two 1st degree relatives	None	4-6 x

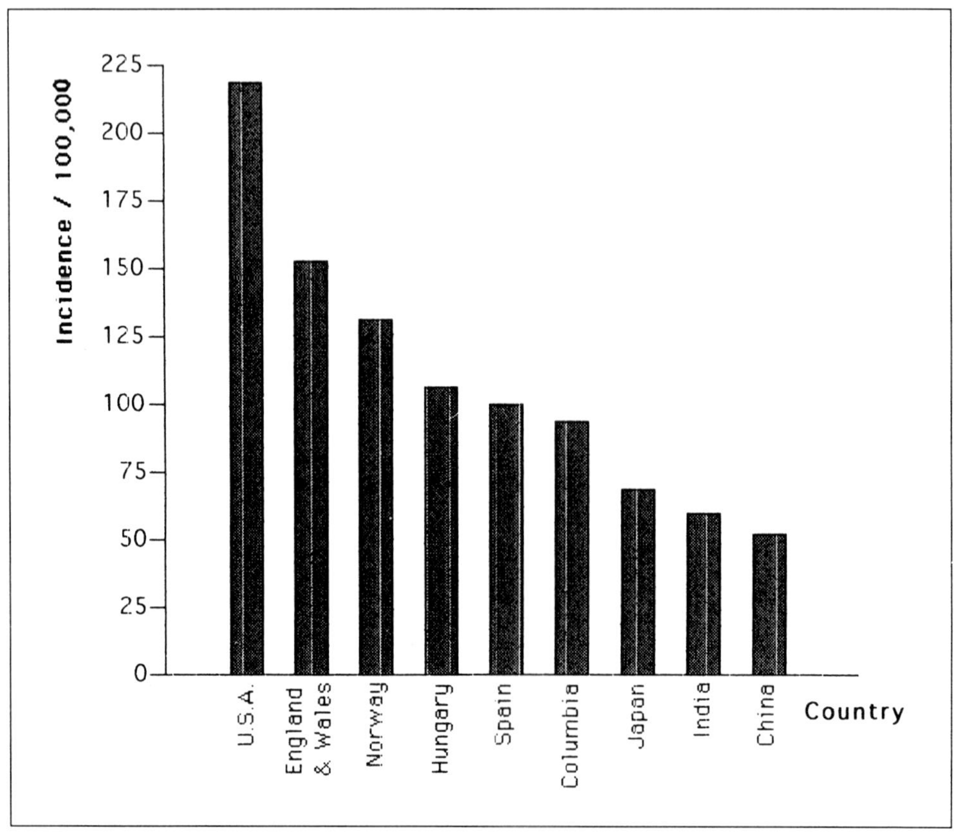

Fig. 1.9. Differences in incidence between geographical localities.

migrating from nations with a low incidence to those with a high incidence are informative and indicate a major non-genetic determinant. Thus, the incidence for Japanese women living in Hawaii appears to be midway between that in Japan and that found among the Japanese community in the USA.[24] Second-generation Japanese women in the USA appear to experience the same risk as their American compatriots.[25] Recently there has been a suggestion that the rate for the disease among Japanese women in Japan has been climbing to that seen among expatriate Japanese living in the USA.[26]

Length of Reproductive Life

An extended reproductive life, either by an early menarche or delayed menopause, increases risk to breast cancer.[27] Conversely an early menopause, whether natural or artificial, seems to protect against breast cancer.[28]

Early age at menarche is a risk factor for breast cancer during both pre-and postmenopausal years. Overall there is a 2-fold increase in risk among those whose menarche occurred before age 12 compared with those who started to menstruate after age 13 and in general there is about a 20% decrease in risk for each year that menarche is delayed.[29] This factor may account for a substantial component of international differences in breast cancer rates,[30] the average age of menarche in the USA being 12.8 years as compared with 17 years in China.

The statistics for menopause are even more striking. Women with a menopause at 55 years or older have twice the risk of those whose menopause occurred naturally before 45 years of age, whereas surgically induced premature menopause is associated with an overall 40% reduction in risk and if performed before the age of 35 years, decreases risk to one third of that in women with a natural menopause.[31] The protection produced by ovariectomy and the hazard of late menopause appear to be life-long, as is reflected by the reduced incidence at induced menopause and later age at natural menopause in breast cancer patients.

Childbearing

Nulliparous women have an increased risk of breast cancer (on average 1.4-fold) as compared with their parous counterparts.[32] However, this statement hides a degree of complexity regarding time of first and last pregnancy, multiparity and ensuing lactations. Age at first pregnancy seems to be important. A first pregnancy within a few years of menarche reduces the risk of subsequent breast cancer by over 50%.[33] The degree of protection diminishes as pregnancy is delayed such that, after the age of 30 years, pregnancy may result in an increased risk of breast cancer compared with that in nulliparous women. This can result in substantial risk differences among parous women— for example that between women having their first baby at 18 and those with a first birth after age 35 is calculated to be 3-fold. The protection seems to require a full-term pregnancy although it need not be followed by lactation.

While age at first full-term pregnancy is an important determinant of risk, there may be additional influences associated with duration of lactation, multiparity and age at last full-term pregnancy.[34,35] Thus it has been suggested that prolonged lactation and high number of pregnancies decrease risk,[36] whereas late last pregnancy increases risk.[37] However, the protective effects of both lactation and multiparity on risk are controversial. The influence of lactation may disappear once parity and age at first delivery are taken into account[36] or be restricted to premenopausal cancers.[38,39] It may be that any effect is particularly associated with prolonged lactation; a population-based case control study in China demonstrated a 30% reduction in breast cancer risk for each 5 years of breast feeding.[40] Multiparity is subject to similar considerations in that it is only in populations with an unusual degree of multiparity that protective influences may be readily seen.[37,41] This would allow rationalization with studies that conclude that the number of births has only a modest influence on the risk of breast cancer after adjustment for the ages of women at the birth of their children[39] (there is a suggestion that, in addition to early age at first birth, early age at second birth is protective[35]).

Life in Utero

Although controversial, there is evidence that perinatal events can influence risk of breast cancer in female off-spring.[42,43] Thus pre-eclampsia/clampsia, which is associated with lowered estrogen levels during pregnancy, appears to reduce incidence[44] whereas mothers with raised estrogen levels during pregnancy may confer higher risk to their daughters.[45] Interestingly, dizygotic twins whose mothers generally have higher levels of estrogen have raised risks of breast cancer.[46]

Obesity/Body Weight and Height

Obesity appears to be associated with increased risk of breast cancer, particularly in postmenopausal women.[47] In terms of weight there is an increased risk for heavier postmenopausal women (a 10 kg increment in weight results in approximately an 80% increase in risk[48]) but a reduced risk for heavier premenopausal women.[49] In relation to height, there is an increased risk of breast cancer in taller premenopausal women.[48,50]

Benign Breast Disease

Most, but not all, studies have reported an increased risk of breast cancer in patients with benign breast disease but the degree of increased risk is variable and usually modest.[51] The exceptions to this are individuals whose benign lesion is associated with atypical hyperplasia or abnormal proliferation.[52] Atypical ductal or lobular hyperplasia is associated with a 4- to 5-fold increase in risk of breast cancer. Among those with a family history of breast cancer risk rises by 8- to 10-fold.[53] Patients with solitary breast cysts do not seem to be predisposed towards breast cancer but multiple cysts, particularly if they are associated with proliferative disease do increase risk.[54] There is also evidence that cysts may be subdivided according to epithelial lining and it is those with apocrine epithelium which are associated with increased risk.[55]

Ionizing Radiation

Japanese women who were exposed to radiation following the atomic bomb attacks on Hiroshima and Nagasaki develop carcinoma of the breast at a higher rate than might be expected from the age-matched control population.[56] The risk of developing these cancers appears to be related to the dose received and age at the time of exposure; those between puberty and 30 years of age were particularly susceptible. Other studies have demonstrated that women who received repeated chest

X-rays during the treatment of tuberculosis are also at a higher risk of developing carcinoma of the breast.[57] There seems little doubt, therefore, that ionizing radiation contributes to the development of breast cancer.

Family History

Women with a first degree relative (mother, grandmother, sister or daughter) who has had breast cancer are at increased risk of breast cancer themselves.[58] While approximately 20% of breast cancer will present with a family history, a distinction should be made between the majority who probably have sporadic breast cancer with a "chance" occurrence in relatives and the one third (7% of all breast cancer patients) who have a true hereditary etiology as determined by medical-genetic scrutiny.[59] Non-hereditary "familial" breast cancer has the same features as non-familial cancer, i.e., it tends to occur in postmenopausal women and to be unilateral whereas the confirmed hereditary form has a distinctive characteristic, in that the disease tends to be associated with other forms of cancer, has an early premenopausal onset[60] and a predisposition to be bilateral.[61] Overall the increased risk associated with a family history of breast cancer is 2- to 3-fold but subgroups can have much greater chances of developing the disease.[62] Thus, a premenopausal woman has a 3- to 5-fold increased risk if her mother had breast cancer; this rises to 5- to 7-fold if her mother and grandmother had the disease and to >10 if bilateral cancer was identified in either or both of the relatives. Indeed by combining factors such as multiple family relatives, early onset, bilaterality and occurrence of other malignancies such as ovarian cancer, it is possible to identify individuals with a very high chance of developing breast cancer but these women form an extremely small group.[63]

ORIGINS

Most breast cancers originate in the primary functional elements of the breast, the terminal-duct lobular units (TDLU)[64] which consist of terminal ductules and acini embedded in groups in connective tissue. Malignancy seems to start in the lining epithelium of the ductules and acini, actively functioning lobules being a prerequisite for development of the disease even in postmenopausal women. Classically it is thought that there are a series of transitional stages through which normal breast progresses before the overt phenotype of invasive cancer is reached (Fig. 1.10). These include "hyperplasia" in which the epithelial cells lining the TDLU proliferate and become several layers thick, "atypia" in which the epithelial hyperplasia becomes excessive and the cells display abnormal features and "ductal carcinoma in situ" in which the cells show the features of unrestrained division and histological abnormalities that characterize malignant cells, but without penetrating the basement membrane (which maintains the integrity of tissue

However, there are minorities in whom disease behaves exceptionally and a substantial effort has been invested in discovering factors which might reflect inherent biological aggressiveness of tumors rather than their stage of advancement. This has resulted in a plethora of indices, most of which have not stood the test of time. Nevertheless, certain factors such as markers of proliferation ("S" phase, Ki67 and other nuclear antigens), differentiation (histological sub-type, mucins), nuclear abnormality (ploidy) metastatic potential (nm23), angiogenesis (vascular counts), products of oncogene/suppressor genes (p53, c-*erb*B-2, H-*ras*, c-*myc*) and growth factor receptors (estrogen receptors, EGF-receptors) are showing promise. If these indices are not only markers of prognosis but program tumor behavior, therapies founded on their biology could be developed.

TREATMENT

The mainstay of treatment of invasive breast cancer, which is apparently confined to the breast, is surgical removal of the tumor with some form of additional axillary surgery.[70] In recent years, there has been a trend to reduce the extent of surgery from radical mastectomy to local excision of tumor, using radiotherapy to eradicate occult malignant cells in residual breast tissue. It is clear from the natural history of breast cancer that the disease presents late but disseminates early so that many women presenting with cancer evident only in the environment of the breast will in fact have distant metastatic disease. It is thus routine practice to offer women with early disease (particularly those with invaded axillary lymph nodes) some form of adjuvant systemic therapy. In those with overt metastatic cancer, systematic therapy is mandatory unless the disease is so advanced that the sole aim is relief of symptoms.

Breast cancer is moderately sensitive to commonly used chemotherapeutic drugs. Adriamycin is the single most effective agent[71] but the current trend is to use drugs in combination to combat the heterogeneity of breast tumors and to avoid early induction of drug-resistance. Details of the use of chemotherapy as a treatment for breast cancer may be found in several recent reviews.[71,72]

In common with cancers of the prostate and endometrium, many breast cancers appear to be dependent upon steroid hormones, the deprivation of which leads to suppression of growth. In premenopausal women this has taken the form of castration, either by ovariectomy or ovarian radiation but drugs such as LHRH agonists are more acceptable and have the advantage of reversibility on discontinuation of treatment. Antiestrogens, progestins and aromatase inhibitors are the endocrine therapies of choice in postmenopausal women and endocrine ablative surgery such as adrenalectomy and hypophysectomy are now redundant procedures. Endocrine manipulation as a mode of therapy for breast cancer is the subject of chapter 8.

REFERENCES

1. Lee PA, Xenakis T, Winer J et al. Puberty in girls: correlation of serum levels of gonadotropins, prolactin, androgens, estrogens and progestins with physical changes. J Clin Endocrinol Metab 1976; 43:775-784.

2. Boyar RM, Wu RHK, Roffwarg H et al. Human puberty: 24-hour estradiol patterns in pubertal girls. J Clin Endocrinol Metab 1976; 43: 1418-1421.

3. Longcope C, Pratt JH, Schneider SH et al. In vivo studies on the metabolism of estrogens by muscle and adipose tissue of normal males. J Clin Endocrinol Metab 1976; 43:1134-1145.

4. Vermeulen A, Verdonck L. Sex hormone concentrations in post-menopausal women. Relation to obesity, fat mass, age and years post-menopause. Clin Endocrinol 1978; 9:59-66.

5. James VHT, Reed MJ, Folkerd EJ. Studies of estrogen metabolism in postmenopausal women with cancer. J Steroid Biochem 1981; 15:235-245.

6. Ruder HJ, Loriaux L, Lipsett MB. Estrone sulfate: production rate and metabolism in man. J Clin Invest 1972; 51:1020-1033

7. MacLusky NJ, Clark CR, Paden CM et al. End-organ metabolism of oestrogens. In: Lewis GP, Ginsburg eds. Mechanisms of steroid action. London: Macmillan 1981:115-132.

8. Fishman J, Boyar RM, Hellman L. The system estradiol-estrone: a sex difference in oxidation of estradiol in man. J Clin Endocrinol Metab 1972; 34:989-996.

9. Fishman J, Hellman L, Zumoff B et al. Effect of thyroid on hydroxylation of estrogen in man. J Clin Endocrinol Metab 1965; 25:365-368.

10. Guerro R, Landgren BM, Montiel R et al. Unconjugated steroids in the human endometrium. Contraception 1975; 11:169-177.

11. Parker M. Mechanism of steroid hormone action. Cancer Surveys 1986; 5:625-633.

12. King RJ. Oestrogen receptors: an overview of recent advances in their structure and function. Proc Roy Soc Edinburgh 1989; 95B:133-144.

13. Greene S, Walter P, Kumar V et al. Human oestrogen receptor DNA: sequence expression and homology to V-erbA. Nature 1986; 320:134-139.

14. Hackenberg R, Turgetto I, Filmer A et al. Estrogen and androgen receptor-mediated stimulation and inhibition of proliferation by androst-5-ene-3-beta, 17-beta-diol in human mammary cancer cells. J Steroid Biochem 1993; 46:597-603.

15. Price KR, Fenwick GR. Naturally occurring oestrogens in foods—a review. FD Addit Contam 1985; 2:73-106.

16. Setchell KDR, Lawson AM, Mitchell FL et al. Lignan formation in man—microbial involvement and possible roles in relation to cancer. Lancet 1981; 2:4-7.

17. Aldercreutz H. Western diet and Western diseases: some hormonal and biochemical mechanisms and associations. Scand J Clin Lab Invest 1990; 50 (Suppl 20):3-23.

18. Ginsburg J. Environmental oestrogens. The Lancet 1994; 343:284-285.
19. Washington Post, January 21, 1990.
20. Boyle P. Epidemiology of breast cancer. Bailliere's Clin Oncol 1988; 2:1-57.
21. Pike MC, Spicer DV, Dahmoush L et al. Estrogens, progestogens normal breast cell proliferation and breast cancer risk. Epidemiologic Reviews (1993); 15:17-35.
22. Muir C, Waterhouse J, Mack T et al. Cancer incidence in five continents. IACR Scientific Publications, Lyon, France 1987; Vol. 5 (No. 8).
23. Waterhouse JAH, Muir CS, Shanmugaratnam K et al. Cancer incidence in five continents. Vol IV, IACR Scientific Publications No.46, Lyon, France 1982; Vol. 4 (No. 46).
24. Henderson IC. Risk factors for breast cancer development. Cancer 1993; 71:2127-2140.
25. Stemmerman GN. Patterns of disease among Japanese living in Hawaii. Arch Environ Health 1970; 20:266-276.
26. Locke FB, King H. Cancer mortality risk among Japanese in the United States. JNCI 1980; 65:1149-1156.
27. MacMahon B, Cole P, Brown J. Etiology of human breast cancer: a review. JNCI 1973; 50:21-42.
28. Feinleib M. Breast cancer and artificial menopause: a cohort study. JNIC 1968; 41:315-329.
29. Kvale G. Reproductive factors in breast cancer epidemiology. Acta Oncol 1992; 31:187-194.
30. Harris JR, Lippman ME, Veronesi U et al. Breast cancer. New Eng J Med 1992; 327:319-328.
31. Trichopoulos D, MacMahon B, Cole P. Menopause and breast cancer risk. JNCI 1972; 48:605-613.
32. White E. Projected changes in breast cancer incidence due to the trend toward delayed childbearing. Am J Public Health 1987; 77:495-497.
33. MacMahon B, Cole P, Lin TM et al. Age at first birth and cancer of the breast. A summary of an international study. Bulletin of the World Health Organization 1970; 43:209-221.
34. Trichopoulos D, Hsieh CC, MacMahon B et al. Age at any birth and breast cancer risk. Int J Cancer 1983; 31:701-704.
35. Ewertz M, Duffy SW, Adami HO et al. Age at first birth, parity and risk of breast cancer: a meta-analysis of 8 studies from the Nordic countries. Int J Cancer 1990; 46:597-603.
36. Kelsey JL, John EM. Lactation and the risk of breast cancer. New Eng J Med 1994; 330:136-137.
37. Kalache A, Maguire A, Thompson SG. Age at last full-term pregnancy and risk of breast cancer. Lancet 1993; 341:32-35.
38. United Kingdom National Care Study Group. Breast feeding and risk of breast cancer in young women. BMJ 1993; 307:17-20.
39. Newcome PA, Storer BE, Longnecker MP et al. Lactation and a reduced risk of premenopausal breast cancer. New Eng J Med 1994; 330:31-37.

40. Yuan JM, Yu MC, Ross RK et al. Risk factors for breast cancer in Chinese women in Shanghai. Cancer Res 1988; 48:1949-1953.
41. Miller WR. Hormonal factors and risk of breast cancer. Lancet 1993; 341:25-26.
42. Hilakivi-Clarke L, Clarke R, Lippman ME. Perinatal factors increase breast cancer risk. Breast Cancer Res Treat 1994; 31:273-284.
43. Anbazhagan R, Gusterson BA. Prenatal factors may influence predisposition to breast cancer. Eur J Cancer 1994; 30A:1-3.
44. Ekbom A, Trichopoulos D, Adami HO et al. Evidence of prenatal influences on breast cancer risk. Lancet 1992; 340:1015-1018.
45. Trichopoulos, D. Hypothesis: does breast cancer originate in utero. The Lancet 1990; 335:939-940.
46. Hsieh CC, Lan S-J, Ekbom A et al. Twin membership and breast cancer risk. Am J Epidemiol 1992; 136:1321-1326.
47. de Waard F, Baanders-van Halewijn EA. A prospective study in general practice on breast cancer risk in postmenopausal women. Int J Cancer 1974; 14:153-160.
48. de Waard F, Cornelis JP, Aoki K et al. Breast cancer incidence according to weight and height in two cities of the Netherlands and in Aichi prefecture, Japan. Cancer 1977; 40:1269-1275.
49. Willett WC. Browne MI, Bain C et al. Relative weight and risk of breast cancer amongst premenopausal women. Am J Epidiol 1985; 122:731-740.
50. Stoll BA, Vattenn LJ, Kvinnsland S. Does early physical maturity influence breast cancer risk? Acta Oncologica 1994; 33:171-176.
51. Webber W, Boyd N. A critique of the methodology of studies of benign breast disease and breast cancer risk. J Natl Cancer Inst 1986; 77:397-404.
52. Page DL, Vander Zwaag R, Rogers LW et al. Relation between component parts of fibrocystic disease complex and breast cancer. J Natl Cancer Inst 1978; 61:1055-1063.
53. Page DL, Dupont WD, Rogers LW et al. Atypical hyperplastic lesions of the female breast. A long-term follow-up study. Cancer 1985; 55: 2698-2708.
54. Bundred NJ, West RR, Dowd JO et al. Is there an increased risk of breast cancer in women who have had a breast cyst aspirated? Br J Cancer 1991; 64:953-955.
55. Dixon JM, Lumsden AB, Miller WR. The relationship of cyst type and risk factors for breast cancer and the subsequent development of breast cancer in patients with breast cystic disease. Eur J Cancer 1985; 21:1047-1050.
56. McGregor H, Land CE, Choi K et al. Breast cancer incidence among atomic bomb survivors, Hiroshima and Nagasaki, 1950-69. J Natl Cancer Inst 1977; 59:799-811.
57. Boice JD Jr, Monson RR. Breast cancer in women after repeated fluoroscopic examinations of the chest. J Natl Cancer Inst 1977; 59:823-832.
58. Kelsey JL. A review of the epidemiology of human breast cancer. Epidemiol Rev 1979; 1:74-109.

59. Lynch HT, Albano WA, Heireck JJ et al. Genetics, biomarkers and control of breast cancer: a review. Cancer Genetics Cytogenetics 1984; 13:43-92.
60. Anderson DE. Familial predisposition. In: Schottenfeld D, Fraumeni JF Jr., eds. Cancer epidemiology and prevention. Philadelphia: WB Saunders, 1982:483-493.
61. Prior P, Waterhouse JAH. Incidence of bilateral tumours in a population-based series of breast cancer patients. I. Two approaches to an epidemiological analysis. Br J Cancer 1978; 37:620-634.
62. Evans DGR, Fentiman IS, McPherson K et al. Familial breast cancer. BMJ 1994; 308:183-187.
63. Eby N, Chang-Claude J, Bishop DT. Familial risk and genetic susceptibility for breast cancer. Cancer Causes & Control 1994; 5:458-470.
64. Anderson TJ. Genesis and source of breast cancer. Br Med Bull 1991; 47:305-318.
65. Wellings SR, Jensen HM, Marcum RG. An atlas of subgross pathology of the human breast with special reference to possible precancerous lesions. J Natl Cancer Inst 1975; 55:231-273.
66. Tabar L, Fagerberg, G, Day N E et al. Breast-cancer-treatment and natural-history—new insights from results of screening. The Lancet 1992; 339:412-414.
67. Baum M. Breast Cancer: the facts. Oxford University Press 1981.
68. Facts on Cancer. Annual Report of the Cancer Research Campaign 1988.
69. Carter CL, Allen C, Henson DE. Relation of tumor size, lymph node status, and survival in 24,740 breast cancer cases. Cancer 1989; 63:181-187.
70. Yarnold JR. Early stage breast cancer: treatment opinions and results. Br Med Bul 1991; 47:372-387.
71. Henderson IC, Harris JR, Kinne DW et al. Cancer of the breast. In: DeVita Jr, S Hellman, SA Rosenberg, eds. Cancer: principles and practice of oncology (3rd Ed). Philadelphia: Lippincott 1989:1197-1267.
72. Gregory WM, Smith P, Richards MA et al. Chemotherapy of advanced breast cancer: outcome and prognostic factors. Br J Cancer 1993; 68:988-995.

ESTROGENS
AND THE NORMAL BREAST

The mammary gland is basically a modified sweat gland.[1] It is composed of epithelial, adipose and fibrous connective tissue elements (Fig. 2.1), the relative proportions of which vary with species and developmental state of the gland.[2] The human gland is unique in that the breast may attain full structural development without the stimulus of copulation or pregnancy. Developmentally, there are however three overlapping phases of activity associated with puberty, ovulatory menstrual cycles and pregnancy. Thus, the breast is relatively quiescent until the onset of puberty when, at a time which may precede menarche by several years, the ductal system proliferates within the adipose stroma. Simultaneously, lobular buds develop although the lobules themselves do not completely form until ovulatory menstrual cycles occur. Cyclical changes have been documented through the menstrual cycle[3] and many women experience premenstrual fullness and pain in their breasts.[4] During pregnancy, both ductal and glandular elements of the breast proliferate massively so that by full-term the organ is composed of a compact mass of lobules comprising multiple alveoli lined by secreting cells. These produce colostrum during pregnancy and milk during lactation. It is only during pregnancy and lactation that the breast achieves full secretory status.

Because the breast develops at puberty but only reaches full maturity during the course of pregnancy and conversely involutionary changes occur postpartum and glandular structures progressively atrophy after the menopause (Fig. 2.2), it seems obvious that ovarian and placental hormones are implicated in breast development. However, it is worth reviewing the evidence that among such endocrine influences estrogens have a crucial role and define the particular processes involved.

ESTROGENS AND BREAST DEVELOPMENT
AT PUBERTY

Estrogen seems to be central to breast development at puberty. Thus, in girls whose breasts do not form because of gonadal dysgenesis,

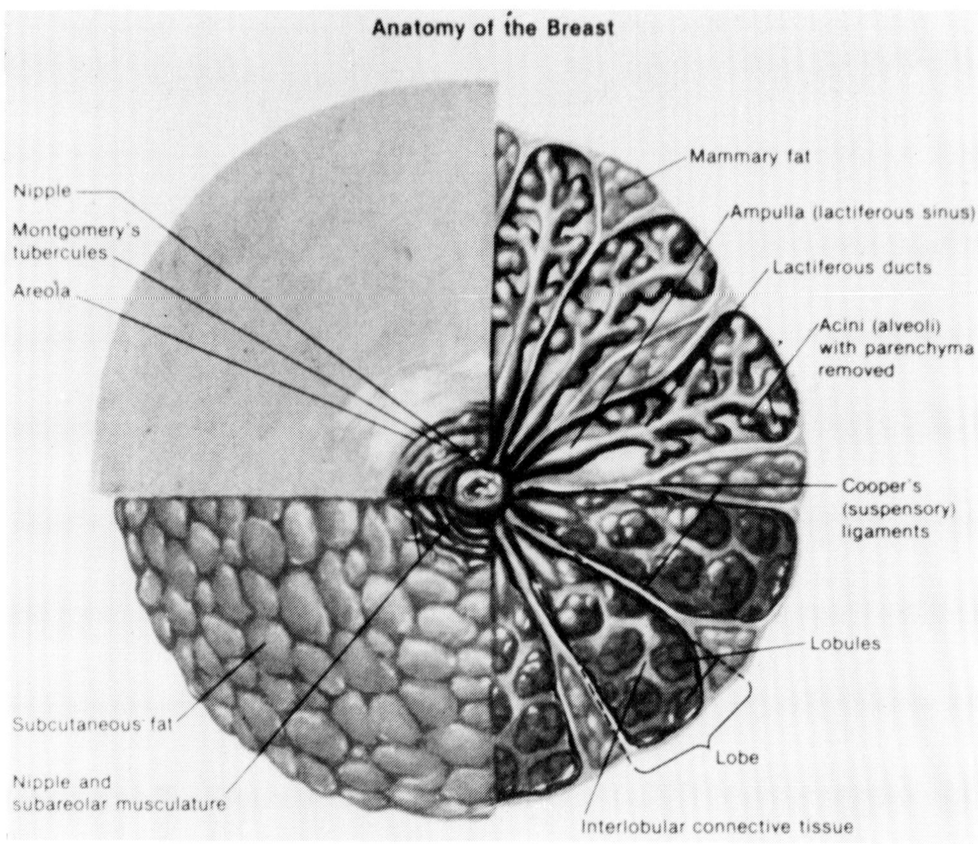

Fig. 2.1. The anatomy of the breast.

full development may be induced by the simple expedient of administering estrogen,[5] although in individuals whose gonadal failure is secondary to pituitary deficiency, it is sometimes necessary to provide pituitary hormones in addition to estrogen. These observations would be totally compatible with the reports that estrogen-secreting tumors in prepubescent girls cause precocious breast development.[6] However, to suggest that estrogen alone can account for breast development would be misleading. At puberty, breast development in girls usually precedes the secretion of major estrogen by the ovary;[7] indeed, levels of estrogen in pubertal girls with substantial breast development may not be higher than in males.[8] Thus, while there is a progressive increase in estradiol and estrone during the course of breast development, individual variations are great and it is only at a stage when the breast is almost mature that levels in females consistently exceed those in males. The correlation between degree of breast development and circulating levels of estrogen is therefore far from perfect.

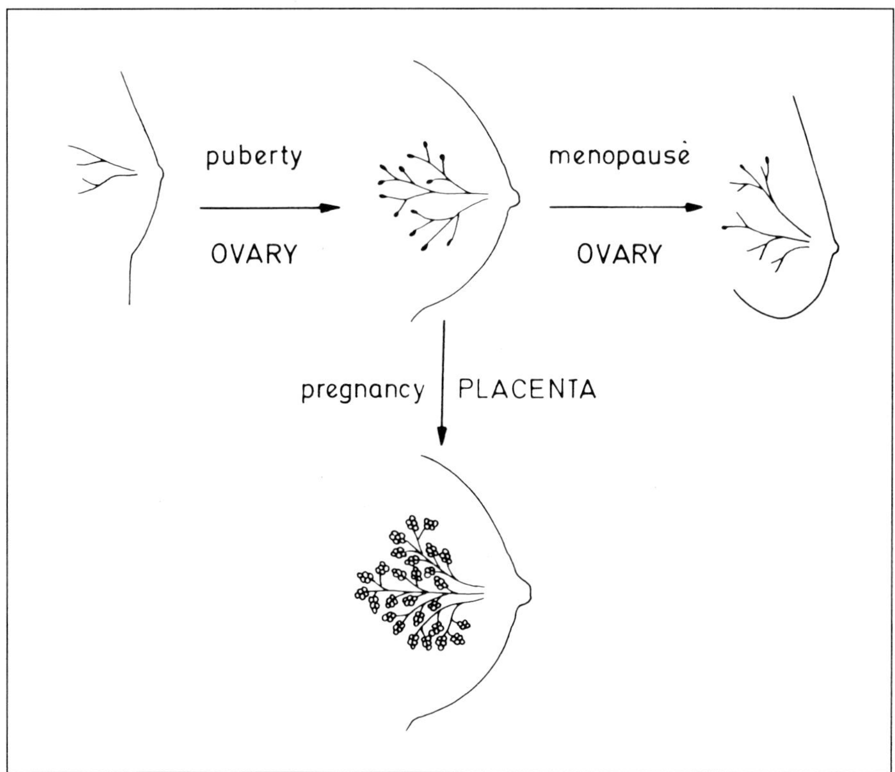

Fig. 2.2. Development changes in the breast.

It may be that adrenal androgens produced at menarche which have estrogenic activity (see chapter 1) induce pubertal development. Other factors, such as local levels of insulin-like growth factors (IGF), may also account for an increased sensitivity of the breast to estrogenic stimulation at puberty and the differential development observed between individuals. Thus, IGF levels peak at puberty and correlate better with breast size than with chronological age[9] or circulating estrogens;[5,7] specific receptors for IGF may also be detected in the normal breast.[10] The relevance of these observations needs to be substantiated, especially since females with hereditary IGF-I deficiency have delayed puberty[11] but normal breast development.[12] It seems reasonable to deduce that normal breast development is dependent upon the permissive presence of estrogen but that the effectiveness of estrogen depends on the simultaneous presence of other factors such as gonadotrophins, glucocorticoids and IGF and tissue receptors for these factors.

THE MATURE RESTING BREAST

Although the adult non-lactating breast is regarded as resting, it does produce limited amounts of secretion which appear to be reabsorbed during travel through the duct system so that fluid does not normally appear in the nipple unless suction is applied.[13] The gland also appears to respond to the cyclic nature of hormones in premenopausal women. Thus, during the menstrual cycle, the normal breast TDLU epithelium exhibits greater proliferation in the luteal than in the follicular phase (Fig. 2.3).[14] While it is tempting to explain this observation on the basis of the generally higher estrogens in the luteal phase, this would be simplistic—when estrogens are at their highest during mid-cycle, mitotic activity in the breast can be low. It has been suggested that the trophic effects of estrogen in the breast may be indirect[1] and dependent upon the presence of other hormones.[15] Progestins have been implicated as a result of the observations that oral contraceptives (particularly progestin-only pills) increase proliferation[16] and a marker of progestin action (fatty acid synthetase) rises parallel with proliferation in breast epithelium.[17] These observations are not totally compatible with findings in model systems. For example, estrogen has a primary proliferative action while progestins are largely ineffective in normal breast maintained as xenografts in immunocompromised mice.[18]

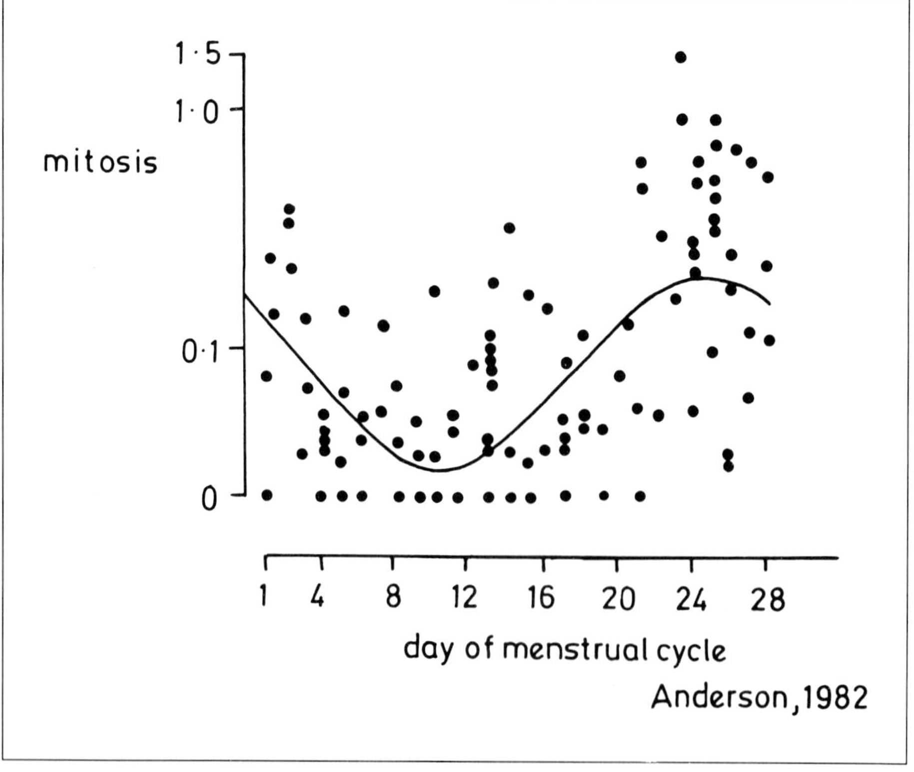

Fig. 2.3. *Mitoses in terminal ductal lobular units of the breast through the menstrual cycle (modified from refs. 3 and 14).*

Since the major effects of estrogen in target organs are mediated through the estrogen receptor and the progesterone receptor is induced by estrogen, it has been of interest to examine levels of these steroid receptors in the normal breast. Although the amounts of estrogen receptor in the normal breast are low in comparison with breast cancer,[19] incidence and level are reduced in the luteal phase of the menstrual cycle and by the use of oral contraceptives.[20,21] Immunohistochemical studies have also shown two different patterns of staining for estrogen receptors—sporadic and uniform.[20] Only the sporadic pattern is reduced during the luteal phase and thereby exhibits classical down-regulation by progesterone. The reduced expression of ER during both the luteal phase and oral contraceptive use are at times of relatively increased proliferation and this is again paradoxical if estrogen is the prime mitogenic stimulus to the resting breast. Against this background, it is interesting that progesterone receptors in the normal breast remain relatively constant during the menstrual cycle which suggests constitutive expression rather than induction by estrogen[20,22] and which contrasts with observations in the endometrium.[23]

The part played by estrogen in the changes occurring in the breast during the menstrual cycle are clearly difficult to define and may be dependent upon a host of other interacting factors. The complexity of this situation is not helped by differing responses in parous and nulliparous breasts, for example, it has been noted that estrogen receptors tend to be low in the breasts of recently parous women.[20]

ESTROGEN AND BREAST INVOLUTION AT MENOPAUSE

Proliferative activity within the breast decreases with age[24] and with the decline of ovarian function breast involution occurs. As a result, the rate of cell proliferation in the postmenopausal breast is considerably less than that in the premenopausal breast.[25] The process may begin before the cessation of menstruation, there often being a preclimacteric phase occurring between 35 and 45 years of age.[26] This involves a decrease in glandular epithelium with some involution of acinar and lobular tissues. In the postclimateric phase there is much more substantial reduction of glandular tissues with a concomitant increase in fat deposits. Loss of lobular and alveolar structures is striking and occasionally only collecting ducts mark the site of a lobule. Eventually the ducts degenerate leaving residual small islands of atrophic parenchyma surrounded by connective tissue and fat (see Plate). As a result, while glandular tissue can constitute about one third of the mature breast in premenopausal women, after the menopause it may represent less than 5%. In contrast, the proportion of fat increases with age and represents the largest component of the postmenopausal breast (Fig. 2.4). However, involution is not a uniform process and frequently one part of the breast may lose all its lobules while another

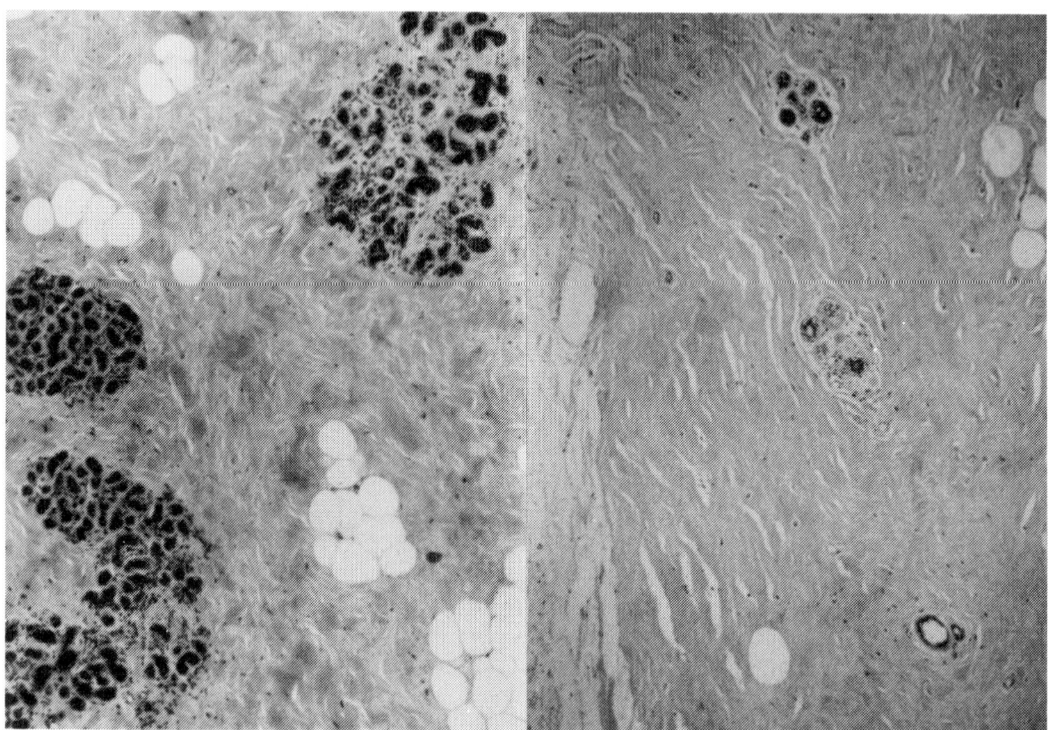

Plate. (left) Groups of normal resting lobules surrounded by fibrous tissue and fat in the breast of a premenopausal woman, (right). Breast tissue from a postmenopausal woman comprising mainly stroma with only occasional atrophic lobules.

retains a normal pattern.[27] It is therefore not unusual to see well-preserved lobules in the breasts of postmenopausal women and indeed the suggestion has been made that this is a risk factor for breast cancer; persistent lobules are found more frequently in the mastectomy specimens obtained after the diagnosis of breast cancer than in breasts examined at routine autopsy.[28]

Given that the major changes at the menopause result from diminished ovarian function and mirror circulating levels of ovarian hormones, it is reasonable to attribute the process of breast involution to estrogen deprivation, although direct mechanistic evidence of this is lacking. However, the practice of treating menopausal symptoms and metastatic breast cancer with hormones does provide the opportunity to determine whether the administration of estrogen to postmenopausal women delays or reverses breast involution. Despite the prevalence of these practices, most of these women do not subsequently have breast biopsies and the majority of observations are therefore somewhat anecdotal although informative. The single largest study is of Husbey and Thomas[29] who examined normal atrophic breasts from patients with advanced breast cancer who were at least five years past their menopause and who had been treated with large pharmacological

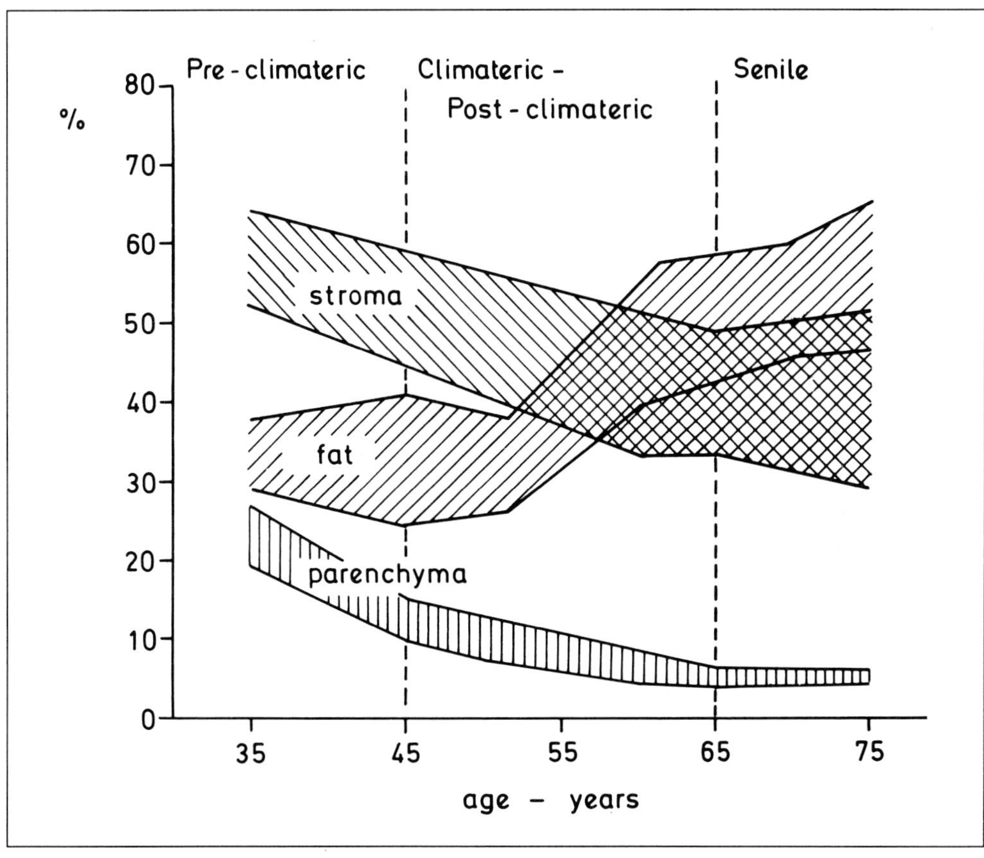

Fig. 2.4. Changes with age in the relative proportions of the principal elements within the breast.

doses of estrogenic hormones for between 1 and 31 months. The appearance of the excised breast tissue was compared with that from untreated patients of a similar age. This and similar studies have potential drawbacks in terms of the normality of the breast tissue examined, the possibility that the presence of cancer or previous treatments may influence normal tissue and the size of the dose of administered estrogen. Nevertheless breast tissue from 34 of 36 patients showed evidence of epithelial stimulation as evidenced by the presence of small ducts, interlobular connective tissue and what appeared to be the formation of new lobules. In 25 patients, new small ducts, an increase in the presence of mitotic figures and occasional secreting lobules were seen. While these changes are the reverse of the atrophic process occurring at the menopause, only in one case had the breast tissue been restored to the premenopausal state. Furthermore, several studies which have examined breast material from postmenopausal women treated with more physiological doses of estrogen for menopausal symptoms or as replacement therapy have generally reported no differences in histological features compared with controls.[30]

Thus, although there is evidence that the administration of high doses of estrogen to post-menopausal women will delay the process of breast involution, the degree of response varies between individuals and rarely constitutes a full reversal of processes following a natural menopause or castration.

SUMMARY

That major developmental events within the breast primarily occur at puberty and during pregnancy and involution takes place at the menopause surely implicates steroids in these processes. Among such hormones, estrogens appear to play a central and permissive role but the simultaneous influence of other factors such as gonadotrophins, glucocorticoids growth factors and their tissue receptors are also important although less well defined.

REFERENCES

1. Anderson TJ, Miller WR. Morphological and biological observations relating to the development and progression of breast cancer. In: Dickson R, Lippman M, eds. Mammary tumorigenesis and malignant progression. Kluwer Academic Publishers 1994:3-27.
2. Miller WR, Anderson TJ. Oestrogens, progestogens and the breast In: Whitehead MI, Studd J, eds. The menopause. Blackwell Scientific Press 1988:234-246.
3. Anderson TJ, Ferguson DJP, Raab G. Cell turnover in the "resting" human breast: influences of parity, contraceptive pill, age and laterality. Br J Cancer 1982; 46:376-382.
4. Gateley CA, Mansel RE. Management of cyclical breast pain. Br J Hosp Med 1990; 43:330-332.
5. Laron Z, Kauli R, Pertzelan A. Clinical evidence on the role of oestrogens in the development of the breast. Proc Roy Soc (Edin) 1989; 95B:13-22.
6. Howell A. Clinical evidence for the involvement of oestrogen in the development and progression of breast cancer. Proc Roy Soc (Edin) 1989; 95B:49-57.
7. Ratcliffe S. The clinical consequences of an extra sex chromosome. Growth Matters 1991; 6:2-4.
8. Bidlingmaier F, Knorr D. Oestrogens—physiological and clinical aspects, pediatric and adolescent endocrinology, Vol 4. Basel: Karger 1978:76-81.
9. Rosenfield RJ, Furlanetto R, Bock D. Relationship of somatomedin C concentration to pubertal changes. J Pediat 1983; 103:723-728.
10. Pekonen F, Partanen S, Makinen T et al. Receptors for epidermal growth factor and insulin growth factor 1 and their relation to steroid receptors in human breast cancer. Cancer Res 1988; 48:1343-1347.
11. Laron Z, Sarel R, Pertzelan A. Puberty in Laron type dwarfism. Eur J Pediatrics 1980; 134:79-83.

12. Laron Z, Prager LR, Dickerman Z. Diagnostic use of LH-RH. In: Vickery BH, Nestor JJ Jr, Hafez ESE, eds. LH-RH and its analogs—contraceptive and therapeutic applications. Lancaster: MTP Press, 1984:367-374.

13. Petrakis NL. Physiologic, biochemical and cytologic aspects of nipple aspirate fluid. Breast Cancer Res Treat 1986; 8:7-19.

14. Anderson TJ, Battersby S. The involvement of oestrogen in the development and function of the normal breast: histological evidence. Proc Roy Soc (Edin) 1989; 95B:23-32.

15. King RJB. A discussion of the roles of oestrogen and progestin in human mammary carcinogenesis. J Steroid Biochem Molec Biol 1991; 39(5B):811-818.

16. Anderson TJ, Battersby S, King RJB et al. Oral contraceptive use influences resting breast proliferation. Human Pathol 1989; 20:1139-1144.

17. Chalbos D, Escot C, Joyeux C et al. Expression of the progestin-induced fatty acid synthetase in benign mastopathies and breast cancer as measured by RNA in situ hybridization. J Natl Cancer Inst 1990; 82:602-606.

18. Laidlaw IJ, Clarke RB, Howell A et al. The proliferation of normal human breast tissue implanted into athymic nude mice is stimulated by estrogen but not progesterone. Endocrinology 1995; 136:164-171.

19. Carpenter S, Georgiade G, McCarty KS Sr et al. Immunohistochemical expression of oestrogen receptor in normal breast tissue. Proc Roy Soc (Edin) 1989; 95B:59-66.

20. Battersby S, Robertson BJ, Anderson TJ et al. Influence of menstrual cycle, parity and oral contraceptive use on steroid hormone receptors in normal breast. Br J Cancer 1992; 65:601-607.

21. Williams G, Anderson E, Howell A et al. Oral contraceptive (OCP) use increases proliferation and decreases oestrogen receptor content of epithelial cells in the normal human breast. Int J Cancer 1991; 48:206-210.

22. King RJB. Estrogen and progestin effects in human breast carcinogenesis. Breast Cancer Res Treat 1993; 27:3-15.

23. Press MF, Greene GL. Localization of progesterone receptor with monoclonal antibodies to the human progestin receptor. Endocrinology 1988; 122:1165-1175.

24. Potten CS, Watson RJ, Williams GT et al. The effect of age and menstrual cycle upon proliferative activity of the normal human breast. Br J Cancer 1988; 58:163-170.

25. Kramer WM, Rush BF. Mammary duct proliferation in the elderly. Cancer 1973; 31:130-137.

26. Vorherr H. Development of the female breast. In: Vorherr H, ed. The breast: morphology, physiology and lactation. New York: Academic Press 1974:1-19.

27. Miller WR, Anderson TJ. Oestrogens, progestogens and the breast. In: Whitehead MI, Studd J, eds. The menopause. Blackwell Scientific Press 1988:234-246.

28. Wellings SR, Jensen HM, Marcum RG. An atlas of subgross pathology of the human breast with special reference to possible precancerous lesions. J Natl Cancer Inst 1975; 55:231-273.
29. Huseby RA, Thomas LB. Histological and histochemical alterations in the normal breast tissues of patients with advanced breast cancer being treated with estrogenic hormones. Cancer 1954; 7:54-74.
30. Fechner RE. Benign breast disease in women on estrogen therapy. Cancer 1972; 29:273-279.

CHAPTER 3

ESTROGENS AND THE RISK OF BREAST CANCER

The evidence linking estrogens with the risk of breast cancer comes from work in many disciplines. In this chapter perspectives will be derived from research based on epidemiology, clinico-pathology, endocrinology, metabolism and molecular biology. Consideration will also be given as to whether estrogens may act as initiators and/or promoters of breast cancer.

EPIDEMIOLOGICAL EVIDENCE

The epidemiological evidence linking estrogens with risk of breast cancer comes from two areas: the general associations between reproductive/menstrual history and breast cancer, and the effects of exogenous estrogens on the incidence of breast cancer.

MENSTRUAL AND REPRODUCTIVE FACTORS

The etiology of breast cancer has a strong hormonal component. Most notably, menstrual status and reproductive history are important determinants of risk to breast cancer.[1] The disease does not occur before puberty and an extended reproductive life, whether by an early menarche or late menopause, increases risk.[2]

The influence of menopause and the age when it occurs are particularly informative. Thus, there is a downward inflection in the incidence rate for breast cancer at the time of menopause and thereafter breast cancer incidence rises more slowly.[3] This implies that the rise prior to age 50 is the result of breast cell proliferation driven by sex-steroids associated with cyclical ovarian activity and menopause saves some who would have otherwise developed breast cancer. It follows therefore that blockade of ovarian function should protect against breast cancer and conversely, delaying menopause should be associated with increased risk. Epidemiological observations support this (Table 3.1). Women with a menopause at 55 years of age or older have almost twice the risk of those whose menopause occurred naturally before 45 years of age and castration early in reproductive life markedly reduces

Table 3.1. The influence of age at menarche and menopause on risk of breast cancer

| Menarche | | Menopause | | | |
| Age (years) | Relative Risk | Natural | | Artificial | |
		Age (years)	Relative Risk	Age (years)	Relative Risk
≤12	1.7	–	–	<35	0.36
13	1.1	–	–	35-39	0.68
14	1.0	<45	1.0	40-44	0.65
15	1.0	45-49	1.3	45-49	0.70
16	0.8	50-55	1.6	>50	1.00
≥17	0.8	>55	1.9	–	–

risk (by two-thirds if performed before 35 years of age).[4] The protection of castration and hazards of late menopause appear to be lifelong as is reflected by the reduced incidence at induced menopause and later age at natural menopause of breast cancer patients compared with the general population.[5] These observations have important implications and suggest that ovarian activity plays a part in the development of at least two thirds of breast cancers in women who undergo a natural menopause and that because the breasts of women at 35 years have already been exposed to over half the normal period of ovarian activity they would normally receive, simple exposure to ovarian hormones is not causative of breast cancer.

Age at menarche is also an influential factor associated with risk (Table 3.1). Those who start to menstruate early have an increased risk and cumulative protection occurs with each year that menarche is delayed. The effects can be significant and it is estimated that the later age at menarche in Japanese girls as compared with their American counterparts might account for at least part of the difference in breast cancer rates between the countries.[6] For menarche to occur it is necessary to attain a critical body mass in relation to height.[7] Height is determined in part genetically and in part by diet whereas weight is largely a dietary determinant. Critical mass has to be maintained for menstruation to continue. Those who lose weight as a result of anorexia nervosa, or as part of strenuous athletic training will develop amenorrhea.[8,9] It is pertinent that there is a reduced incidence of breast cancer among women who were former college athletes.[10]

As is shown in Table 3.2, these findings have led to two different theories as to why prolonged reproductive life should increase risk—either there must be a cumulative effect of menstrual cycles or something special about those early and late in life which impart a particular sensitivity to the breast.

In terms of the latter it has been postulated that, at each end of reproductive life, menstrual cycles are irregular and there are major

Table 3.2. Alternative theories used to explain the high risk of breast cancer conferred by prolonged reproductive life

Hypothesis	Premise	Consequence	Supportive Data
Cumulative and extended exposure to menstrual cycles	Ovulatory Cycles are bad for risk	Breast is exposed to combined trophic effects of estrogen and progestogen	1. Early establishment of regular menstrual cycles increases risk 2. Premature menopause decreases risk 3. Increased proliferation within breast during luteal phase
Luteal phase insufficiency "estrogen windows"	Anovulatory cycles are bad for risk	Breast is exposed to estrogen unopposed by progestogen	1. Late menopause associated with increased frequency of irregular cycles 2. Anovulatory cycles major cause of infertility (nulliparity increases risk of cancer) 3. The presence of critical susceptible periods

periods of anovulation during which the breast is exposed to estrogen unopposed by progesterone (estrogen windows).[11] This may be true prior to the menopause when there is a variable period of time (as long as eight years) during which menstrual cycles are irregular, longer and apparently anovulatory.[12,13] There is also a suggestion that women with a late menopause have an increased frequency of longer and presumably anovulatory menstrual cycles than those with an early menopause.[13] Anovulatory cycles are a major cause of infertility/subfertility, the incidence of which is reported to be high among women with breast cancer.[14]

However, there are also epidemiological data against the estrogen window hypothesis. Thus, a cohort follow-up of infertile women has not shown a clear excess of breast cancer among those with anovular cycles.[15] There are also reports that breast cancer patients establish regular menstrual cycles more rapidly than controls[16] and that frequent ovular cycles impart greater risk for breast cancer than anovular cycles.[17] Additionally, longitudinal studies in schoolgirls have failed to confirm that those with an early menarche have more anovular cycles than those with a later menarche.[18] Indeed, girls who have an early menarche appear to develop ovulatory cycles more rapidly so that during their second decade they have higher circulating levels of estradiol and lower sex hormone-binding globulin (SHBG) levels.[19] Similarly, a study of young girls in which both the time of onset of menstruation and that at which regular periods became established were recorded showed that, for a fixed age at menarche, establishment of regular menstrual cycles within one year of first menstrual period more than doubled the risk of breast cancer when compared to women with a five year or longer delay for menstruation to regularize.[20] Furthermore, women with a menarche at age 12 or younger and rapid establishment of periods had an almost 4-fold increased risk when compared with women with menarche at later years and long duration of irregular menses.

It seems more likely that increased risk results from the cumulative effects of regular menstrual cycles and the persistent trophic exposure of the breast to cycling ovarian hormones,[16] estrogens and progestogens acting in concert to promote the proliferation of cells making them susceptible to the effects of carcinogenesis. Certainly there is a consensus that the normal breast is more likely to be stimulated by estrogen in the presence of progestogen than in its absence (as evidenced by the higher level of proliferation in the luteal phase compared with the follicular phase of the menstrual cycle[21] and following the use of combined estrogen-progestin contraceptive pills[22]). Prolonged and cumulative expression of the breast to regular menstrual cycles therefore appears hazardous.

Increased risk caused by the cumulative effects of ovulatory menstrual cycles would also be compatible with the protective influence of pregnancy (especially if multiple, early in life and followed by prolonged lactational amenorrhea). This would break up the pattern of regular cyclic exposure of the breast to trophic hormones while at the same time causing stem cells to differentiate.

It is appropriate at this stage to consider body weight, another risk factor which might be mediated by estrogen. While body weight has little influence on the risk of premenopausal breast cancer, heavier women seem to be at greater risk in the postmenopausal period.[23] It is thus relevant in postmenopausal women that estrogen is largely derived from the extraglandular conversion of adrenal androgens[24] and that the rate and degree of this conversion increases with body weight.[25] It is also pertinent that the geographical differences in breast cancer risk are most marked in the postmenopausal period[26] and postmenopausal women in Westernized societies tend to be more overweight than their counterparts in less industrialized countries.[6,27] Indeed, using a theoretical model, Pike suggested that this factor might account for 85% of the difference in breast cancer rates between Japanese and American postmenopausal women.[28]

THE EFFECTS OF EXOGENOUS ESTROGEN

If estrogens influence risk of breast cancer it might be expected that women given exogenous estrogen would have a higher incidence of cancer. There are three sets of circumstances in which estrogens have been administered to women on a relatively large scale. These are (a) during pregnancy in an attempt to prevent miscarriage; (b) at and after the menopause to relieve menopausal symptoms and (c) during child-bearing years to prevent conception.

Exogenous estrogen during pregnancy
Particularly in the USA, very high doses of diethylstilbestrol were given in the 1950s and 1960s to pregnant women who either had a history of abortion, were threatening to abort, or had other complications. It was thus tragic that the therapy was not only ineffective but associated with increased incidence of clear cell adenocar-cinoma of the vagina and cervix in the daughters and of breast cancer in the mothers themselves.[29] The increased risk of breast cancer is about 35% and seems to be independent of other risk factors for breast cancer. However the particular salient point of these observations is the long latency period between exposure and the appearance of breast cancer, 20 years elapsing before the risk became apparent (Table 3.3). There was an excess of both large and small tumors which would seem to exclude heightened surveillance as a cause of increased incidence in the treatment group.

Exogenous estrogen at menopause
Treatment to relieve osteoporosis and hot flushes at the menopause by estrogen replacement therapy usually involves the use of conjugated estrogens such as premarin. While there is unequivocal evidence that such therapy can cause endometrial cancer,[30] effects on breast cancer are much more controversial despite a considerable amount of study (Fig. 3.1). Intuitively it might be expected that as estrogen is being given at the time of the menopause or following castration to relieve the symptoms of hormone deprivation, the therapy would be associated with the known hazard of a delayed menopause and abolish the protective effect of castration on breast cancer risk. While some case-control studies have indeed shown an increased risk with estrogen replacement therapy (ERT)[31,32] and one investigation demonstrated that ERT obliterated the protective effect of bilateral oophorectomy,[33] these reports are somewhat exceptional and several recent meta-analyses[33-36] have failed to confirm increased risk with the possible exception of women with a longer duration of exposure to estrogen.

Table 3.3. Breast cancer risk according to time since exposure to stilbestrol during pregnancy

Time since exposure (years)	Relative risk (95% CI)
0-9	1.0 (0.3-3.0)
10-19	1.1 (0.7-1.8)
20-29	1.6 (1.0-2.4)
30-39	2.5 (1.1-5.8)

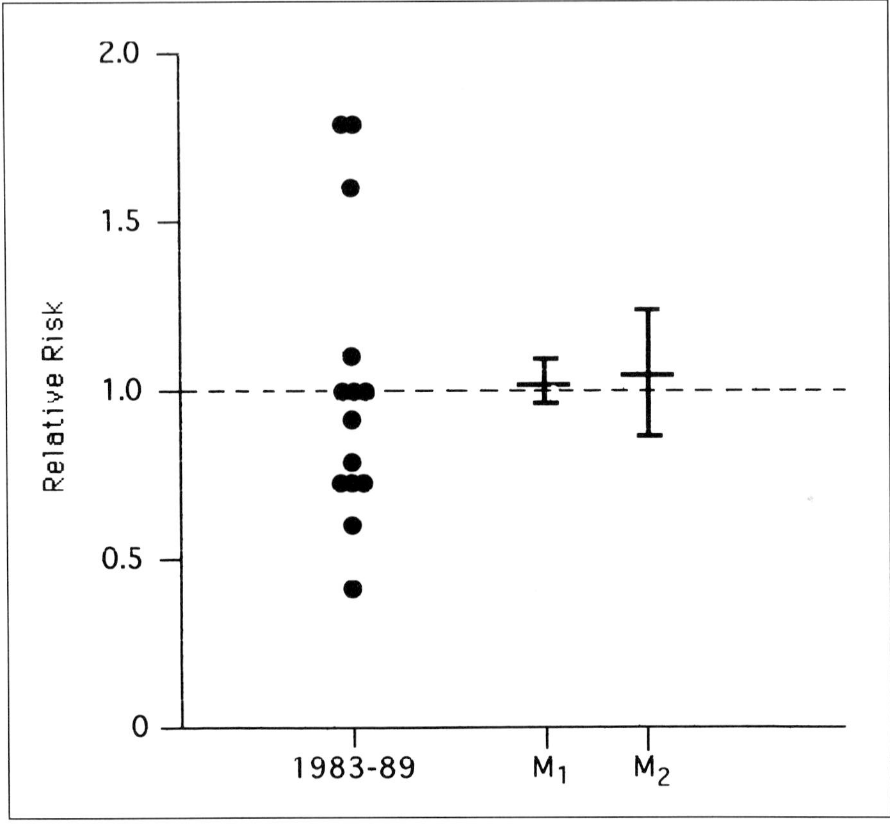

Fig. 3.1. Relative risk of breast cancer following use of ERT. Column 1 represents case-control studies between 1983 and 1985. M_1 represents the meta-analysis described in reference 33 and M_2 represents a subset of studies in which either high dose or long duration of estrogen treatment has been assessed.

Because of the importance of these observations in terms of direct evidence of estrogen increasing risk of postmenopausal breast cancer, it is worth considering in more detail specific aspects of these studies which are potentially informative. First of all, there are confounding factors relating to women who are prescribed estrogen replacement therapy.[31,37] For example obesity is positively correlated with postmenopausal cancer but negatively with menopausal estrogen use (possibly reflecting the propensity of thin women to suffer more severe menopausal symptoms).[36] Secondly it may be that while short-term administration of estrogen is without risk, extended use is more hazardous. There is evidence to support this concept.[37-40] In one study in Sweden[38] the relative risk of breast cancer increased from 0.7 in short term use to 1.7 for more than nine years of use (see Table 3.4). These data are consistent with meta-analyses which have addressed the issue and found no detrimental effects for overall use of ERT but significantly increased risk in women having in excess of 15 years of use.[35] Interestingly, while there is the suggestion that the length of exposure may increase risk most investigations have failed to find a positive relationship between dose of estrogen and risk.[33,34] A third factor is the type of estrogen used (See Table 3.5). Most ERT utilize conjugated estrogen but non-conjugated estrogens have been employed, particularly in Europe. It is thus interesting that Bergkvist et al[38] have reported that the use of estradiol for six or more years was associated with a substantial increase in risk while conjugated estrogens were not. Three case-control studies have also found some evidence of higher risk associated with non-conjugated estrogens,[40-42] particularly diethylstilbestol. This may be particularly pertinent given the findings referred to earlier that administration of the same estrogen during pregnancy is also hazardous. Finally, certain subgroups of women may be more susceptible to the effects of ERT; particularly those at increased risk of breast cancer for other reasons. However, results on family history, benign breast disease and obesity are not conclusive and can be complicated.[32,33,43-45] For example one study suggested that ERT might protect against breast cancer in patients with a previous history of benign breast conditions but enhanced risk if used before the diagnosis of benign breast disease.[46]

Table 3.4. Observed and expected numbers of cases of breast cancer, with relative risks and 95% confidence intervals, according to the duration of estrogen treatment

Months of Treatment	Relative Risk (Confidence Interval)
≤ 6	0.7 (0.4-1.0)
7-36	1.1 (0.9-1.4)
37-72	1.0 (0.8-1.4)
73-108	1.3 (0.9-1.9)
≥ 109	1.7 (1.1-2.7)
Any treatment	1.1 (1.0-1.3)

Table 3.5. Formulation of ERT and risk of breast cancer

Formulation	Relative risk (95% C.I.)	
Never	1.0	
Conjugated estrogen	1.4	(1.2-1.7)
Estrogen/progestin	1.5	(0.99-2.4)
Other estrogens	1.1	(0.7-1.8)
Estrogen/Androgen	2.5	(0.95-6.4)

The above considerations relate to risk of breast cancer but figures relating to survival from breast cancer are also interesting and suggest that patients given ERT have an improved survival from breast cancer.[32,38,47] This may be because of the more favorable staging of breast cancers in ERT patients compared with other women. If so, some of the excess risk in women receiving ERT may be attributable to earlier diagnosis of breast cancer (due to greater surveillance). This would then further weaken the case that ERT substantially increases risk of breast cancer (apart from a modest effect associated with prolonged use). In view of the protective effect of the menopause these results are surprising and may reflect the differences between ERT and natural menstrual cycles in terms of the types of estrogens involved and their presentation to the breast.

Exogenous estrogen during reproductive years

Estrogens administered in the form of oral contraceptive pills usually consist of synthetic estradiol-17b derivatives (ethinyl estradiol or its 3-methyl ether, mestranol) and one of a number of progestogens. Oral contraceptive pills were first introduced in the USA in the 1960s and in the UK shortly thereafter. Initially they were used for family spacing by women in the middle of their fertile years (25-40 years of age). The large number of studies on these women have been reassuring in that none have suggested any significant increase in risk apart from the occasional report of a positive association between breast cancer risk and total duration of oral contraceptive use. However, anxieties have been expressed about possible harmful effects of oral contraceptive when used either before first full-term pregnancy or before age 25[49-51] and there is now evidence of trends between risk and duration of oral contraceptive use (Table 3.6).[51,52] There are further complications in assessing influences of oral contraceptives in terms of inherent biases of case-control studies, the varying types and doses of steroids used, latency of effect and the background against which these steroids are being prescribed.[53] Although there is no hard evidence of a risk effect associated with particular pill formulations, relative risks have been reported as being significantly higher for preparations containing at least 50 mg estrogen compared with lower dose combined oral contraceptives[54] and hence the trend for modern pills to contain lower doses of estrogen. Latency of effect deserves special mention since time intervals between exposure to risk and diagnosis of cancer can be considerable as evidenced by the time-gap between menarche and first appearance of breast cancer;[20] no cases of breast cancer were diagnosed in the first 10 years following exposure to irradiation from the bombing Hiroshima and Nagasaki and significant effects were not demonstrated for 20 years;[55] and the time interval between administration of diethylstibestrol in pregnancy and significantly increased incidence of breast cancer has been 20-40 years.[26,56] Short term follow-up is therefore likely to yield negative results and

***Table 3.6. Relative risk of breast cancer by duration and pattern
of use of oral contraceptives***

Type of use	Duration of use (months)	Relative Risk (95% CI)	
Never	0	1.00	
Continuous	1-48	0.86	(0.55, 1.33)
	49-96	1.25	(0.72, 2.16)
	97+	2.57	(1.31, 5.05)
Interrupted only	1-48	1.07	(0.59, 1.94)
by pregnancy	49-96	1.70	(1.04, 2.79)
	97+	1.65	(0.99, 2.78)
Intermittent	1-48	1.00	(0.63, 1.58)
	49-96	1.34	(0.87, 2.06)
	97+	1.53	(0.95, 2.45)

the potential influences of the widespread use of contraceptive estrogens which started in the 1970s may only now become apparent.

Finally, the effects of oral contraceptives need to be considered against the background of ovarian steroid production; it is conceivable that contraceptive steroids could be either protective or have deleterious effects on the breast depending upon the nature and regularity of ovarian activity in particular women.

SUMMARY

The epidemiological evidence linking estrogens with risk of breast cancer is provocative but not conclusive. Menarche and menopause are influential in the etiology of breast cancer and their effects are likely to be mediated by estrogen. Similarly, findings relating to exposure to exogenous estrogens during pregnancy and at the menopause are suggestive, but not unequivocal, of increased risk of breast cancer; the data on the oral contraceptives, while largely reassuring, are still too immature to be totally convincing but long-term use in young women is a matter of concern.

CLINICO-PATHOLOGICAL EVIDENCE

The clinico-pathological evidence linking estrogen with risk of breast cancer is indirect, partly because of the difficulties of separating effects from those of other hormones and partly because of the ethics of performing appropriate investigations to prove cause or effect.

The histological evidence that estrogens may stimulate proliferation of normal breast epithelium has already been reviewed (chapter 2). Such stimulatory influences have relevance for risk of breast cancer

because proliferation may increase the number of target cells susceptible to malignant transformation[3,57] and proliferating cells appear more
susceptible to carcinogenesis than quiescent cells.[58,59] It is thus relevant
that the breasts of young women (which have higher labelling indices
than those from older women[60]) appear more sensitive to cancer initiation resulting from irradiation. This evidence is derived from women
exposed to irradiation either at Hiroshima or after multiple chest
fluoroscopies; girls in their teens were more likely to develop breast
cancer than those exposed at a later age.[54,61,62]

Clinical observations in males subject to relative or absolute estrogenic excess are also informative. Thus, men with Klinefelter's syndrome have a gonadal abnormality which results in low androgen in
the presence of normal or raised estrogen. This relative estrogen excess
may cause gynaecomastia and a 20 times increased incidence of mammary cancer over that in the general male population.[63,64] Pharmacological doses of estrogen given to young men have been linked to breast
cancers. Symmers[65] reported on two transvestite males who had been
exposed to estrogen for five years and subsequently died from metastatic breast cancer early in life. This may be contrasted with the low
evidence of mammary cancer reported in men treated with estrogen
for carcinoma of the prostate (who are generally older and exposed to
estrogen for comparatively short periods).[66,67]

The last piece of indirect clinico-pathological evidence which suggests that estrogens may promote the development of breast cancer
comes from a pathological examination of breast tissue in which tissue
from both breasts of 110 consecutive women (who had autopsies for
medico-legal reasons) were carefully scrutinized for precursor lesions
of cancer. These results reveal a decrease in the incidence of both atypical
ductal hyperplasia and carcinoma in situ after the menopause suggesting that ovarian hormones were required to maintain these putative
precursors of invasive cancers.

ENDOCRINOLOGICAL EVIDENCE

Considerable efforts have been expended in attempts to show that
women at high risk of breast cancer and/or those who subsequently
develop the disease, have abnormal endocrine profiles and more specifically may be subject to hyperestrogenization. It is worth summariz-
ing the data, if only to illustrate the problems associated with such an
exercise.

The following synopsis excludes studies of patients presenting with
breast cancer since it is possible that the presence of disease, particularly at an advanced stage, might itself affect endocrine profiles and
given the long latent period that may have elapsed before the clinical
appearance of cancer, hormonal status may have changed radically from
that which was initially associated with risk. Even with these major
exclusions, there are complexities in deciding how to assess estrogenic

status in terms of which body fluid to assay, which estrogen to measure and how to take into account the variation within and between menstrual cycles, in premenopausal women.

Urine

Initially, measurements of endogenous estrogens were hampered by the lack of sensitive assays and early studies were performed on urine which allowed the extraction of large sample volumes. However, population studies of high and low risk groups and familial studies (see Table 3.7) did not yield consistent evidence that any individual urinary estrogen was associated with increased risk,[69] although one group observed *lower* estradiol glucuronide in women at risk for familial cancer.[70,71] As this was also associated with elevated estrone sulfate,[71] it was postulated that this reflected an abnormality in estrogen conjugation. There have also been suggestions that while individual urinary estrogens are not associated with risk, an imbalance in the ratio of the three major urinary estrogens might be important.[74] Thus, the estriol quotient (estriol: estrone plus estradiol) has been reported to be higher in Oriental women than in Caucasians[73] and in parous women compared to nulliparous.[74] Since the balance is in favor of relatively higher levels of estriol in the low risk group, this led to the hypothesis that estriol was protective and impeded the biological actions of more powerful estrogens such as estradiol and estrone. However, except during pregnancy, negligible amounts of estriol are found in the blood[75] and in any case the urinary ratio does not reflect estrogenic status.[76] In particular, it has been shown that estrogen levels in blood, production rates and metabolic clearance rates are not correlated with the proportion of estrone, estradiol and estriol found in the urine.[77]

Interestingly the evidence that subsequent breast cancer can be predicted by urinary steroids is stronger for androgens than for estrogens. Of particular importance was the prospective study initiated by Bulbrook in 1961 on the Island of Guernsey in which urine specimens were collected from 5000 normal women.[78] When a case of breast

Table 3.7. Urinary estrogens and risk of breast cancer (positive findings only)

Risk Factor	Estrogen	Finding	Ref
Family History	Estradiol glucuronide	Lower levels in women at risk	Fishman et al. Science 1979; 204:1089. Fishman et al. Cancer Res 1983; 43:1884.
	Estrone sulfate	Higher levels in women at risk	Fishman et al. Cancer Res 1983; 43:1884.
Geographical Environment	Estriol quotient	Higher in Oriental than Caucasian women	MacMahon et al. Int J Cancer 1974; 14:161.
Parity	Estriol quotient	Higher in parous (cf nulliparous)	Cole et al. Lancet 1976; 2:596.

cancer was subsequently diagnosed, the patient's specimen was retrieved from storage together with up to 10 matched controls. Assays for androsterone, etiocholanolone and dehydroepiandrosterone were then carried out. Within 10 years, 27 women had developed breast cancer and their excretion of androsterone and etiocholanolone was significantly lower than that of the controls, this being present up to nine years before onset of the disease. The abnormality was found mainly in premenopausal women (A similar study by De Waard and Banders-van Halewun[79] failed to show subnormal androgen excretion in postmenopausal women). Twenty-five years of follow-up are now available in Guernsey and it is apparent that while cases of breast cancer occurring in the early years of the study had a low excretion of androgen metabolites, women in whom tumors appeared late in life had a higher excretion of these steroids.[80] In other words, androgen excretion is related to age at diagnosis and not to absolute risk.[81]

BLOOD

With the advent of radioimmunoassays, estrogens could be measured in blood. This provided a more direct estimate of the levels of hormones to which target tissues were exposed and allowed a re-evaluation of the hypothesis that the breasts of women who were at increased risk to cancer may be exposed to more estrogen than those who were not.

Results were however no more consistent (Table 3.8). Serum estradiol was reported to be substantially lower in Oriental premenopausal women maintaining a traditional life-style (as compared with women from Western societies with an increased risk).[82] In contrast others have reported levels of estrogens in the blood of Japanese women to be normal.[83]

The effect of menarche on hormone profiles also came under scrutiny. Thus, a longitudinal study of 200 healthy schoolgirls, showed that those with early menarche (at high risk of breast cancer) had increased serum estradiol and significantly lower sex hormone-binding globulin (SHBG).[8,84] This was already apparent at 10 years of age and persisted for up to five years after menarche. High estradiol: SHBG ratios would be expected to result in increased amounts of free estradiol, since SHBG is the major protein which binds estradiol in the circulation (see the section below on biologically available estrogen).

In an attempt to determine a hormonal basis for the protective effect of first birth on breast cancer risk, plasma and urinary hormonal profiles were measured in premenopausal nulliparous women and their parous sisters.[85] No differences were found in either estrone or estradiol levels. However, parous women had significantly shorter cycle lengths than the nulliparous group and when women with similar cycle lengths were compared the parous subjects had significantly lower levels of estradiol but higher levels of sex hormone-binding globulin (without differences being evident in levels of biologically available estradiol).[85,86]

Table 3.8. Estrogens in blood and risk of breast cancer

Risk Factor	Estrogen	Finding	Ref.
Familial History	Estrone plus estradiol	Increased levels in daughters (not sisters)during luteal (not follicular) phase	Henderson et al. New Eng J Med 1975; 293:790.
	Estrone, estradiol and estriol	No difference between family history group and cohorts	Boffard et al. Eur J Cancer Clin Oncol 1981;17:1071. Fishman et al. Cancer Res 1983; 43:1884. Fishman et al. Cancer Res 1978; 38:4006.
Geographic Environment	Estradiol	Lower cases in Oriental premenopausal women (cf Western women)	Key et al. Br J Cancer 1990; 62:631.
	Estradiol/Estrone	Normal levels in premenopausal Japanese women	Bulbrook et al. Eur J Cancer Clin Oncol 1976; 12:725.
	Estrone	Lower levels in postmenopausal Japanese women	Pike et al. Nature 1983; 303:767.
Parity	Estrone/Estradiol	Similar levels in nulliparous/parous sisters (correcting for cycle length lower levels of estradiol in parous subjects)	Bernstein et al. JNCI 1985; 74:741.
Menarche	Estradiol	Increased levels in girls with early menarche	Frisch et al. J Amer Med Assoc1981; 246:1559. Vihko et al. Rev Endo Related Cancer 1986; 23:11.
Benign breast disease	Estrone/Estradiol	No consistent results	England et al. Br J Cancer 1974; 30:571. Martin et al. J Steroid Biochem 1978; 9:1251. Wang et al. Br Cancer Res Treat 1985; 6:5.
Obesity	Estrone, Estrone sulfate	Higher levels in obese women	Vermeulen et al. Clin Endocrinol 1978; 9:59. James et al. J Steroid Biochem 1981; 15:235.

Results on estrogen levels in patients with benign breast disease have been contradictory.[87-89] Values for estradiol have been reported to be either normal or elevated during the luteal phase in premenopausal women with benign breast disease but none of these studies have really taken into account the wide variety of conditions encompassed within the term "benign"; neither has any study singled out benign conditions associated with proliferative change within the breast. Given the unusually high concentrations of conjugated estrogens within the breasts of women with certain benign conditions (see chapter 6), it may be that circulating estrogens are not particularly informative.

Obesity in postmenopausal women is associated with raised circulating estrogens[90] and several studies have reported positive correlations between the degree of overweight and levels of plasma estrogen.[91,92] As these women have an increased risk of breast cancer, these data can be taken as evidence of hyperestrogenaemia in this particular risk group. The low postmenopausal weight of Japanese women also leads to low estrogen levels[93] and possibly accounts for their low risk of breast cancer.

Several groups have measured circulating levels of estrogen in women at increased risk because of a family history of breast cancer. Henderson and colleagues[94] assayed total blood estrogens (estrone plus estradiol) in daughters and sisters of women with breast cancer and matched controls. They found that the daughters (but not the sisters) of breast cancer patients had marginally but significantly increased levels of estrogens during the luteal phase but not during the follicular phase of the menstrual cycle. In a similar study performed by Boffard et al[95] serum estrogen levels were measured in 52 adolescent girls with a family history of breast cancers and 90 girls without a history but no differences were found between the groups. Furthermore, Fishman's group[96,97] reported that estrogens measured through the menstrual cycle of 30 women at risk for familial breast cancer were not different from those in an equal number of matched controls.

These results on estrogens circulating in the blood do not provide particularly convincing evidence that women at risk for subsequent breast cancer are exposed to states of hyperestrogenaemia. However, as indicated in the introductory chapter, between 40-50% of estradiol in blood is bound with high affinity to sex hormone-binding globulin (SHBG), most of the remainder being bound non-specifically with low affinity to albumin and only a small fraction is free. Recently attention has focused on this latter fraction since there is evidence that free steroids are freely diffusible into cells whereas those bound to SHBG are not.[98] The biological availability of the albumin-bound fraction of estradiol has not been studied extensively but because of the virtually instantaneous dissociation of steroids that bind to albumin[99] this may also have easy access to cells. The most recent measurements on blood have therefore attempted to measure "free" estrogens either directly by equilibrium dialysis or indirectly by determining levels of SHBG (Table 3.9). In terms of the latter there is an inverse relationship between SHBG levels and body weight, with grossly obese women having low SHBG levels.[100] In postmenopausal women this would reinforce the estrogenic effects of their higher levels of estrone. Similarly, Japanese women appear to have more of their estradiol bound to SHBG than do their (higher-risk) British counterparts.[101] However, when the amounts of estradiol bound to albumin, SHBG, or unbound to transport proteins were compared in five racial groups living in Hawaii no differences were found in spite of a 5-fold range in incidence rates of

Table 3.9. "Free Estrogens" and sex hormone binding globulin (SHBG) and risk of breast cancer

Risk Factor	Finding	Ref.
Geographical environment	Greater proportion of estradiol bound to SHBG Japanese women (cf British women).	Moore et al. Int J Cancer 1986; 38:625.
	No difference in racial groups in Hawaii	Goodman et al. Eur J Cancer Clin Oncol 1988; 24:1855.
Obesity	Inverse correlation between SHBG and body weight	Kopelman et al. Clin Endocr 1980; 12:363.
Subsequent development of Breast Cancer	Early development associated with high 'Free Estradiol' (and low SHBG in postmenopausal patients)	Bulbrook et al. Annals NY Acad Sci 1986; 464:373.
	Late development of cancer not associated with significant abnormalities	Bulbrook et al. Annals NY Acad Sci 1988; 538:248.

breast cancer.[102] Perhaps the most illuminating observation has come from the investigation referred to earlier in relation to urinary androgens in which Bulbrook and co-investigators[78] carried out a prospective study on the Island of Guernsey. Blood was obtained from 5000 ostensibly normal women who were then screened for breast cancer by mammography and clinical examination. Preliminary results on the first 13 women to develop breast cancer showed that they had a much higher proportion of their serum estradiol in the non-protein bound fraction than the controls, at a significance level of p,0.00005.[103] The sex hormone-binding globulin levels were correspondingly at the lower end of the normal range in the postmenopausal (but not the premenopausal) precancerous patients. Despite the absolute amounts of estrogen involved being small, the conclusion drawn from these findings was that women with high amounts of biologically available estradiol in their blood were at greater risk of breast cancer. However, as the study matured, the new cases of breast cancer were found to have SHBG levels within the normal range and eventually the difference between cases and controls became insignificant. It was therefore proposed that the time between a negative screen and the diagnosis of breast cancer reflected tumor growth rates;[104] low SHBG levels and high proportions of free estradiol were associated with rapidly growing tumors which appeared in the first few years of the study. Later cases whose tumors grew more slowly were associated with SHBG levels in the upper part of the normal range.

BREAST FLUID AND TISSUE

The levels of estrogen in urine and plasma only provide an indirect and not necessarily accurate indication of those within the breast and more information may be obtained on the estrogenic environment by performing measurements on breast-derived fluids and tissue. There is no doubt that amounts of estrogen in such material can differ substantially from those in the circulation and do not always reflect levels in either plasma or urine.[105,106] This phenomenon has its own particular interest and is the subject of chapter 6. Without pre-empting the topic, it is sufficient to say that, with the exception of certain sub-sets of cyst fluids, there is little to suggest that measurements of estrogen within breast-derived material will help identify women at particular risk of subsequent breast cancer.

From the above considerations it is difficult to come to any other conclusion than that there is no consistent evidence derived from measurements of endogenous estrogens to support the concept that abnormal levels are associated with increased risk to subsequent breast cancer (although it may be that a hyperestrogenic environment can stimulate occult tumors so that they become quickly apparent). Despite this negative conclusion, it is unwise to dismiss endogenous estrogens as risk factors for breast cancer and it is still necessary to consider that any hormone abnormality may be transient, being present only at certain critical inductive times, that cumulative exposure is important and small differences in estrogen levels, which are difficult to detect, become critical if maintained over a long period of time, that pattern of presentation of estrogen may be crucial such that cyclicity or periodicity assumes more importance than absolute levels, and that phytoestrogens, catechol estrogens and other estrogenic compounds have been relatively ignored (it may be relevant that a recent prospective cohort study involving 14,000 women found that those in the top percentile for serum levels of DDE as estimated 8 years before diagnosis had 4-fold greater risk of developing breast cancer than those in the bottom percentile).[107] We must also consider that the influence of estrogen may be modified by the effect of other hormones, and that susceptibility to endogenous estrogens may vary within risk groups. Finally general and local metabolism of estrogens within the body should not be ignored. This aspect will now be reviewed.

METABOLIC EVIDENCE

The two principle pathways of estrogen metabolism appear to be hydroxylation at C2 and C16. However, the reactions appear to be mutually exclusive and virtually never occur on the same molecule. Because 16α-hydroxylase and 2-hydroxylase compete for the same substrate, estrone, significant enhancement of 2-hydroxylation will be biologically equivalent to decreased 16α-hydroxylation. Bradlow, Fishman and colleagues have developed in vivo methods of assessing the activities of these pathways by incorporating ^3H into the metabolically reactive site of the estrogen molecule, administering the labeled steroid to individuals and then determining the release of ^3H into body water.[108,109] Although there is very little difference in metabolic patterns between pre- and postmenopausal women (which suggests that metabolism is largely time-invariant[108]) other studies have yielded interesting results. For example, the extent of 16α-hydroxylation appears to be elevated in women at high risk of breast cancer for familial reasons.[109,110] Organ culture studies have also shown that 16α-hydroxylation in terminal ductal lobular units (TDLU) derived from mastectomy specimens is significantly increased compared to that in TDLU from mammoplasty specimens.[111] Asian women also generally have low levels of 16α-hydroxyestrone but high levels of 2-hydroxyestrone[112]—the lower levels of 2-hydroxyestrone in Western women may be caused by their relative obesity, which decreases 2-hydroxylation.[113] The significance of these studies lies in the properties of 16α-hydroxyestrone, which, despite low affinity for the estrogen receptor, binds irreversibly to the receptor and thus permanently activates it.[114] This estrogen also does not bind to SHBG so that most of that circulating is available for biological action. Unlike 16α-hydroxyestrone, 2-hydroxyestrone (2OHE$_1$) is peripherally inactive.[115]

As elevated levels of 16α-hydroxyestrone may promote cancer and because of the refractory nature of 16α-hydroxylation to interventions in humans, the possibility of altering the risk of hormone-dependent cancers by dietary or pharmacological stimulation of 2-hydroxylation becomes an interesting strategy.

MOLECULAR EVIDENCE

To put into perspective the evidence that at a molecular level estrogens are capable of increasing risk of cancer, it is necessary to have an understanding of the molecular processes that occur during carcinogenesis. Although knowledge of this is accumulating at a rapid rate, neither the number nor the exact nature of the steps leading to malignant transformation is known. Experimental data and epidemiological evidence suggest more than one rate-limiting step is entailed in the transformation process[116] and both genetic aberrations and defects in the kinetics of tissue growth and differentiation are involved.[117] Accepted dogma suggests that every cell possesses tissue-specific proto-oncogenes,[118] which are important in normal growth and differentiation and are normally turned off by diploid pairs of regulator genes or anti-oncogenes (or more imaginatively termed tumor suppressor genes[118,119]). Malignant transformation occurs when an oncogene is inappropriately turned on or suppressor genes are lost or turned off. Recent experimentation indicates that different oncogenes may cooperate in malignant transformation[120] and suggests that there has to be at least two "hits" to initiate the cancer process.[118,121] To interpret the action of estrogen it is necessary to consider the concepts of initiation and promotion. There is a general consensus that initiators are mutagens and that initiation involves mutations or similar abnormalities at specific genetic loci.[122] The mechanism of promotion is ill-defined in terms of target cells. Classically promotion involves the clonal expansion of initiated cells but it may also encompass the processes by which pools of susceptible stem cells are enlarged.

ESTROGENS AS INITIATORS

In the standard assays for mutogens, most naturally occurring estrogens give negative results,[123] although the synthetic estrogen diethylstilbestrol may test positive results in certain systems (cell cultures exposed to estrogen can display an increased frequency of genetic abnormalities but this is probably a phenomenon associated with a concomitant increase in proliferative activity[125]).[124] The one class of natural estrogens which may be exceptional are catechol estrogens. Thus, catechol estrogens such as 2-hydroxy- and 4-hydroxyestrone may be metabolized into O-quinone intermediates which are capable of producing free radicals and causing DNA damage.[126] 16α-hydroxyestrone forms adducts with DNA, which can lead to mistranslation.[127] The physiological significance of these observations in relation to breast carcinogenesis still requires to be clarified. It may also be relevant that many non-steroid compounds which have estrogenic characteristics can also function as mutagens[128] but it is unclear at this stage whether mutagenesis results from estrogenic or genotoxic activity. This clearly complicates the interpretation of the mechanism of such chemicals in breast cancer risk.

ESTROGENS AS CO-INITIATORS/PROMOTERS

Studies on chemical carcinogenesis have identified substances which induce cancer in bio-systems but are themselves not genotoxic.[129] Many of these compounds appear to act as carcinogens merely by increasing cell proliferation and there is a molecular basis for the view that cell division is essential for the genesis of human cancer.[130] Cell division increases the risk of genetic mistakes[130,131] and may cause disjunction of chromosomes and convert damaged single-stranded DNA into gaps or mutations. As a result proto-oncogenes may be activated or overexpressed; conversely, tumor suppressor genes may be lost or inactivated. Estrogens are capable of stimulating cell division in target tissues[132] and, as indicated earlier, cells which are subject to the proliferative effects of estrogen are also prone to genetic errors which might occur during the process of DNA copying in cell division. Estrogens may profoundly influence the expression of proto-oncogenes such as c-*fos* and c-*myc* which are key regulators of cell division.[133]

Whether estrogens act as "co-initiators" by increasing the chances of genetic damage during the course of replication in the breast is unresolved. However the fact that estrogens are capable of inducing proliferation in both normal breast and invasive cancers suggests that they may also do so in intermediate or transformed cells. If this is the case estrogens would fit the classical definition of tumor promoters on the basis that they can expand the pool of cells susceptible to a second genetic hit. Consequently most experts regard the role of estrogen in carcinogenesis classically as one of a promoter.

CONCLUSIONS

The notion that estrogens increase risk to breast cancer feels intuitively correct. After all, the breast is a target organ for estrogens which cause it to grow at puberty and estrogens may delay atrophic processes and maintain epithelial proliferation if given at the menopause. Furthermore, many of the known risk factors for breast cancer are linked with life-time exposure to estrogen and the profound protective effect of ovariectomy early in life cannot be ignored and imply that ovarian estrogens are important in the genesis of most breast cancers. Additionally trophic effects of estrogens on proliferation within the breast are compatible with the role of a tumor promoter—increased frequency of cell division could result in DNA copying errors, which in turn would lead to the genetic or epigenetic aberrations necessary for neoplastic transformation. Intuition, however, is not proof and there is a counter-perspective. The classical risk factors for breast cancer (such as early menarche, late menopause, postmenopausal obesity) are rarely associated with more than a 2-fold increase in risk and exposure to exogenous estrogens (although increasing risk) does not have the same strength of relationship as is found between estrogen use and other endocrine-related malignancies such as endometrial cancer. Finally measurements of endogenous estrogens in women either at risk or subsequently developing breast cancer have not shown them to be different from controls. These paradoxes cannot be totally resolved at present but some further comment may be helpful. First, it is necessary to consider the possibility that estrogens are essentially permissive, i.e., their presence is necessary for the genesis of cancer but relatively minor changes in level do not markedly affect risk. The influence of estrogen on breast cancer risk may only manifest itself at crucial periods of high proliferation/sensitivity such as at puberty or result from prolonged and sustained exposure. It is interesting therefore that the levels of proliferation in the "resting" breast are substantially lower than those in the endometrium. This may reflect a lower threshold of estrogen sensitivity to stimulus within the breast and correspondingly lower susceptibility to malignant change. The epidemiology and endocrinology associated with early menarche and prolonged reproductive life would be compatible with this concept. Given that only 30% of breast cancers arise in women with reproductive risk factors, it had been hoped that measurements of endogenous estrogen would identify women at increased risk of developing breast cancer on account of their raised levels of estrogens. This has not proven to be the case but problems surround the assessment of estrogenic status in the context of critical time periods, cumulative exposure and the type of estrogen to be measured. In terms of the latter there is a current awareness that classical estrogens are not the whole story and environmental chemicals, although they have considerably less estrogenic potency than estradiol, may build up in the food chain, may be stored in breast fat and through cumulative combined exposure, may have a role in breast cancer risk. It is also necessary to consider not only the effects of estrogen but the factors which influence differential susceptibility to estrogen within the breast. These may include estrogens themselves which have been implicated both in prenatal imprintation which primes estrogen responsiveness and programs metabolic pathways regulating the synthesis and disposition of estrogens. Finally like other malignancies, risk to breast cancer will be multifactorial and estrogens represent only one factor which has to be considered in the context of others. While data on the protective effects of castration suggest estrogen is important in risk of most breast cancers, the effects of ovariectomy are dramatic in comparison with endocrine influences associated with other reproductive risk factors or the use of current exogenous hormone regimes. These considerations are summarized in Figure 3.2. The complex nature of this figure also serves to explain why the transition from intuition to specific proof for the involvement of estrogen in the risk for breast cancer has proven to be tortuous.

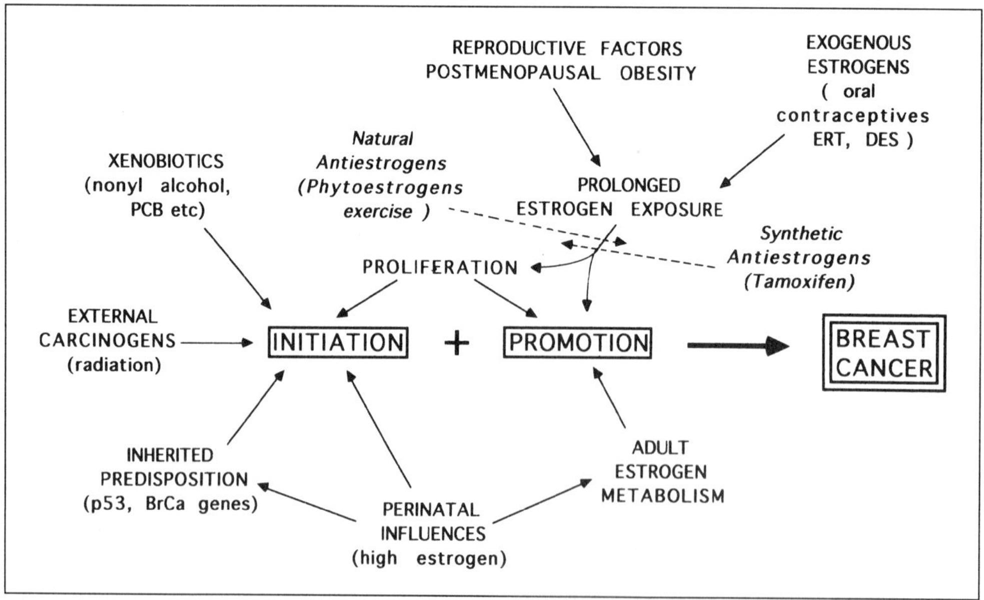

Fig. 3.2. *Complexity of interactions between estrogenic and other factors in the development of breast cancer. Plain text represents stimulatory influences; italic text represents inhibitory effects.*

REFERENCES

1. Boyle P. Epidemiology of breast cancer. Bailliere's Clin Oncol 1988; 2:1-57.
2. MacMahon B, Cole P, Brown J. Etiology of human breast cancer: a review. JNCI 1973; 50:21-42.
3. Moolkgavkar SH. Hormones and multistage carcinogenesis. Cancer surveys 1986; 5:635-648.
4. Trichopoulos D, MacMahon B, Cole P. Menopause and breast cancer risk. JNCI 1972; 48:605-613.
5. Wienfeld AM. The relationship of cancer of female breast to artificial menopause and menstrual status. Cancer 1956; 9:927-936.
6. Pike MC, Spicer DV, Dahmoush L et al. Estrogens, progestogens, normal breast cell proliferation, and breast cancer risk. Epidemiologic Revs 1993; 15:17-35.
7. Kvale G. Reproductive factors in breast cancer epidemiology. Acta Oncol 1992; 31:187-194.
8. Frisch RE, Gotz-Welbergen AV, McArthur JW et al. Delayed menarche and amenorrhea of college athletes in relation to age of onset of training. J Amer Med Assoc 1981; 246:1559-1563.
9. Bernstein L, Ross RK, Lobo RA et al. The effects of moderate physical activity on menstrual cycle patterns in adolesence, implications for breast cancer prevention. Br J Cancer 1987; 55:681-685.
10. Frisch RE, Wyshak G, Albright NC et al. Lower prevalence of breast cancer and cancers of the reproductive system among former college athletes compared to nonathletes. Br J Cancer 1985; 82:885-891.
11. Korenman SG. Oestrogen window hypothesis of the aetiology of breast cancer. Lancet 1980; i:700-701.
12. LaVecchia C, Decarli A, DiPietro S et al. Menstrual cycle patterns and the risk of breast disease. Eur J Cancer Clin Oncol 1985; 21:417-421.
13. Wallace RB, Sherman BM, Bean JA et al. Menstrual cycle patterns and breast cancer risk factors. Cancer Res 1978; 58:4021-4024.
14. Gilliam AG. Fertility and cancer of the breast and of the uterine cervix: comparisons between rates of pregnancy in women with cancer at these and other sites. J Natl Cancer Inst 1951; 12:287-304.
15. Ron E, Lunenfeld B, Menezer J et al. Cancer incidence in a cohort of infertile women. Am J Epidemiol 1987; 125:780-790.
16. Henderson BE, Pike MC, Casagrande JT. Breast cancer and the estrogen window hypothesis. Lancet 1981; 2:363-364.
17. Henderson BE, Ross RK, Judd HL et al. Do regular ovulatory cycles increase breast cancer risk? Cancer 1985; 56:1206-1208.
18. Apter D, Vihko R. Early menarche, a risk factor for breast cancer indicates early onset of ovulatory cycles. J Clin Endocrinol Metab 1983; 57:82-86.
19. Vihko RK, Apter DL. The epidemiology and endocrinology of the menarche in relation to breast cancer. Cancer Surveys 1986; 5:561-571.
20. Henderson BE, Bernstein L. The international variation in breast cancer rates: an epidemiological assessment. Breast Cancer Res Treat 1991; 18:S11-S17.

21. Going JJ, Anderson TJ, Battersby S et al. Proliferative and secretory activity in human breast during natural and artificial menstrual cycles. Proc Am J Pathol 1988; 130:193-204.

22. Anderson TJ. The involvement of oestrogen in the development and function of the normal breast: histological evidence. Proc Roy Soc Edin 1989; 95B:23-32.

23. de Waard F, Baanders-van Halewijn EA. A prospective study in general practice on breast cancer risk in postmenopausal women. Int J Cancer 1974; 14:153-160.

24. Vermeulen A, Verdonck L. Sex hormone concentrations in post-menopausal women. Relation to obesity, fat mass, age and years post-menopause. Clin Endocrinol 1978; 9:59-66.

25. James VHT, Reed MJ, Folkerd EJ. Studies of estrogen metabolism in postmenopausal women with cancer. J Steroid Biochem 1981; 15:235-245.

26. Barber HRK. Cancers of breast, uterus and ovary. In: Stoll BA, ed. Risk factors and multiple cancer. John Wiley & Sons Ltd. 1984: 315-330.

27. De Waard F, Cornelis JP, Aoki K et al. Breast cancer incidence according to weight and height in two cities in the Netherlands and in Aichi Prefecture, Japan. Cancer 1977; 40:1269-1276.

28. Pike MC, Krailo MD, Henderson BE et al. "Hormonal" risk factors, "breast tissue age" and the age-incidence of breast cancer. Nature 1983; 303:767-770.

29. Colton T, Greenberg R, Noller K et al. Breast cancer in mothers prescribed diethylstilbestrol in pregnancy. JAMA 1993; 269:2069-2100.

30. Weiss NS, Ure CL, Ballard JH et al. Decreased risk of fractures of the hip and lower forearm with postmenopausal use of estrogen. New Eng J Med 1980; 303:1195-1198.

31. Henrich JB. The postmenopausal estrogen/breast cancer controversy. JAMA 1992; 268:1900-1902.

32. Bluming AZ. Hormone replacement therapy: benefits and risks for the general postmenopausal female population and for women with a history of previously treated breast cancer. Seminars in Oncol 1993; 20:662-674.

33. Armstrong BK. Estrogen therapy after the menopause: boon or bane? Med J Aust 1988; 148:213-214.

34. Dupont WD, Page DL. Menopausal estrogen replacement therapy and breast cancer. Arch Intern Med 1991; 151:67-72.

35. Steinberg K, Thacker SB, Smith J et al. A meta-analysis of the effect of estrogen replacement therapy on the risk of breast cancer. JAMA 1991; 265:1985-1990.

36. Colditz GA, Egan KM, Stampfer MJ. Hormone replacement therapy and risk of breast cancer: results from epidemiologic studies. Am J Obstet Gynecol 1993; 168:1473-1480.

37. Brinton LA, Schairer C. Estrogen replacement therapy and breast cancer risk. Epidemiologic Revs 1993; 15:66-79.

38. Bergkvist L, Adami HO, Persson I et al. The risk of breast cancer after estrogen and estrogen-progestin replacement. N Engl J Med 1989; 321:293-297.

39. Ewertz M. Influence of non-contraceptive exogenous and endogenous sex hormones on breast cancer risk in Denmark. Int J Cancer 1988; 42:832-838.

40. Brinton LA, Hoover R, Fraumeni JF Jr. Menopausal oestrogens and breast cancer risk: an expanded case-control study. Br J Cancer 1986; 54:825-832.

41. Kelsey JL, Fisher DB, Holford TR et al. Exogenous estrogens and other factors in the epidemiology of breast cancer. JNCI 1981; 67:327-333.

42. Hiatt RA, Bawol R, Friedman GD et al. Exogenous estrogen therapy and breast cancer after bilateral oophorectomy. Cancer 1984; 54:139-144.

43. Mills PK, Beeson L, Phillips RL et al. Menopausal estrogens and breast cancer. N Engl J Med 1976; 295:401-405.

44. Colditz GA, Stampfer MJ, Willett WC et al. Type of postmenopausal hormone use and risk of breast cancer: 12-year follow-up from the Nurses' Health Study. Cancer Causes Control 1992; 3:433-439.

45. Yang CP, Daling JR, Band PR et al. Noncontraceptive hormone use and risk of breast cancer. Cancer Causes Control 1992; 3:475-479.

46. Dupont WD, Page DL, Rogers LW et al. Influence of exogenous estrogens, proliferative breast disease and other variables on breast cancer risk. Cancer 1989; 63:948-957.

47. Hunt K, Vessey M, McPherson K. Mortality in a cohort of long-term users of hormone replacement therapy: an updated analysis. Br J Obstet Gynaecol 1990; 97:10860-10866.

48. La Vecchia C. Oral contraceptives and breast cancer. The Breast 1992; 2:76-81.

49. Pike MC, Henderson BE, Casagrande JT et al. Oral contraceptive use and early abortion as risk factors for breast cancer in young women. Br J Cancer 1981; 43:72-76.

50. Pike MC, Henderson BE, Krailo MD et al. Breast cancer in young women and use of oral contraceptives: possible modifying effect of formulation and age at use. Lancet 1983; ii:926-930.

51. McPherson K, Vessey MP, Neil A et al. Early oral contraceptive use and breast cancer: results of another case-control study. Br J Cancer 1987; 56:653-660.

52. Chilvers CED, Smith SJ et al. The effect of patterns of oral contraceptive use on breast cancer risk in young women. Br J Cancer 1994; 67:922-923.

53. Chilvers CED, Deacon JM. Oral contraceptives and breast cancer. Br J Cancer 1990; 61:1-4.

54. UK national case-control study group. Oral contraceptive use and breast cancer risk in young women. Lancet 1989; i:973-982.

55. Tokunaga M, Norman JE, Asano M. Malignant breast tumours among atomic bomb survivors, Hiroshima and Nagasaki. J Natl Cancer Inst 1979; 62:1347-1359.

56. Greenberg ER, Barnes AB, Resseguie L et al. Breast cancer in mothers given diethylstilbestrol in pregnancy. N Eng J Med 1984; 311:1393-1397.

57. Thomas DB. Do hormones cause breast cancer? Cancer 1984; 53:595-604.

58. Frei JV, Harsono T. Increased susceptibility to low doses of a carcinogen of epidermal cells in stimulated DNA synthesis. Cancer Res 1967; 27:1482-1484.

59. Marquardt H. Cell cycle dependence of chemically-induced malignant transformation in vitro. Cancer Res 1974; 34:1612-1615.

60. Potten CS, Watson RJ, Williams GT et al. Cell proliferation in the normal human breast. The effect of age and menstrual cycle upon proliferative activity of the normal breast. Br J Cancer 1988; 58:163-170.

61. Howell A. Clinical evidence for the involvement of oestrogen in the development and progression of breast cancer. Proc Roy Soc (Edin) 1989; 95B:49-57.

62. Hrubec Z, Boice JD, Monson RR et al. Breast cancer after multiple fluoroscopies—2nd followup of Massachusetts women with tuberculosis. Cancer Res 1989; 49:229-234.

63. Harnden DG, Maclean N, Langlands AO. Carcinoma of the breast and Klinefelters syndrome. J Med Gen 1971; 8:460-461.

64. Scheike O, Svenstrup B, Fransden VA. Male breast cancer. II. Metabolism of oestradiol-17 beta in men with breast cancer. J Steroid Biochem 1973; 4:489-501.

65. Symmers WS. Carcinoma of the breast in transexual individuals after surgical and hormonal interferene with the primary and secondary sex characteristics. Br Med J 1968; 2:82-85.

66. Benson WR. Carcinoma of the prostate with metastases to breasts and testis; critical review of the literature and a report of a case. Cancer 1957; 10:1235-1245.

67. O'Grady WP, McDivitt RW. Breast cancer in a man treated with diethylstilbestrol. Archives of Path 1969; 88:162-165.

68. Neilsen M, Thomsen JL, Primdahl S et al. Breast cancer and atypia among young and middle-aged women. A study of 110 medicolegal autopsies. Br J Cancer 1987; 56:814-819.

69. Fentiman IS. The endocrine dimension. In: Prevention of Breast Cancer. RG Landes Company, Austin 1993.

70. Fishman J, Fukushima DK, O'Connor J et al. Low urinary estrogen glucuronides in women at risk of familial breast cancer. Science 1979; 204:1089-1091.

71. Fishman J, Bradlow HL, Fukushima DK et al. Abnormal estrogen conjugation in women at risk for familial breast-cancer at the periovulatory stage of the menstrual-cycle. Cancer Res 1983; 43:1884-1890.

72. MacMahon B, Cole P, Brown JB et al. Urine oestrogen profiles of Asian and North American women. Lancet 1971; 2:900-902.

73. MacMahon B, Cole P, Brown JB et al. Urine oestrogen profiles of Asian and North American Women. Int J Cancer 1974; 14:161-167.

74. Cole P, Brown JB, MacMahon B. Oestrogen profiles of parous and nulliparous women. Lancet 1976; 2:596-599.

75. Lipsett MB. Oestrogen profiles and breast cancer. Lancet 1971; ii:1378.

76. Zumoff B, Fishman J, Bradlow HL et al. Hormone profiles in hormone-dependent cancers. Cancer Res 1975; 35:3365-3368.

77. Longcope C, Pratt JH. Blood production rates of oestrogens in women with differing ratios of urinary oestrogen conjugates. Steroids 1977; 29:483-492.

78. Bulbrook RD, Hayward JL, Spicer CC. Relation between urinary androgen and corticosteroid excretion and subsequent breast cancer. Lancet 1971; 2:395-397.

79. De Waard F, Banders-van Halewun EA. A prospective study in general practice on breast cancer risk in postmenopausal women. Int J Cancer 1974; 14:153-160.

80. Bulbrook RD, Hayward JL. Wang DY et al. Identification of women with a high risk of breast cancer. Breast Cancer Res Treat 1986a; 7(Suppl):5-10.

81. Bulbrook RD, Thomas BS. Hormones are ambiguous risk factors for breast cancer. Acta Path Scand 1989; 28:841-848.

82. Key TJA, Chen J, Wang DY et al. Sex hormones in women in rural China and in Britain. Br J Cancer 1990; 62:631-636.

83. Bulbrook RD, Swain MC, Wang DY et al. Plasma oestradiol-17β, oestrone and progesterone and their urinary metabolites in normal British and Japanese women. Eur J Cancer Clin Oncol 1976; 12:725-728.

84. Vihko R, Apter D. Hormonal profile and disposition to breast cancer. Rev Endocrine Related Cancer 1986; 23:11-15.

85. Bernstein L, Pike MC, Ross RK, et al. Estrogen and sex hormone-binding globulin levels in nulliparous and parous women. J Natl Cancer Inst 1985; 74:741-745.

86. Moore JW, Key TJ, Bulbrook RD et al. Sex hormone binding globulin and risk factors for breast cancer in a population of normal women who had never used exogenous sex hormones. Br J Cancer 1987; 56:661-666.

87. England PC, Skinner LG, Cottrell KM et al. Serum oestradiol-17β in women with benign and malignant breast disease. Br J Cancer 1974; 30:571-576.

88. Martin PM, Kuttenn F, Serment H et al. Studies on clinical, hormonal and pathological correlations in breast fibroadenomas. J Steroid Biochem 1978; 9:1251-1255.

89. Wang DY, Fentiman IS. Epidemiology and endocrinology of benign breast disease. Breast Cancer Res Treat 1985; 6:5-36.

90. Kirschner MA, Schneider G, Ertel NH et al. Obesity, androgens, estrogens, and cancer risk. Cancer Res 1982; 42(Suppl):3281s-3285s.

91. Vermeulen A, Verdonck L. Sex hormone concentrations in post-menopausal women. Relation to obesity, fat mass, age and years post-menopause. Clin Endocrinol 1978; 9:59-66.

92. JamesVHT, Reed MJ, FolkerdEJ. Studies of estrogen metabolism in postmenopausal women with cancer. J Steroid Biochem 1981; 15:235-245.

93. Shimizu H, Ross RK, Bernstein L et al. Serum oestrogen levels in postmenopausal women: comparison of American whites and Japanese in Japan. Br J Cancer 1990; 62:451-453.

94. Henderson BE, Gerkins V, Rosario I et al. Elevated serum levels of estrogen and prolactin in daughters of patients with breast cancer. N Engl J Med 1975; 293:790-795.

95. Boffard K, Clark CMG, Irvine JBD et al. Serum prolactin, androgens, oestradiol and progesterone in adolescent girls with or without a family history of breast cancer. Eur J Cancer Clin Oncol 1981; 17:1071-1077.

96. Fishman J, Bradlow HL, Fukushima DK et al. Abnormal estrogen conjugation in women at risk for familial breast cancer at the periovulatory stage of the menstrual cycle. Cancer Res 1983; 43:1884-1890.

97. Fishman J, Fukushima D, O'Connor J et al. Plasma hormone profiles of young women at risk for familial breast cancer. Cancer-Res 1978; 38:4006-4011.

98. Anderson DC. Sex-hormone-binding globulin. Clin Endocrinol 1974; 3:69-96.

99. Pardridge WM, Mietus LJ, Frumar AM et al. Effects of human serum on transport of testosterone and estradiol into rat brain. Am J Physiol 1980; 239:E103-E108.

100. Kopelman PG, Pilkington TRE, White N et al. Abnormal sex steroid secretion and binding in massively obese women. Clin Endocr 1980; 12:363-369.

101. Moore JW, Hoare SA, Millis RR et al. Binding of oestradiol to blood proteins and the aetiology of breast cancer. Int J Cancer 1986; 38:625-630.

102. Goodman MJ, Bulbrook RD, Moore JW. The distribution of estradiol in the sera of normal Caucasian, Chinese, Filipino, Hawaiian and Japanese women living in Hawaii. Eur J Cancer Clin Oncol 1988; 24:1855-1960.

103. Bulbrook RD, Moore JW, Clark GMG et al. Relation between risk of breast cancer and bioavailability of estradiol in blood: prospective study in Guernsey. In: Angelli A, Bradlow HL, Dogliotti L eds. Endocrinology of the breast: basic and clinical aspects. Annals of the New York Acad of Sci 1986; 464:373-388.

104. Bulbrook RD, Moore JW, Allen BS et al. Sex-hormone-binding globulin and the natural history of breast cancer. An NY Acad Sci 1988; 538:248-256.

105. Rose PR, Lahti H, Laakso K et al. Serum and breast duct fluid prolactin and estrogen levels in healthy Finnish and American women and patients with fibrocystic disease. Cancer 1986; 57:1155-1554.

106. Petrakis NL. Oestrogens and other biochemical and cytological components in nipple aspirates of breast fluid: relationship to risk factors for breast cancer. Proc Roy Soc (Edin) 1989; 95B:169-181.

107. Wolff MS, Paolo G, Toniolo P et al. Blood levels of organochlorine residues and risk of breast cancer. J Natl Cancer Inst 1993; 85:648-652.

108. Fishman J, Bradlow HL, Schneider J et al. Radiometric analysis of oxidation in man: sex differences in estradiol metabolism. Proc Nat Acad Sci USA 1980; 77:4957-4960.

109. Bradlow HL, Hershcopf RJ, Martucci CP et al. 16α-hydroxylation of estradiol: a possible risk marker for breast cancer. Ann NY Acad Sci 1989; 464:138-151.

110. Osborne MP, Karmali RA, Hershcopf RJ et al. Omega-3 fatty acids: modulation of estrogen metabolism and potential for breast cancer prevention. Cancer Invest 1988; 8:629-631.

111. Osborne MP, Bradlow HL, Wong GYC et al. Upregulation of estradiol C16α-hydroxylation in human breast tissue: a potential biomarker of breast cancer. JNCI 1993; 85:1917-1920.

112. Lemon HM, Heidel JW, Rodriguezsierra JF. Increased catechol estrogen metabolism as a risk factor for non-familial breast cancer Cancer 1992; 69:457-465.

113. Schneider J, Bradlow HL, Strain G et al. Effect of obesity on estradiol metabolism: decreased formation of nonuterotropic metabolites. J Clin Endocrinol Metab 1983; 56:973-978.

114. Swaneck G, Fishman J. Covalent binding of the endogenous estrogen 16α-hydroxy-estroneo estradiol receptor in human breast cancer cells: characterization and intranuclear localization. Proc Natl Acad Sci USA 1988; 85:7831-7835.

115. Martucci C, Fishman J. Impact of continuously administered catechol estrogens on uterine growth and LH section. Endocrinol 1979; 105:1288-1292.

116. Moolgavkar SH. Hormones and multistage carcinogenesis. Cancer Surveys 1986; 5:635-648.

117. Moolgavkar SH, Knudson AG Jr. Mutation and cancer: a model for human carcinogenesis. JNCI 1981; 66:1037-1052.

118. Knudson AG. Hereditary cancer, oncogenes and antioncogenes. Cancer Res 1985; 45:1437-1443.

119. Stanbridge EJ. Identifying tumor suppressor genes in human colorectal cancer. Science 1990; 247:12-13.

120. Land H, Parada LF, Weinberg RA. Tumorigenic conversion of primary embryo fibroblasts requires at least two cooperating oncogenes. Nature 1983; 304:596-601.

121. Hecker E. Three stage carcinogenesis in house skin—recent results and present status of an advanced model system of chemical carcinogenesis. Toxicol Pathol 1987; 15:245-248.

122. Weinstein IB. The origins of human cancer: molecular mechanisms of carcinogenesis and their implications for cancer prevention and treatment—Twenty-seventh GHA Clowes Memorial Award Lecture. Cancer Res 1988; 48:4135-4143.

123. World Health Organization/International Agency for Research on Cancer: Genetic and related effects: an IARC monographs on the evaluation of carcinogenic risks to humans. 1987; Suppl 250-256; 293-295; 369-371; 426-433; 437-443.

124. Li JJ, Li SA. Estrogen carcinogenesis in hamster tissues: a critical review. In: Negro-Vilar A, Horwitz KB, eds. Endocrine aspects of cancer. Endocrine Reviews. The Endocrine Society Press 1990; 86-93.

125. Preston-Martin S, Pike MC, Ross RK et al. Increased cell division as a cause of human cancer. Cancer Res 1990; 50:7415-7421.

126. Nutter LM, Wu Y-Y, Ngo EO et al. An o-quinone form of estrogen produces free radicals in human breast cancer cells; correlation with DNA damage. Chem Res Toxicol 1994; 7:23-28.

127. Suto A, Bradlow HL, Wong YC et al. Experimental down-regulation of intermediate biomarkers of carcinogenesis in mouse mammary epithelial cells Breast Cancer Res Treat 1993; 27:193-202.

128. Butterworth BE. Nongenotoxic carcinogens in the regulatory environment. Regul Toxicol Pharmacol 1989; 9:244-256.

129. Ames BN. Mutagenesis and carcinogenesis: endogenous and exogenous factors. Environ Mutat 1989; 13:1-12.

130. Cohen SM, Ellwein LB. Cell proliferation in carcinogenesis. Science 1990; 249:1007-1011.

131. Ames BN, Gold LS. Too many rodent carcinogens: mitogenesis increases mutagenesis. Science 1990; 249:970-971.

132. Freeman CS, Topper YJ. Progesterone and glucocorticoid in relation to the growth and differentiation of mammary epithelium. J Toxicol Environ Health 1978; 4:269-282.

133. Sekeris CE. Hormonal steroids act as tumour promoters by modulating oncogene expression. J Cancer Res Clin Oncol 1991; 117:96-101.

CHAPTER 4

ESTROGEN AND TUMOR BEHAVIOR

This chapter considers the weight of evidence that estrogens may influence (or be influenced by) the natural history of breast cancer from the same standpoints that were considered for risk in chapter 3.

EPIDEMIOLOGICAL EVIDENCE

While the classical risk factors for breast cancer have a strong hormonal component and have direct relevance in associating estrogens with development of breast cancer, they are less helpful in implicating estrogen in the behavior of established tumors.

However, there is a suggestion that survival rates from breast cancer are higher among women in areas where breast cancer rates are low[1] and it has been hypothesized that factors which determine tumor development may also affect the course of the disease.[2] For example, not only is breast cancer incidence lower in Japan compared with that in the USA but the disease tends to run a more benign course in Japan.[2] Higher survival rates in Japan are not explained by differences in age, stage, histology, parity or age at first full-term pregnancy but an influence of dietary fat intake can not be excluded. Dietary consumption of fat is related to obesity and obese women are more likely to develop metastasis and have a short survival. For example, Abe and colleagues reported a five year survival rate of 56% in obese women compared with 80% in non-obese women[3] and others have found that among breast cancer risk factors, body weight was the only parameter associated with survival.[4] Effects of obesity are likely to be mediated at least in part by estrogens, because obese women have elevated levels of non-protein bound and total estrogens[5] and adipose tissue is a major site of estrogen biosynthesis in postmenopausal women.[6]

Patients with an early onset of disease may develop tumors with a more aggressive phenotype[7] which is more likely to be estrogen receptor-negative.[8] Ottman and coworkers[9] found that estrogen receptor levels were significantly lower in postmenopausal women who had a family history of breast cancer than those who did not, but there was no difference in estrogen receptor levels among pre- and perimenopausal women who had no family history of breast cancer nor was there a difference in estrogen receptor levels between familial and non-familial premenopausal patients.

The influence of pregnancy on the natural history of breast cancer is also potentially informative, because estrogen levels are at least 10 times higher during pregnancy than at other periods. It is a pity therefore that no consensus exists as to whether pregnancy at the time of diagnosis of breast cancer confers a different prognosis as compared with non-pregnant patients of a similar age and stage of disease[10] (although a very recent study has detected a significantly poorer survival for pregnant women under 30 years of age at diagnosis).[11] Neither is evidence consistent that patients diagnosed during pregnancy derive benefit from termination of pregnancy;[12] indeed one study reported an adverse effect on survival for patients who had a termination of pregnancy.[13] Furthermore, while there are concerns that the elevated levels of circulating estrogen associated with pregnancy after diagnosis for breast cancer might stimulate micrometastatic disease, most studies have failed to show any detriment in survival for patients who become pregnant after mastectomy.[10] Indeed there are indications of a survival advantage for patients who become pregnant after primary treatment compared with those who do not.[10,14]

The epidemiology associated with the administration of exogenous estrogens to breast cancer patients ought to be more definitive. There are now considerable data relating to the use of estrogen replacement therapy in postmenopausal patients after their primary treatment for breast cancer. Instinctively it might be expected that if estrogens are growth promoting, hormone replacement therapy would increase the risk of recurrence by reactivating growth of residual breast cancer cells; and by stimulating proliferative activity in mammary epithelial cells which have undergone transformation. In fact there are few data to support this belief. If anything, results suggest the opposite; so much so that one case-control study which showed no adverse effect on cancer outcome positively recommended prospective studies of ERT in postmenopausal breast cancer patients. It is also well-established that pharmacological doses of estrogen can cause regression of tumor in advanced disease and prevent relapse in patients with earlier forms of the disease.[16] However, studies in experimental animals suggest that the estrogen receptor system in mammary tumors is refractory to pharmacological dose of estrogen.[17] This contrasts with the stimulating effects of physiological doses of estrogen which have been used in the clinical studies to recruit cancer cells before the use of chemotherapy (see below).[18]

CLINICO-PATHOLOGICAL EVIDENCE

That certain breast cancers require estrogen for their continued growth is the basis for the use of endocrine deprivation as treatment for breast cancer (see chapter 8). Thus, ovariectomy and LHRH agonists will cause regression in about 30% of breast cancers in premenopausal women[19] and adrenalectomy, hypophysectomy, aromatase inhibitors, antiestrogens and pharmacological amounts of steroids will cause remissions in a similar proportion of postmenopausal patients.[20] While these therapies may have effects on several hormones, there is reason to implicate estrogens in particular. Thus, as is shown in Table 4.1, all procedures have in common the ability either to reduce tumor levels of estrogen, or to antagonize the mechanism of estrogen action. Additionally, the major beneficial effects of such therapies seem to be associated with cancers which possess high affinity receptors for estrogen.[21] Furthermore, administration of estrogen to women with breast cancer can increase cellular proliferation within tumors. Thus Dao and co-workers measured labelling-index (LI) in skin metastases before and during treatment with ethinyl estradiol and progesterone given daily for 3-9 days and demonstrated that LI increased in seven of the 10 tumors.[22] Similar results have been reported by others following the daily administration of diethylstilbestrol.[23] This concept has been used clinically to recruit cells into cell division by stimulation with estrogen before the use of chemotherapy.[18]

An interesting clinical observation which may be linked to estrogen action is that timing of surgery in premenopausal women can influence prognosis.[24] Although controversial, it has been suggested that breast cancer patients who have breast surgery during the first half of

---

Table 4.1. Major endocrine therapies—effects on estrogen biosynthesis/action

Therapy	Potential mechanism of action
Ovariectomy	Ablation of major source of estrogen in premenopausal women
Adrenalectomy	Eliminates major source of androgen precursor of estrogen in postmenopausal women
Hypophysectomy	Removes pituitary hormones trophic to ovarian and adrenal biosynthesis of estrogenic hormones
LHRH-agonists	Down-regulate LHRH drive for ovarian production of estrogens
Aromatase inhibitors	Prevent biosynthesis of estrogens from androgens
Antiestrogens	Block action of estrogen at its receptor
Pharmacological doses of steroids (e.g., diethylstilbestrol)	Down-regulate estrogen receptors

the menstrual cycle have a poorer prognosis than those having the procedure in the second half of the cycle. It is hypothesized that factors including estrogen aid tumor spread through vasculature in the follicular phase.[25] In support of this, estrogens may have effects on the endothelium[26] and conversely antiestrogen and specific metabolites such as 2-methoxyestrone may be anti-angiogenic.[27] Estrogens will also stimulate estrogen receptor-positive tumor cells to produce and synthesize proteases which can break down basement membrane and facilitate metastasis.[28]

ENDOCRINOLOGICAL EVIDENCE

Considerable effort has been expended on measuring estrogen levels in urine, blood and saliva, either as individual estrogens, total estrogens or non-protein-bound estrogen in both pre- and postmenopausal women with breast cancer in an attempt to show that these are abnormal in women with cancer, could maintain tumor growth and may predict for tumor behavior and response to therapy.[29,30] This is despite the possibility that any abnormality detected might not be specific and simply reflect the stress of having cancer and in patients with advanced disease might be secondary to effects of metastases on, for example, liver function.

In the event, no convincing correlations were derived from early studies which sought to link urinary estrogen concentrations with clinical course of breast cancer after mastectomy and response to endocrine treatment (Table 4.2).[31] It was of interest, however, that estrogen could still be detected in the urine of some women following endocrine ablation[32] (which says something about sources of estrogen) and conversely certain women who failed to respond occasionally had no measurable estrogen in their urine (which says something about hormone-responsiveness of their disease).[33]

Comparisons between levels of estrogen in the blood between breast cancer cases and controls are equally confused and not particularly convincing.[31,34-37] Thus, while studies have shown that estradiol levels

Table 4.2. Urinary estrogens in case-cohort studies of breast cancer

Findings	Reference
Reduced levels in cases	Lemon. J Surg Oncol 1972; 4:255-273.
Normal levels	Arguelles et al. Lancet 1973; i:165-167.
Normal levels in premenopausal women	Cole et al. Cancer Res 1978; 38:745-750.
Elevated levels in cases	Hellman et al. J Clin Endo Metab 1971; 33:138-142.
Elevated levels in postmenopausal cases	Thijssen et al. J Steroid Biochem 1974; 6:729-734. Morreal et al. JNCI 1979; 63:1171-1174.

in premenopausal women and both estradiol and estrone levels in post-menopausal patients are higher in cases as compared with controls, it is equally possible to cite similar studies which fail to find significant differences.[31] Results on bio-available "free" (or non-protein-bound) estrogens are more consistent (Table 4.3). Thus, five case-control studies have shown that women with breast cancer have significantly more estradiol in the free fraction than the controls.[38-42] Two of these studies[41-42] also showed an increase in the albumin-bound fraction in breast cancer patients. Percentages of free and albumin-bound estradiol were negatively correlated with the SHBG concentration. In two studies[39,42] the increase in the bioavailable fraction could be attributed partially to diminished SHBG levels. A case-control study carried out in Holland[43] showed no significant differences in free estradiol. These authors have shown, however, that the proportion of free estradiol is significantly correlated with free fatty acid levels in the blood.[44] Salivary estradiol is thought to reflect the concentration of unbound estradiol in the blood but Wang and co-workers[45] could detect no differences in salivary estradiol between disease-free patients and controls throughout the entire menstrual cycle.

Although percentages of free estradiol have not been measured in relation to the clinical course of breast cancer, several groups have measured SHBG capacities. Significant positive correlations between tumor estradiol receptor status and the SHBG-binding capacity in Japanese women with breast cancer were observed;[46,47] high SHBG-binding capacities were also associated with a long disease-free period.[48] It was concluded that the SHBG-binding capacity might be a surrogate marker of tumor hormone dependence. However, Harris and co-workers[49] were unable to confirm the relationship between SHBG and disease recurrence in British women and others[50,51] have found no obvious relationship between SHBG-binding capacity and tumor estrogen receptor status. The possibility arises that the positive findings apply only to Japanese women.

The prospective study carried out by Bulbrook and colleagues[52] on the Island of Guernsey has already been referred to in the context of

Table 4.3. Bio-available estrogen in case-cohort studies of breast cancer

| Free E$_2$(%) | | | Relative | |
Case	Control	Ratio	SHBG	Reference
2.15	1.52	1.41	=	Siiteri et al. In: Hormones & Breast Cancer 1981.
2.17	1.67	1.30	↓	Moor et al. Int J Cancer 1982; 29:17-21.
1.85	1.52	1.21	=	Reed MJ et al. Cancer Res 1983; 43:3940-43.
1.72	1.44	1.19	↓	Ota et al. Cancer 1986; 57:558-62.
2.25	2.02	1.11	=	Langley et al. JNCI 1985; 75:823-29.
1.47	1.54	0.95	=	Bruning et al. Br J Cancer 1985; 51:479-84.

risk but their observations also have implications with regard to the nature of the tumors appearing. This is because women who developed breast cancer in the early years of the investigation had a higher proportion of their circulating estradiol in the non-protein-bound fraction than the controls, whereas women developing their cancers later did not. If the time between a negative screen and diagnosis of breast cancer was a reflection of growth rates, those with early cancers could be supposed to have both rapidly growing tumors and a higher proportion of biologically active estrogen. While the association could be casual, it equally could be causal with estrogen accelerating the growth of occult breast cancer so that clinically detectable lesions appear earlier.

METABOLIC EVIDENCE

There is no direct evidence that the metabolism of estrogen influences the behavior of breast cancer or is itself influenced by the presence, stage or progression of the disease. Although 16α-hydroxylation of estrogens is elevated in breast cancer patients, it is suggested that the activity is time-invariant[53] and would therefore be present before the overt appearance of the disease. Indeed, as is discussed earlier, 16α-hydroxylation may be an important factor in risk and promotion of breast cancer.

MOLECULAR EVIDENCE

At a molecular level, the single most important parameter linking estrogens with the behavior of breast cancers is the estrogen receptor. As will be discussed in more detail later, the major effects of estrogen are mediated through these intracellular proteins.[54] It is thus relevant that there are profound changes in tissue levels of estrogen receptors (ER) in the breast with the progression from "normal" breast to hyperplasia to non-invasive malignancy to invasive cancers.[55] In comparison with invasive tumors, estrogen receptor levels are on average a 10-fold magnitude lower in the normal breast.[56] Levels in hyperplastic lesions and non-invasive cancer are matters of debate; certain workers have suggested that the cells in these lesions are uniformly ER-positive[57] whereas others have emphasized that levels and incidence are still substantially lower than those in invasive cancers even when corrected for cellularity.[58] That levels of ER in invasive cancers are much in excess of those found in other breast tissues is suggestive of an increased sensitivity to and a greater dependence upon estrogen. Upregulation of estrogen receptors in breast cancer may also be associated with deregulation of controls; for example, it has been more difficult to show that cancer ER levels vary through the menstrual cycle,[59] as has been observed in both the normal breast[60] and endometrium.[61] Parallel data have been found for an ER-related protein (27 kD heat shock protein),[62] levels being low in the normal breast, high in hormone-sensitive tumors and intermediate (with a heterogeneous staining pattern) in carcinoma in situ.[63]

The presence of ER in invasive cancers potentially relates to tumor behavior conferring both increased likelihood of response to endocrine treatment and a differentiated more benign phenotype. Both these aspects will be discussed in more detail later but suffice to indicate at this stage that 60-70% of ER-positive cancers respond to hormone treatment compared with 5-10% of ER-negative cancers[21,64] and that ER are more likely to be present in early-stage, well-differentiated cancers (Table 4.4). Increased incidence in elderly postmenopausal patients would also be compatible with slow growth.[65]

CONCLUSIONS

Clinical experience that endocrine deprivation therapy is associated with tumor regression in at least one third of patients strongly suggests that these cancers require hormones for their continued growth. That these same tumors possess high-affinity estrogen receptors implies that estrogen is the specific trophic agent involved. Experimentation with cell lines derived from breast cancers would be consistent with these observations. While withdrawal of estrogen causes tumor regression, the evidence for supplementation of estrogen increasing growth is not totally convincing. Epidemiological data suggest that increased estrogen levels as experienced by premenopausal women during pregnancy or by postmenopausal women undergoing hormone replacement therapy are neither associated with accelerated growth of primary tumors nor the early appearance of recurrent disease. However administration of estrogen under controlled conditions (for example when trying to increase susceptibility to chemotherapeutic drugs), has been associated with increased proliferation in tumor cells. Many clinicians also have anecdotal examples of how individual patients have experienced accelerated tumor growth following the inadvertent use of preparations containing estrogens. It is thus considered almost unethical to administer estrogen to women with breast cancer especially as estrogens are capable of influencing the processes associated with metastatic spread and tumor advancement in experimental systems. These are the subjects of further chapters.

Table 4.4. Estrogen receptor status and size/grade of invasive breast cancers

Size of Primary Tumor	ER + ve (%)	p value
< 2 cm	81	
2-5 cm	78	
≥ 5 cm	70	< 0.0001
Tumor Grade		
I	91	
II	80	
III	0.48	< 0.001

Derived from Thorpe & Rose. Cancer Surveys 1986; 5:505-25.

REFERENCES

1. Haenszel WM. Contributions of end results data to cancer epidemiology. In: Cutler SJ, ed. International Symposium on End Results of Cancer Therapy. NCI Monograph 1974; 15:21-33.
2. Chlebowski RT, Rose D, Buzzard M et al. Adjuvant dietary fat intake reduction in postmenopausal breast cancer patient management. Breast Cancer Res Treat 1991; 20:73-84.
3. Abe R, Kumagai N, Kimagai M. Biological characteristics of breast cancer in obesity. Tohoku J Exp Med 1976; 120:351-359.
4. La Vecchia C. Nutritional factors and cancers of the breast, endometrium and ovary. Eur J Cancer Clin Oncol 1989; 25:1945-1951.
5. Ingram D, Nottage E, Ng S et al. Obesity and breast disease. Cancer 1989; 64:1049-1053.
6. Simpson ER, Mendelson CR. Effect of aging and obesity on aromatase activity of human adipose cells. Am J Clin Nutr 1987; 45:290-295.
7. Caleffi M, Fentiman IS, Birkhead BG. Factors at presentation influencing the prognosis in breast cancer. Eur J Cancer Clin Oncol 1989; 25:51-56.
8. Fentiman IS. Breast cancer prevention with tamoxifen. The role of tamoxifen in the prevention of breast cancer. Eur J Cancer 1990; 26:655-656.
9. Ottman R, Hoffman P, Lagios M. Difference in estrogen receptor levels between familial and nonfamilial breast cancer patients. Am J Epidemiol 1978; 108:230.
10. Bluming AZ. Hormone replacement therapy: benefits and risks for the general postmenopausal female population and for women with a history of previously treated breast cancer. Seminars in Oncol 1993; 20:662-674.
11. Guinee VF, Olsson H, Möller T et al. Effect of pregnancy on prognosis for young women with breast cancer. Lancet 1994; 343:1587-1589.
12. Barnavon Y, Wallack MK. Management of the pregnant patient with carcinoma of the breast. Surg Gynecol Obstet 1990; 171:347-352.
13. King RM, Welch JS, Martin JK Jr et al. Carcinoma of the breast associated with pregnancy. Surg Gynecol Obstet 1985; 160:228-232.
14. Hubay CA, Barry FM, Murr CC. Pregnancy and breast cancer. Surg Clin North Am 1978; 58:819-831.
15. Wile AG, Opfell RW, Margileth DA et al. Hormone replacement therapy does not affect breast cancer outcome. Proc Am Soc Clin Oncol 1991; 10:58 (abstr).
16. Haddow A, Watkinson JM, Paterson E. Influence of synthetic oestrogens upon advanced malignant disease. Br Med J 1944; 2:393-398.
17. Klinge CM, Bambara RA, Zain S et al. Estrogen receptor binding to nuclei from normal and neoplastic rat mammary tissues in vitro. Cancer Res 1987; 47:2852-2859.
18. Conte P, Pronento P, Rubagatti A et al. Conventional versus cytokinetic polychemotherapy with estrogenic recruitment in metastatic breast cancer: results of a randomised cooperative trial. J Clin Oncol 1987; 53:339-347.

19. Nicholson RI, Walker KJ. Use of LH-RH agonists in the treatment of breast disease. Proc Roy Soc (Edin) 1989; 95B:271-281.

20. Forrest APM. Endocrine management of breast cancer. Proc Roy Soc (Edin) 1989; 95B:1-10.

21. Hawkins RA, Roberts MM, Forrest APM. Oestrogen receptors in breast cancer: current status. Br J Surg 1980; 67:153-169.

22. Dao TL, Sinha DK, Nemoto T et al. Effect of estrogen and progesterone on cellular replication of hukman breast tumours. Cancer Res 1982; 42:359-362.

23. Conte PF, Fraschini G, Drewinko B. Estrogen induced expansion of the growth fraction in receptor negative human breast cancer. J Steroid Biochem 1985; 23, 6B:1169-1172.

24. Badwe RA, Gregory WM, Chaudary MA et al. Timing of surgery during menstrual cycle and survival of premenopausal women with operable breast cancer. Lancet 1991; i:1261-1264.

25. Badwe RA, Richards MA, Fentiman IS et al. Surgical procedures, menstrual cycle phase and prognosis in operable breast cancer. Lancet 1991; 338:815-816.

26. Fukuda M, Maekawa J, Hosokawa Y et al. Hormone-dependent changes of blood vessels in DMBA-induced rat mammary carcinoma and its regression studied by 3H-thymidine autoradiography. Basic Appl Histochem 1985; 29:21-43.

27. Fotsis T, Zhang Y, Pepper MS et al. The endogenous oestrogen metabolic 2-methoxyoestradiol inhibits angiogenesis and suppresses tumour growth. Nature 1994; 369:237-239.

28. Rochefort H, Augereau P, Briozzo P et al. Oestrogen-induced pro-cathepsin D in breast cancer: from biology to clinical application. Proc Roy Soc Edin 1989; 95B:107-118.

29. Leclercq G, Heuson JC. Therapeutic significance of sex-steroid hormone receptors in the treatment of breast cancer. Eur J Cancer 1977; 13:1205-1215.

30. Lippman ME, Allegra JC. Estrogen receptor and endocrine therapy of breast cancer. New Eng J Med 1978; 299:930-933.

31. Moore JW, Thomas BS, Wang DY. Endocrine status and the epidemiology and clinical course of breast cancer. Cancer Surveys 1986; 5:537-559.

32. Bulbrook RD, Greenwood FC. Persistence of urinary oestrogen excretion after oophorectomy and adrenalectomy. Br Med J 1957; 1:662-666.

33. Greenwood FC, Bulbrook RD. Effect of hypophysectomy on urinary oestrogen in breast cancer. Br Med J 1957; 1:666-668.

34. England PC, Skinner LG, Cottrell KM et al. Sex hormones in breast disease. Br J Surg 1975; 62:806-809.

35. Sherman BM, Wallace RB, Jochimsen PR. Hormonal regulation of the menstrual cycle in women with breast cancer: effect of adjuvant chemotherapy. Clin Endocrinol 1979; 10:287-296.

36. Adami HO, Johansson EDB, Vegelius J et al. Serum concentrations of estrone, androstenedione, testosterone and sex-hormone-binding globulin in postmenopausal women. Uppsala J Med Sciences 1979; 84:259-274.

37. Drafta D, Schindler AE, Milcu St M et al. Plasma hormones in pre- and postmenopausal breast cancer. J Steroid Biochem 1980; 13:793-802.

38. Siiteri PK, Hammond GL, Nisker JA. Increased availability of serum estrogens in breast cancer: a new hypothesis. In: Pike MC, Siiteri PK, Welsch CW. Hormones and breast cancer, Banbury Report 8. Cold Spring Harbor NY: Cold Spring Harbor Laboratory 1981.

39. Moore JW, Clark GMG, Bulbrook RD et al. Serum concentrations of total and non-protein-bound oestradiol in patients with breast cancer and in normal controls. Int J Cancer 1982; 29:17-21.

40. Reed MJ, Cheng RW, Noel CT et al. Plasma levels of estrone, estrone sulphate and estradiol and the percentage of unbound estradiol in postmenopausal women with and without breast cancer. Cancer Res 1983; 43:3940-3943.

41. Langley MS, Hammond GL, Bardsley A et al. Serum steroid binding proteins and the bioavailability of estradiol in relation to breast diseases. JNCI 1985; 75:823-829.

42. Ota DM, Jones LA, Jackson GL et al. Obesity, non-protein-bound estradiol in the sera of breast cancer patients. Cancer 1986; 57:558-562.

43. Bruning PF, Bonfrer JMG, Hart AAM. Non protein-bound estradiol, sex-hormone-binding-globulin, breast cancer and breast cancer risk. Br J Cancer 1985; 51:479-484.

44. Bruning PF, Bonfrer JMG. Free fatty acid concentrations correlated with the available fraction of estradiol in human plasma. Cancer Res 1986; 46:2606-2609.

45. Wang DY, Fantl VE, Hahibollahi F et al. Salivary oestradiol and progesterone levels in premenopausal women with breast cancer. Eur J Cancer Clin Oncol 1986; 22:427-433.

46. Murayama Y, Sakuma T, Udagawa H et al. Sex hormone binding globulin and estrogen receptor in breast cancer: technique and preliminary clinical results. J Clin Endocrinol Metab 1978; 46:998-1006.

47. Murayama Y, Utsonomiya J, Ansano K et al. Sex hormone binding globulin and recurrence after mastectomy. Gann 1979; 70:715-716.

48. Murayama Y, Utsonomiya J, Takahashi I et al. Sex hormone binding globulin as a reliable indicator of hormone dependence of breast cancer. Annals Surg 1979; 190:133-137.

49. Harris AL, Smith IE, Dowsett M et al. Sex hormone binding globulin level and prognosis in early breast cancer. Lancet 1981; 1:279.

50. Mason RC, Miller WR, Hawkins RA et al. Plasma sex hormone binding globulin and tumour oestrogen receptor status in breast cancer patients. Lancet 1981; 1:617.

51. Sulkes A, Fuks Z, Gordon A et al. Sex hormone binding globulin (SHBG) and breast cancer: a correlation with obesity but not with estrogen receptor status. Eur J Cancer Clin Oncol 1984; 20:19-23.

52. Bulbrook RD, Moore JW, Clark GM et al. Relation between risk of breast cancer and bioavailability of estradiol in blood: prospective study in Guernsey. In: Agnelli A, Bradlow HL, Dogliotto L, eds. Endocrinology of the breast: basic and clinical aspects. Annals NY Acad Sci 1986; 464:373-388.

53. Moore JW, Clark GMG, Hoare SA et al. The binding of oestradiol to blood proteins and the aetiology of breast cancer. Int J Cancer 1986; 38:625-630.

54. Fishman J, Bradlow HL, Schneider J et al. Radiometric analysis of oxidation in man: sex differences in estradiol metabolism. Proc Nat Acad Sci USA 1980: 4957-4960.

55. Howell A. Clinical evidence for the involvement of oestrogen in the development and progression of breast cancer. Proc Roy Soc Edin 1989; 95B:49-57.

56. Carpenter S, Georgiade G, McCarty Sr KS et al. Immunohistochemical expression of oestrogen receptor in normal breast tissue. Proc R Soc Edin 1989; 95B:59-66.

57. Nenci I, Marchetti E, Querzoli P. Commentary on human mammary preneoplasia. The estrogen receptor promotion hypothesis. J Steroid Biochem 1988; 30:105-106.

58. Hawkins RA, Tesdale AL, Ferguson WA et al. Oestrogen receptor activity in intraduct and invasive breast carcinoma. Breast Cancer Res Treat 1987; 9:129-133.

59. King RJB. A discussion of the roles of oestrogen and progestin in human mammary carcinogenesis. J Steroid Biochem Molec Biol 1991; 39:811-818.

60. Anderson TJ, Battersby S. The involvement of oestrogen in the development and function of the normal breast: histological evidence. Proc Roy Soc Edin 1989; 95B:23-32.

61. Ferenczy A, Bertrand G, Gelfand MM. Proliferation kinetics of human endometrium during the normal menstrual cycle. Am J Obstet Gynec 1979; 133:859-867.

62. King RJB, Finley JR, Coffer AE et al. Characterization and biological relevance of a 29-kDa, oestrogen receptor-related protein. J Steroid Biochem 1987; 27:471-475.

63. Canno A, Coffer AI, Adatia R et al. Histochemical studies with an estrogen receptor-related protein in human breast tumors. Cancer Res 1986; 46:6475-6480.

64. McGuire WL, Carbone PP, Sears ME et al. Estrogen receptors in human breast cancer: an overview. In: McGuire WL, Carbone PP, Vollmer EP, eds. Estrogen receptors in human breast cancer. New York: Raven Press 1975.

65. Thorpe SM, Rose C. Oestrogen and progesterone receptor determinations in breast cancer: technology and biology. Cancer Surveys 1986; 5:505-525.

CHAPTER 5

SOURCES OF ESTROGEN AND SITES OF BIOSYNTHESIS

Given that estrogens may promote the development of breast cancer and that a subset of tumors requires these hormones for their continued growth, it has been important to define the sources by which the breast and its tumors obtain estrogen. There appears to be three major sources—exogenous supplies, and extraglandular synthesis and glandular synthesis of estrogen. The relative contribution of each varies according to menopausal status, body characteristics and, in patients with breast cancer, whether endocrine treatment has been administered. Thus (as is shown in Fig. 5.1) in premenopausal women, glandular synthesis by the ovary is largely responsible for circulating levels of estrogen and their fluctuation through the menstrual cycle. Nevertheless, at certain time-points during the menstrual cycle, particularly during the early follicular phase, the absence of a large developing follicle means that extraglandular production provides a substantial proportion of synthesized estrogen.[1]

Extraglandular synthesis increases in obese women[2] and this can either supplement glandular production of estrogen or in the case of amenorrhoeic premenopausal women assume a primary role.[3]

Until recently, the influence of exogenous dietary estrogens on premenopausal women has been regarded as marginal but lately evidence has accumulated that this may not be necessarily so.[4] It has also been suggested that detergents and certain by-products of industrial pollution have characteristics of estrogens and these may contribute to an estrogenic environment.[5] There is epidemiological support for this. Feminization of males is becoming more prevalent and, for example, sperm counts are decreasing while the incidence of undescended testis is increasing.[6] These effects are not immediately reconcilable with estrogenic effects in premenopausal females in whom circulating levels of natural estrogens are substantially higher and more potent than synthetic chemicals. However, this may not be the case after the menopause when glandular production of estrogen has ceased. At this time

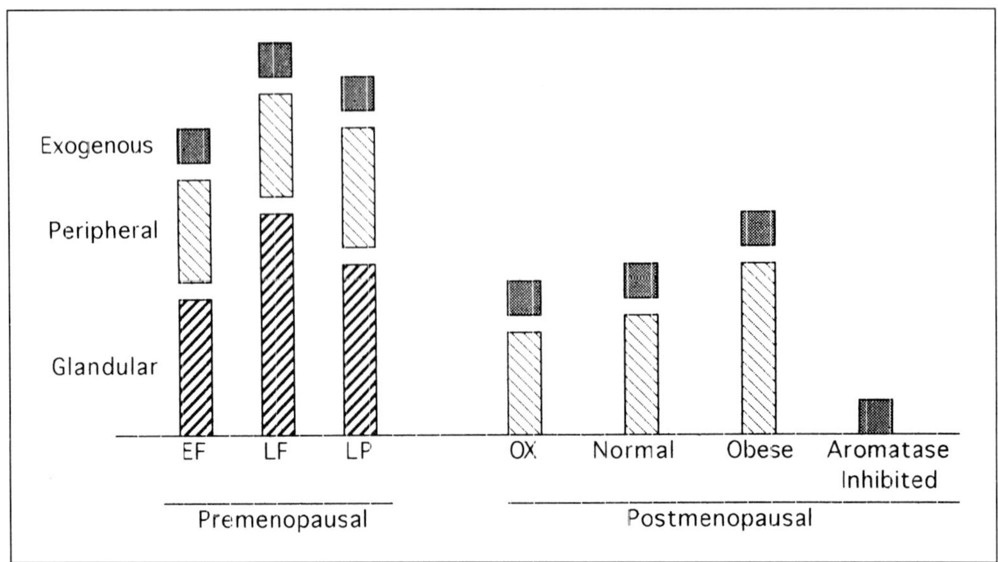

Fig. 5.1. Sources of estrogenic influence in pre- and postmenopausal women.

extraglandular synthesis of estrogens in peripheral tissues assumes greater importance. However, if this is blocked by the use of aromatase inhibitors or by endocrine ablative procedures which remove the source of androgen precursors (i.e., adrenalectomy) the residual estrogenic environment may be derived largely from exogenous sources. The next sections consider the specific sources of estrogens in more detail.

EXOGENOUS SOURCES OF ESTROGENS

There are potentially two major sources of exogenous estrogens, i.e., plants and synthetic chemicals. Extracts of many plants contain agents which are capable of inducing estrus in animals and hence can be classically defined as being "estrogenic."[7] However the principle mammalian estrogens, estrone and estradiol, occur naturally in very few plants and the major classes of plant estrogens are isoflavones, lignans, coumestins and the resorcylic acid lactones.[8] All possess a phenolic ring (see chapter 1). This seems to be a prerequisite for their estrogenic activity which is 500- to 1000-fold less potent than estradiol (Table 5.1). Indeed, the compounds may act also as antiestrogens, presumably by competing with natural ligands for the estrogen receptor (Table 5.2). While both the concentration and potency of these plant estrogens are relatively low, ingestion of their food source, particularly in large quantities, may produce biological effects. The precedent for this comes from animal studies. Thus, the isoflavones, daidzein and genistein which are present in high concentrations in soya increase uterine weight when given to hypophysectomized rats.[9] Similar effects

Table 5.1. Potencies of phytoestrogens

(Phyto)estrogen	Potencies
Estradiol	100
Coumestrol	5
Genistein	0.9
Equol	0.4
Daidzein	0.1

Data based on relative competitive protein binding in uterus as reported by DA Shutt & RI Cox. J Endocrinol 1972; 52:299-310.

Table 5.2. Biological effects of phytoestrogens

Estrogenic

Increase uterine weight in hypophysectomized/ovariectomized/immature rats
Bind to estrogen receptor protein
Induce estrogen-related markers (progesterone receptor in uterine cells and in breast cancer cells)
Stimulate alkaline phosphase activity and prostaglandin output in endometrial cells
Stimulate breast cancer cells in vitro

Antiestrogenic

Prolong follicular phase/length of menstrual cycle and suppresses mid-cycle gonadotrophin peak
Reduce incidence of rodent mammary tumors
Inhibit growth of hormone-dependent mammary tumors
Inhibit proliferation of estrogen-sensitive breast cancer cell lines
Reduce estrogen receptor levels in rodent mammary tumors
Inhibit aromatase enzyme system

have been noted in immature or ovariectomy rats following the administration of the phytoestrogen, coumestrol.[10] Daidzein, equol and enterolactone will also induce biological markers of estrogen action in breast cancer cell lines.[11] These dietary estrogens can be detected in humans and the lignans, (enterolactone and enterodiol), and the isoflavones, (genistein, daidzein equol), have been routinely measured in human urine (Table 5.3).[12] The compounds result from metabolism of dietary precursors by bacteria in the gastrointestinal tract. In common with steroid hormones, these bacterial metabolites may be absorbed from the gastrointestinal tract, undergo conjugation in the liver and enter the enterohepatic circulation. Interestingly, following ingestion of soya protein, concentrations of equol can exceed endogenous estrogens by >1000-fold.[13] Long-term ingestion of soya protein can significantly prolong the follicular phase and overall length of the menstrual cycle in women and suppress mid-cycle peaks of circulating gonadotrophins.[14] Since similar effects can be produced by the

Table 5.3. Comparative excretion of phytoestrogens

(Phyto)estrogen	Oriental	European	American
Estradiol (postmenopausal)	0.76	0.94	–
Genistein	3,440	32.1	–
Daidzein	2,600	40.5	216
Equol	2,600	44.2	63

antiestrogen, tamoxifen,[15] it has been suggested that many of the effects of isoflavones are antiestrogenic and may protect against breast cancer.[16] In keeping with this concept, soya beans reduce estrogen receptor levels and inhibit the growth of mammary cancers in experimental animals.[17] Daidzein and genistein also have anti-proliferative effects on breast cancer cell lines,[17,18] although stimulatory effects have been observed using other phytoestrogens such as equol.[19] Oriental populations (with a lower incidence of breast cancer and better prognosis) consume larger proportions of soy in their diet with daily intakes being within the range which delays appearance of mammary tumors in rodents.[20] These same concentrations are also able to inhibit the aromatase enzyme responsible for estrogen biosynthesis.[21]

The other main sources of exogenous estrogens are synthetic chemicals such as nonylphenols, chlorinated organics, polycyclic aromatic hydrocarbons and related substances, which are added to herbicides, pesticides, detergents and toiletries.[22] These compounds which are estrogenic in fish, birds and animals[5,23] can enter and accumulate in food chains.[5] Although there is no direct evidence that such compounds either cause or accelerate the growth of breast cancer, polychlorated biphenyls and other organochlorides have been reported to be present in higher concentrations in breast cancers than in normal breast tissue[24] and as well as in breast fat of patients with breast cancer as compared with that derived from women without the disease (Table 5.4).[25]

GLANDULAR SYNTHESIS OF ESTROGEN

In the ovary, the developing follicle and corpus luteum are responsible for the synthesis of estrogen. Synthesis is primarily controlled by the gonadotrophins, FSH and LH—hence the use of GnRH agonists and antagonists as agents by which to switch off estrogen production in premenopausal women. The process of estrogen biosynthesis in the ovary is complex and complicated by cooperation between two cell types—thecal cells which are the site of synthesis of androgen precursors and granulosa cells which are the site of aromatization of androgen into estrogen (Fig. 5.2). Thus, thecal cells express the crucial enzyme in androgen synthesis, 17-hydroxylase C17-20 lyase (but not aromatase) whereas granulosa cells possess aromatase (but not

Table 5.4. Comparative levels of organochlorines in breast tissues

Malignant versus Normal Tissue

		Malignant Tissue	Adjacent Tissue	Adipose Tissue
pp-DDT	mean	4.39	1.42	0.75
	range	1.3-6.4	0.3-2.8	0.1-1.4
Total PCBs	mean	9.1	2.7	0.9
	range	4.3-14.2	1.3-4.2	0.2-1.4

Comparison in Breast Adipose Tissue

	Controls	Breast Cancer	
		ER-positive	*ER-negative*
DDE	765 ± 527	2,132 ± 2,050	609 ± 339
Total PCBS	397 ± 162	405 ± 131	332 ± 75

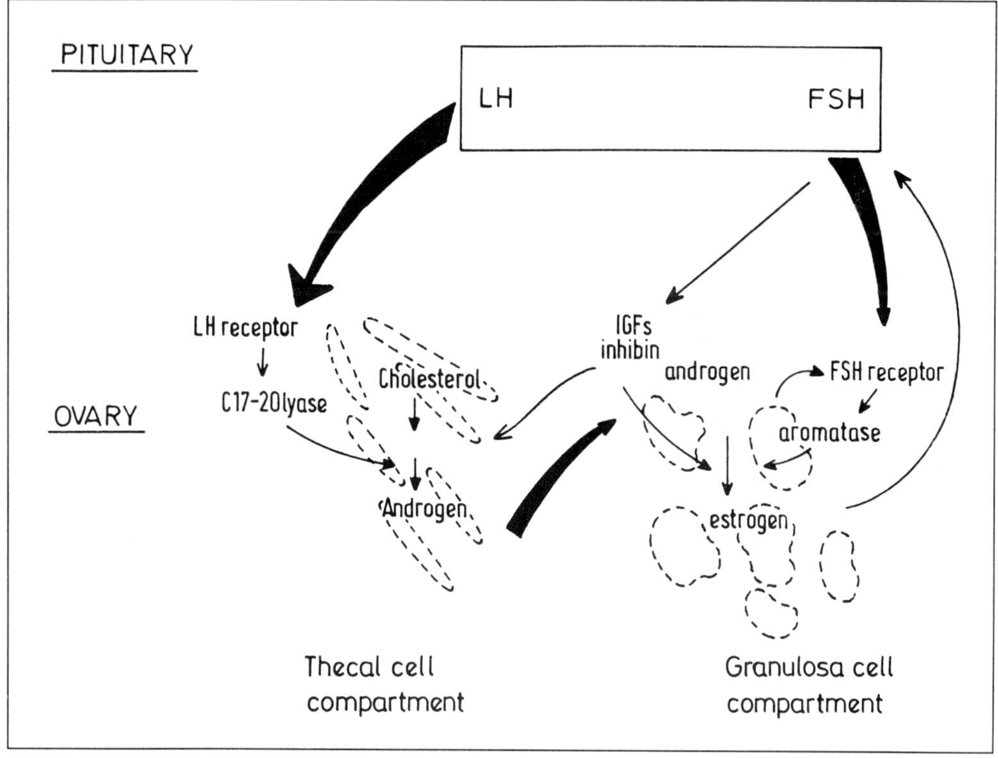

Fig. 5.2. Ovarian estrogen biosynthesis and its control.

17-hydroxylase C17-20 lyase). The combined influence of FSH and LH in controlling estrogen biosynthesis in the ovary lies primarily in the abilities of LH to induce 17-hydroxylase C17-20 lyase in thecal cells and of FSH to induce aromatase in granulosa cells. However, these tonic influences of gonadotrophin are also subject to fine tuning by local factors including ovarian steroids and growth factors. This results in a complex series of autocrine, paracrine and endocrine inter-relationships which coordinate estrogen biosynthesis in the developing follicle (see Fig. 5.2).[26] Thus while LH primarily controls androgen production via 17α-hydroxylase C17-20 lyase, the enzyme activity is also modulated by local factors generated in granulosa cells under the stimulus of FSH; these principles include insulin-like growth factors and members of the inhibin family.[27] Such paracrine communication is necessary because the granulosa cells in developing follicles are required to produce estrogen in quantities which are orders of magnitude higher than in their non-ovulatory counterparts and therefore need correspondingly more androgen substrate—it is thus rational that the androgen supplies from thecal cells should be influenced by the demands of the granulosa cells. Similar fine tuning exists in the granulosa cells whose proliferation and functional differentiation is primarily regulated by FSH. However differentiation is associated with not only induction of the aromatase enzyme but the appearance of LH receptors;[28] consequently granulosa cells in mature follicles can also respond to LH. The LH receptor seems to be functionally coupled to aromatase activity and inhibin synthesis and LH can simultaneously influence aromatization of androgens to estrogens and inhibin production.[27,29] Inhibin potentially completes a paracrine loop by augmenting androgen synthesis in thecal cells (LH can therefore affect estrogen biosynthesis by directly and indirectly stimulating androgen production in thecal cells and by facilitating estrogen formation in mature granulosa cells). To add to the complexity, granulosa cells also express androgen receptors and thecal-derived androgen not only is used as substrate for estrogen but has the potential to modulate responses to FSH. Indeed, the earliest evidence of paracrine communication within the ovary was the observation that FSH induction of aromatase activity was augmented by androgen through an androgen receptor-mediated mechanism.[30] Thus the potential exists for a reciprocal interaction between granulosa-derived inhibin and thecal-derived androgen which gives rise to developmentally related increases in estrogen biosynthesis. Additionally, estrogen itself and other factors such as IGFs and inhibin induced by FSH may act locally to modulate estrogen biosynthesis. These factors may markedly increase the responsiveness of granulosa cell aromatase activity to FSH which occurs during preovulatory follicular development,[31] allowing the follicle to grow and secrete estrogen during the late follicular phase of the menstrual cycle when FSH levels are declining. Estradiol secreted by the mature follicle can also stimulate its own formation by positive feedback control of pituitary LH release.[32] Conversely granulosa-derived estrogen may act as a negative regulator of thecal cell function and suppress thecal androgen synthesis in response to the mid-cycle LH surge.

ADRENAL CORTEX

Although removal of the adrenal causes a fall in circulating estrogens, measurements of arterio-venous differences across the adrenal suggest that the organ produces negligible amounts of estrogen.[33] However, the gland does produce large quantities of Δ4-androstenedione[33,34] which may be aromatized in peripheral tissues. Additionally the adrenal cortex synthesizes and secretes substantial amounts of Δ5-androgens, such as dehydroepiandrosterone (DHA).[35] These are interesting steroids because they circulate in relatively large amounts even in postmenopausal women (Table 5.5) and are capable of interacting with estrogen receptors to elicit estrogenic responses.[36] Indeed, in the absence of estrogen, both Δ5-androstenediol and DHA may maintain the growth of hormone-dependent breast cancer cells.[37] It has thus been postulated that in postmenopausal women, particularly those treated with aromatase inhibitors, these compounds might be responsible for continued growth.[38] The converse case has also been made that these Δ5-steroids may behave as antiestrogens, competing with estradiol for the estrogen receptor.[39,40]

EXTRAGLANDULAR SYNTHESIS

Although the ovary is responsible for the cyclic patterns of estrogens through the menstrual cycle, at certain times, for example during the early follicular phase, extraglandular production can account for about one half of circulating levels.[1] Furthermore, the ovary ceases to produce substantial amounts of estradiol after the menopause[41] and circulating levels of estrogens in postmenopausal women are primarily derived from extraglandular aromatization of adrenal androgens[1,2,41] (Fig. 5.3) which in the form of androstenedione is secreted in amounts approximating to 1 mg per day.[42] Several factors, including stress, obesity and age influence both adrenal production of androgen substrate and level of aromatase and thereby affect the amounts of estrogen produced in postmenopausal women.[42-44]

Table 5.5. Levels and estrogenic activities of Δ5-androgens

| | Concentrations (nM) | | |
	Plasma	Tumor	Relative Binding to ER
E_2	0.02-0.1	0.2-2.6	100
Δ5	1-4	0.3-30	2.5
DHA	5-25	5-500	0.003

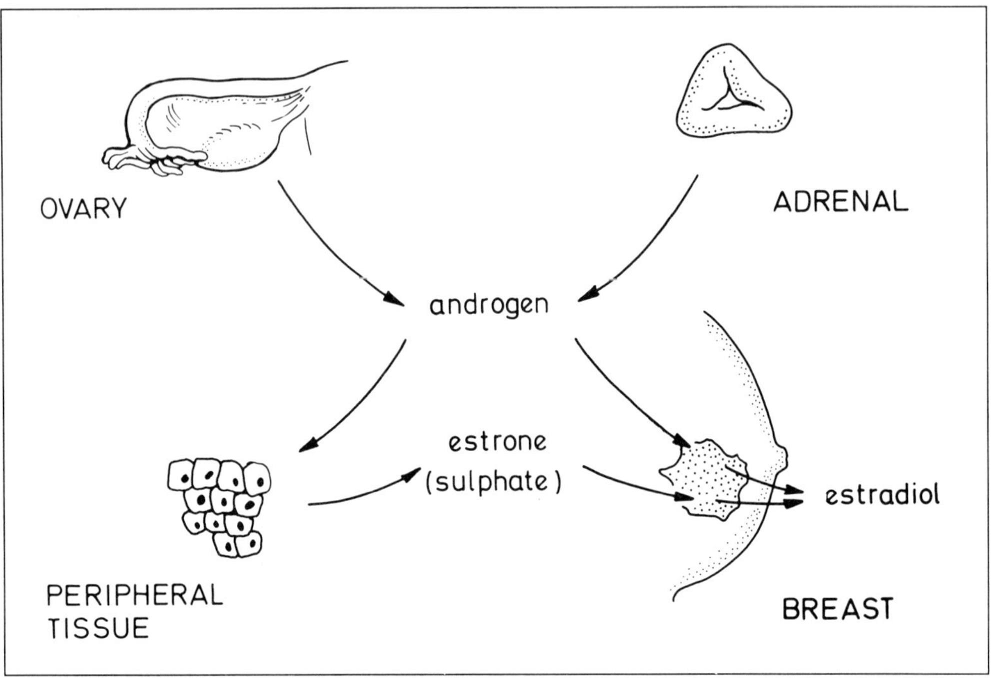

Fig. 5.3. Estrogen production in postmenopausal women.

In vivo isotopic techniques suggest that aromatization of androstenedione to estrone can range from 0.5% to 10% in postmenopausal women.[45] The aromatase enzyme has been found in several extraglandular tissues but predominantly in fat,[46] muscle,[47] skin[48] and liver[49] (and as is addressed in more detail below, in breast carcinoma tissue).[50-51]

The body mass of muscle and adipose tissue dictate that these are major sources of circulating estrogens and there are good correlations between circulating estrogens and indices of body weight in postmenopausal women[2,52] (Fig. 5.4). Interestingly within adipose tissue, the stromal pre-adipocyte compartment seems to be the major site of production rather than adipocytes themselves.[53]

The factors which regulate aromatase activity in peripheral tissues are largely undefined. In vivo administration of ACTH and/or glucocorticoids does not increase aromatase.[54] However, aromatase in cultured stroma cells from adipose tissue may be enhanced by glucocorticoids, insulin like growth factor-I (in the presence of gluco-corticoid), cyclic nucleotides and phorbol esters[55] whereas growth factors such as EGF, TGFα and TGFβ are inhibitory.[56] In contrast no significant influences of prolactin or gonadotrophins have been observed.[57,58]

The capacity for aromatase activity may vary between adipose tissue from different parts of the body. Adipose tissue of the buttocks contains much higher levels of mRNA transcripts for aromatase than that in either abdomen or thighs.[59] Aromatase activity may also be

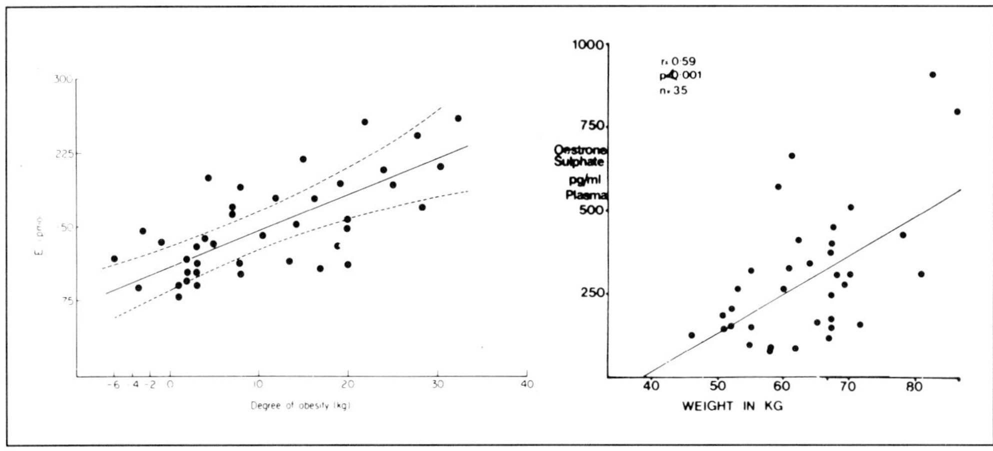

Fig. 5.4. Estrogen levels and body mass in postmenopausal women.

found in adipose tissue derived from the breast.[60] This may have implications with regard to the development and local growth of cancers within the breast—compared with other glands in the body, the adult breast is unusual in being invested in an abundance of adipose tissue.[61] It is thus of interest that aromatase activity has been reported to be significantly higher in mammary adipose tissue from breast cancer patients as compared with that from patients with benign conditions.[62] Furthermore, within the breasts of cancer patients, levels of aromatase activity and mRNA transcripts are higher in adipose tissue from tumor-bearing quadrants as compared with non-involved quadrants (Fig. 5.5).[63,64] These influences seem to be specific to aromatase since other steroid metabolizing enzymes do not show this variation.[63] The reason for enhanced aromatase activity in adipose tissue in the proximity of breast cancers is undefined—it could be inherent (and it has been suggested that the proportion of stromal cells to adipocytes is increased in these specimens[64]) or it could be that tumor-derived growth factors are secreted into the local environment inducing aromatase activity, thuscompleting a paracrine loop similar to that in the ovary. Irrespective of the underlying reason, it is possible that this phenomenon gives rise to locally elevated concentrations of estrogen (see chapter 6) thereby promoting tumor development or growth at this site. At the molecular level it has been recently shown that the increased expression of aromatase in breast adipose tissue results from the preferential utilization of certain upstream regulatory regions of the gene.[65]

About 70% of breast cancers also have the ability to synthesize estrogen from androgen precursors.[51] Although activities are low, they are comparable to those in other peripheral tissues[60,66] and if reflected in vivo would represent pmol amounts of estrogen being produced locally within the breast.[67] The exact site of biosynthesis within

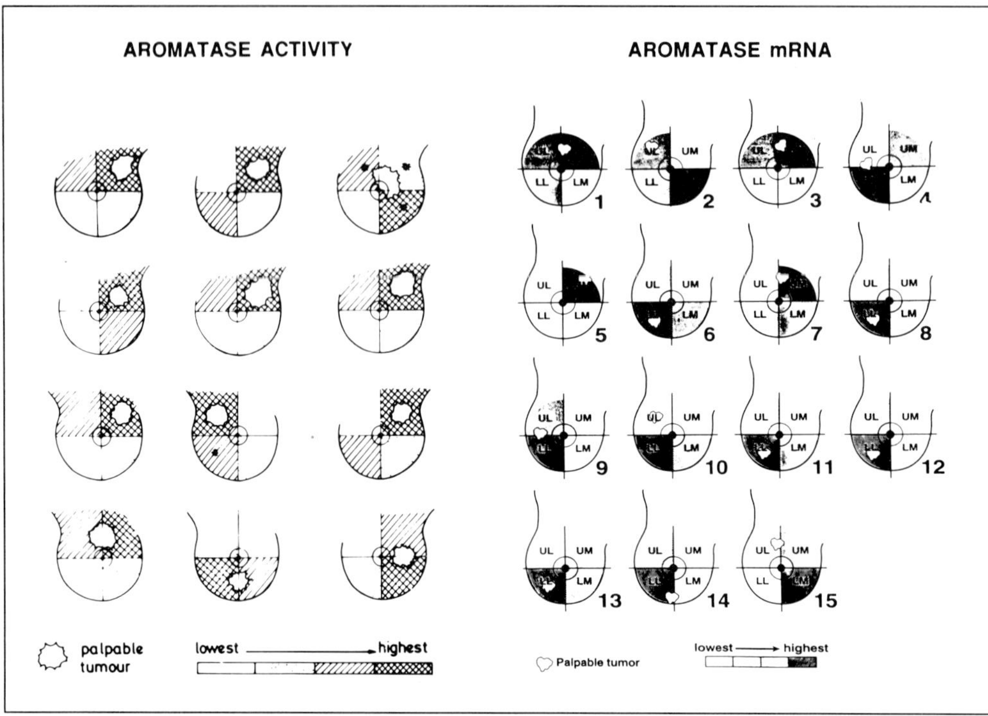

Fig. 5.5. Aromatase activity and mRNA in adipose tissue from breast quadrants in relation to tumor location.

cancers of the breast is still a matter of some controversy; certain immunohistochemical studies suggest that aromatase activity is predominately within tumor epithelial cells[68] but others place the enzyme within the stromal component.[69] Other fundamental issues still to be resolved are whether such local biosynthesis of estrogen within breast cancers can elicit biological responses (such as maintaining tumor growth) and/or contribute towards endogenous levels of estrogen within the breast. Aromatase activity has been detected in both estrogen receptor-positive and receptor-negative tumors,[70] although if it is to be of biological significance it seems more likely to be in estrogen-receptor positive tumors which possess the mechanism by which to process any synthesized estrogen. To address the question of whether estrogen production in breast cancers maintains tumor growth, two studies[71,72] have examined the relationship between aromatase activity and clinical response to aminoglutethimide, a drug which inhibits the aromatase enzyme (see chapter 8). Both studies showed that cancers with aromatase activity were more likely to respond to the inhibitor. No significant associations have been found between tumor in vitro activity and endogenous estrogens,[73,74] but it is possible that in vitro assays do not precisely reflect activity in vivo. Infusion studies in which patients with breast cancer are infused with radioactively labelled androgen precursor and estrogen are potentially more informative. These studies suggest that local estrogen biosynthesis contributes to estrogens within the majority of breast cancers.[75] It should be noted that the infusion experiments do not identify the site of local biosynthesis within the breast which could be primarily in adipose tissue rather than the tumor.

Because of results from steroid perfusion studies, the positive association between tumor aromatase and response to amino-glutethimide as well as the relationship between aromatase in mammary fat and the presence of breast cancer, local estrogen biosynthesis may influence events within the breast—particularly in postmenopausal women in whom the ovary is no longer the primary source of estrogenic hormones. It will thus be important to define the factors which regulate aromatase activity in the breast.

While the above review has concentrated upon the extraglandular synthesis of estrogen, it is also possible that levels of biologically active estrogen may be regulated by other enzyme activities acting locally within mammary tissue and breast cancers. The most important pathways are depicted in Figure 5.6 and illustrate that an alternative source of estradiol is estrone sulfate and that lipoidal estradiol may act as long-acting stores of estrogens. These enzyme activities may account for why estradiol levels are disproportionately high in breast tissue even after the menopause when estrone and its sulfate predominate over estradiol in the circulation.

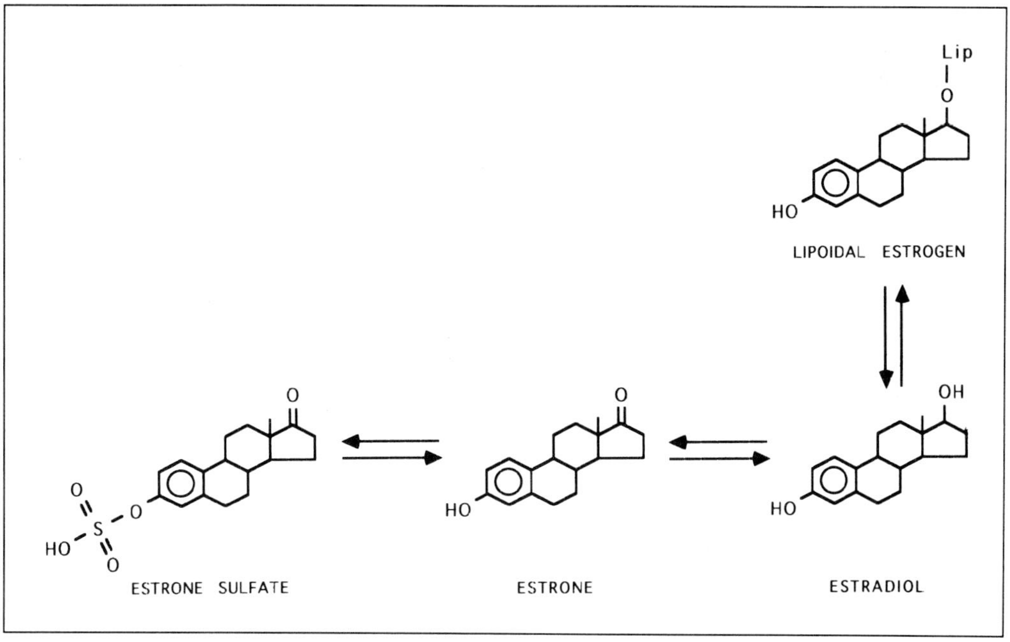

Fig. 5.6. Pathways leading to local estrogen synthesis within the breast.

Estrogen sulfatase is a ubiquitous enzyme which catalyzes the hydrolysis of estrone sulfate to estrone. Activity is readily demonstrable in breast cancers, benign tumors and breast fat.[76] In vitro studies confirmed that estrone sulfate can generate estrogenic responses in human mammary cancer cells as a result of its metabolism.[77] Indeed the estrone sulfate pathway may be a primary route of local estrogen production. Based on in vitro estimates it is calculated that 10-fold more estrone is synthesized via sulfatase than via aromatase under conditions of limited substrate availability.[78] However others have indicated that sulfatase is inhibited by DHEA sulfate and when both estrone sulfate and DHEA sulfate are added to cancer cells at concentrations found in the blood of postmenopausal patients (2 nM and 1 µM respectively), hydrolysis of estrone sulfate is largely inhibited.[79] It is also necessary to take into account the enzyme activity associated with the reverse reaction. The conversion of estrone to estrone sulfate is catalyzed by an estrogen sulfokinase. Sulfokinase activity is found in most breast tissues although there appear to be different forms of the enzyme differing in substrate specificity.[80,81] Interestingly, estradiol sulfate (E_2S) formation is a major route of estradiol metabolism when physiological concentrations of the hormone, are incubated with estrogen receptor (ER)-positive human mammary cancer cell lines.[82] Conversion of E_2 to E_2S is either very low, or absent, when similar experiments are performed with ER-negative human mammary cancer cell lines.[83] In vitro experiments also suggest that enzyme is under the control of estrogen in ER-positive cells.[84] These data on estrogen sulfotransferase and ER expression are in keeping with studies on human mammary cancer tissue. While the exact role of estrogen sulfotransferase in human mammary cancer cells is still unknown, its regulation by E_2 or E_1 suggests that it may protect nuclear ER against excess estrogen. These considerations thus suggest that sulfotransferase activity may be more relevant in determining the state of the E_1S/E_1 axis. However, it would be unwise to dismiss E_1S as a major source of biologically active estrogen within the breast and current research is endeavoring to discover inhibitors of sulfotransferase to develop as therapy for breast cancer.[85]

Whether estrogen is derived from Δ4-androstenedione or from estrone sulfate, the immediate product is estrone. For maximum biological activity this needs to be converted into estradiol by the action of a 17β-hydroxysteroid dehydrogenase (EDH). There may be several forms of the enzyme differing in their co-factor requirements, kinetics of reaction and subcellular distribution.[86] Patterns of enzyme activities may also vary in different types of breast tissue.[87] The position of equilibrium between estrone and estradiol is also unclear; in vitro studies support the direction towards estrone[88] whereas perfusion studies suggest that the breast favors the conversion of estrone to estradiol (Fig. 5.7).[89]

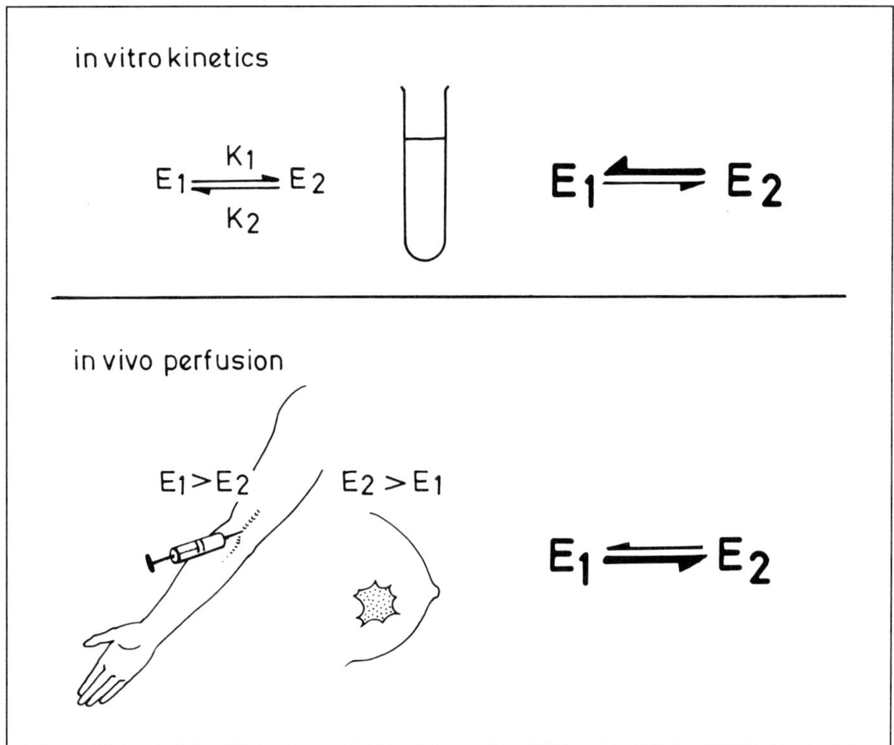

Fig. 5.7. Interconversion of estradiol to estrone.

In vitro studies also suggest that conversion of E_2 to E_1 is higher in ER-poor breast tumors as compared to ER-rich tumors[90] and in ER-negative compared to ER-positive breast cancer cell lines.[83] However in ER-positive cell lines, estrogen seems to activate 17β-hydroxysteroid dehydrogenase by an estrogen inducible factor which influences enzyme activity in only the reductive direction.[91] Interestingly activation of EDH exclusively in the reductive direction can be induced in breast tissues and cells by a number of known growth factors and by conditioned media from fibroblasts (illustrating the potential for paracrine interaction[92]). Progestins also appear to influence EDH activity. For example, in mammary tumors removed from premenopausal women with breast cancer, EDH activity is higher when excised in the luteal phase than in the follicular phase.[93] Furthermore, in postmenopausal women treated with progestins, EDH activity is stimulated in ER-positive, progesterone receptor-positive tumors, but not in tumors lacking both these receptors.[93] In contrast to the effects of estrogens, progesterone seems to increase both the reductive and oxidation directions of the reaction.

Human mammary tumors and other estrogen-responsive tissues, when incubated with the estradiol in vitro, have the ability to synthesize long chain fatty acid esters linked to E_2 at the 17β-position.[94-96] These so-called lipoidal estrogens (E_2-L) which may be composed of a number of individual fatty acid esters remain exclusively within the cell,[96] in contrast to other conjugated metabolites of E_2 which are rapidly eliminated. However, if cultured cells which have been allowed to accumulate E_2-L are transferred to fresh medium lacking E_2, regeneration of E_2 occurs. The enzyme responsible for formation of E_2-L is fatty acyl CoA: estradiol-17β acyl transferase. It appears to be present in both ER-positive and -negative tumors and formation of E_2-L is unrelated to ER and progesterone receptor status.[97] However, the composition of E_2-L formed by ER-positive and -negative breast cancer cell lines is different.[98] Consequently, in ER-negative cell lines there are high rates of accumulation of E_2-L which contain a greater percentage of E_2-17β stearate. This difference appears to be caused by the presence in ER-negative cells of high levels of the E_2-L esterase which hydrolyzes unsaturated fatty acid esters of E_2 at a greater rate than saturated fatty acid esters.[98] Although E_2-L have little affinity for the estrogen receptor,[99] they can behave as long-acting estrogens because of their slow hydrolysis resulting in release of estradiol.[100,101] The precise function of E_2-L within human breast cancer cells is still a matter of speculation[102]—they do not appear to function as a mechanism for delivering estradiol to nuclear receptors, but they may capture estradiol as an intracellular metabolite which can be regenerated later.

SUMMARY

The origin of estrogenic agents which might support estrogen-dependent growth of breast cancers are varied, including glandular synthesis, extraglandular production and exogenous sources. Their relative contribution may differ between and within groups of premenopausal and postmenopausal women. Furthermore, in terms of production of estradiol within the body there are multiple routes of biosynthesis whose contribution to trophic influences on the breast again may differ between individual women according to their physiological state. It follows therefore that strategies which are designed to deprive breast cancers of their estrogenic stimulus may be equally varied and that the optimization of effect will depend upon knowledge of the source and mechanism by which individual tumors maintain their growth. This is discussed in more detail in chapters 6 and 8.

REFERENCES

1. Kirschner MA, Schneider G, Ertel NH et al. Obesity, androgens, estrogens and cancer risk. Cancer Res (Suppl) 1982; 42:3281S-3285S.
2. MacDonald PC, Edman CD, Hemsell DL et al. Effect of obesity on conversion of plasma androstenedione to estrone in postmenopausal women with and without endometrial cancer. Am J Obstet Gynecol 1978; 130:448-455.

3. Sherman BM, Wallace RB, Bean JA. Cyclic ovarian function and breast cancer. Cancer Res (Suppl) 1982; 42:3286S-3288S.

4. Ginsburg J. Environmental oestrogens. Lancet 1994; 343:284-285.

5. Davis DL, Bradlow LHL, Wolff M et al. Medical hypothesis: xenoestrogens as preventable causes of breast cancer. Environ Health Perspect 1993; 101:372-377.

6. Sharpe RM, Skakkebaek NE. Are oestrogens involved in falling sperm counts and disorders of the male reproductive tract? Lancet 1993; 341:1392-1395.

7. Price KR, Fenwick GR. Naturally occurring oestrogens in foods—a review. Fd Addit Contam 1985; 2:73-106.

8. Setchell KDR. Naturally occurring non-steroidal estrogens of dietary origin. In: McLachlan J, ed. Estrogens in the environment: influence on development. New York: Elsevier 1985:69-85.

9. Whitten PL, Naftolin F. Dietary oestrogens: a biologically active background for estrogen action. In: Hochbert R, Naftolin F, eds. The new biology of steroid hormones. New York: Raven Press 1991:155-167.

10. Burroughs CD, Mills KT, Bern HA. Long term genital tract changes in female mice treated neonatally with coumestrol. Reprod Toxicol 1990; 4:127-135.

11. Sathyamoorthy N, Wang TTY, Phang JM. Stimulation of pS2 expression by diet-derived compounds. Cancer Res 1994; 54:957-961.

12. Setchell KDR, Lawson AM, Borriello SP et al. Lignan formation in man—microbial involvement and possible roles in relation to cancer. Lancet 1981; ii:4-7.

13. Setchell KDR, Borriello SP, Hulme P et al. Non-steroidal oestrogens of dietary origin: possible roles in hormone dependent disease. Am J Clin Nutr 19984; 40:569-578.

14. Cassidy A, Bingham S, Setchell KD. Biological effects of a diet of soy protein rich in isoflavones on the menstrual cycle of premenopausal women. Am J Clin Nutr 1994; 60:333-40

15. Golder MP, Phillips EA, Fahmy DR et al. Plasma hormones in patients with advanced breast cancer treated with tamoxifen. Eur J Cancer 1976; 12:719-723.

16. Adlercreutz H. Lignans and phytoestrogens: possible preventive role in cancer. In: Pozen P, ed. Frontiers of gastrointestinal research, vol 14. Basel, Switzerland: S Karger 1988:165-176.

17. Barnes S, Grubbs C, Setchell KDR. Chemoprevention by powdered soybean chips (PSC) of mammary tumors in rats. Breast Cancer Res Treat 1988; 12:128.

18. Pagliacci MC, Smacchia M, Migliorati G et al. Growth-inhibitory effects of the natural phyto-oestrogen Genistein in MCF-7 human breast cancer cells. Eur J Cancer 1994; 30A:1675-1682.

19. Welshons WV, Murphy CS, Koch R et al. Stimulation of breast cancer cells in vitro by the environmental estrogen enterolactone and the phytoestrogen equol. Breast Cancer Res Treat 1987; 10:169-175.

20. Adlercreutz H, Fotsis T, Heikkinen R et al. Diet and urinary excretion of lignans in female subjects. Med Biol 1981; 59:259-261.

21. Adlercreutz H, Bannwart C, Wähälä K et al. Inhibition of human aromatase by mammalian lignans and isoflavonoid phytoestrogens. J Steroid Biochem Molec Biol 1993; 44:147-153.

22. Houghton DL, Ritter L. Organochlorine residues and risk of breast cancer. J Am Coll Toxicol 1995; 14:71-89.

23. Colborn T, Clement C. Chemically induced alterations in sexual and functional development: the wildlife/human connection. In: Advances in modern environmental toxicology, vol 21. Princeton, New Jersey: Princeton Scientific Publishing 1992.

24. Wasserman M, Nogueira DP, Tomatis L et al. Organochlorine compounds in neoplastic and adjacent apparently normal breast tissue. Bull Environ Contam Toxicol 1976; 15:478-484.

25. Dewailly E, Dodin S, Verreault R et al. High organochlorine body burden in women with estrogen receptor-positive breast cancer. JNCI 1994; 86:232-234.

26. Hillier SG. Paracrine control of follicular estrogen synthesis. Sem Reprod Endocrinol 1991; 9:332-340.

27. Hillier SG, Whitelaw PF, Smyth CD. Follicular oestrogen synthesis: the 'two-cell, two-gonadotrophin' model revisited. Molec Cellular Endocrinol 1994; 100:51-54.

28. Whitelaw PF, Smyth CD, Howles CM et al. Cell-specific expression of aromatase and LH receptor mRNAs in rat ovary. J Mol Endocrinol 1992; 9:309-312.

29. Hillier SG. Current concepts of the roles of follicle stimulating hormone and luteinizing hormone in folliculogenesis. Human Reprod 1994; 9:188-191.

30. Hillier SG, Yong EL, Illingworth PI et al. Effect of recombinant activin on androgen synthesis in cultured human thecal cells. J Clin Endocrinol Metab 1991; 72:1206-1211.

31. Zeleznik AJ, Kubik CJ. Ovarian responses in macaques to pulsatile infusion of follicle-stimulating hormones (FSH) and luteinizing hormone: Increased sensitivity of the maturing follicle to FSH. Endocrinol 1986; 119:2025-2032.

32. Yen SSC. The human menstrual cycle. In: Yen SCC, Jaffe RB. Reproductive Endocrinology 2nd ed. Saunders, New York 1986:33-74.

33. Baird DT, Uno A, Melby JC. Adrenal secretion of androgens and oestrogens. J Endocrinol 1969; 45:135-136.

34. Rivarola MA, Saez JM, Meyer WJ et al. Metabolic clearance rate and blood production rate of testosterone and androst-4-ene-3, 17-dione under basal conditions, ACTH and HCG stimulation. J Clin Endocrinol Metab 1966; 26:1208-1218.

35. Nieschlag E, Loriaux DL, Ruder HJ et al. The secretion of dehydroepiandrosterone and dehydroepiandrosterone sulphate in man. J Endocrinol 1973; 57:123-134.

36. Adams J, Garcia M, Rochefort H. Estrogenic effects of physiological concentrations of 5-androstene-3β-17β-diol and its metabolism in MCF-7 human breast cancer cells. Cancer Res 1981; 41:4720-4726.

37. Poulin R, Labrie F. Stimulation of cell proliferation and estrogenic response by adrenal C19-5-ene-steroids in the ZR-75-1 human breast cancer cell line. Cancer Res 1986; 46:4933-4937.

38. Miller WR, Hawkins RA, Mullen P et al. Aromatase inhibition: determinants of response and resistance. Endocrine Related Cancer 1995; 2:73-85.

39. Boccuzzi G, Brignardello E, DiMonaco M et al. Influence of dehydroepiandrosterone and 5-en-androstene-3β,17β-diol on the growth of MCF-7 human breast cancer cells induced by 17β-estradiol. Anticancer Res 1992; 12:799-804.

40. Ebeling P, Koivisto VA. Physiological importance of dehydroepiandrosterone. Lancet 1994; 343:1479-1481.

41. Judd HL, Judd GE, Lucas WE et al. Endocrine function of the postmenopausal ovary: concentration of androgens and estrogens in ovarian and peripheral vein blood. J Clin Endocrinol Metab 1974; 39:1020-1024.

42. Meldrum DR, Davidson BJ, Tataryn IV et al. Changes in circulating steroids with aging in postmenopausal women. Obst Gynecol 1981; 57:624-628.

43. Kirschner MA. The role of hormones in the development of human breast cancer. In: Breast cancer, advances in research and treatment Current Topics Vol 3. Ed WL McGuire. Plenum Press New York 1979; 119-226.

44. James VHT, Folkerd EJ, Bonney RC et al. Factors influencing estrogen production and metabolism in postmenopausal women with endocrine cancer. J Endocrinol Invest 1982; 5:335-345.

45. Longcope C, Kato T, Horton R. Conversion of blood androgens to estrogens in normal adult men and women. J Clin Invest 1969; 48: 2191-2201.

46. Perel E, Killinger DW. The interconversion and aromatization of androgens by human adipose tissue. J Steroid Biochem 1979; 10:623-627.

47. Longcope C. Methods and results of aromatization studies in vivo. Cancer Res 1982; 42(Suppl):3307S-3311S.

48. Schweikert HU, Milewich L, Wilson JD. Aromatization of androstenedione by cultured human fibroblasts. J Clin Endocrinol Metab 1976; 43:785-795.

49. Smuk M, Schwers J. Aromatization of androstenedione by human adult liver in vitro. J Clin Endocrinol Metab 1977; 45:1009-1012.

50. Miller WR, Forrest APM. Oestradiol synthesis from C19 steroids by human breast cancer. Br J Cancer 1974; 33:16-18.

51. Miller WR, Anderson TJ, Jack WJL. Relationship between tumour aromatase activity, tumour characteristics and response to therapy. J Steroid Biochem 1990; 37:1055-1059.

52. Vermeulen A, Verdonck L. Sex hormone concentrations in postmenopausal women. Clin Endocrinol 1978; 9:59-66.

53. Price T, Aitken J, Head J et al. Determination of aromatase cytochrome P450 messenger RNA in human breast tissues by competitive polymerase chain reaction (PCR) amplification. J Clin Endocrinol Metab 1992; 74:1247-1252.

54. Longcope C. Peripheral aromatization: studies on controlling factors. Steroids 1987; 50:253-267.
55. Mendelson CR, Corbin CJ, Smith ME et al. Growth factors suppress and phorbol esters potentiate the action of dibutyryl adenosine 3',5'-monophosphate to stimulate aromatase activity of human adipose stromal cells. Endocrinol 1986; 118:968-973.
56. Simpson ER, Mendelson CR. The regulation of oestrogen biosynthesis in human adipose tissue. Proc Roy Soc Edin 1989; 95B:153-159.
57. Simpson ER, Cleland WH, Mendelson CR. Aromatization of androgens by human adipose tissue in vitro. J Steroid Biochem 1983; 19:707-713.
58. Folkerd EJ, Jacobs HS, van der Spuy Z et al. Failure of FSH to influence aromatization in human adipose tissue. Clin Endocrinol 1982; 16:621-625.
59. Bulun SE, Mahendroo MS, Price T et al. A link between breast cancer and local estrogen biosynthesis suggested by quantification of breast adipose tissue aromatase cytochrome P450 transcripts by competitive PCR. J Clin Endocrinol Metab 1993a; 77:1622-1628.
60. Perel E, Wilkin D, Killinger DW. The conversion of androstenedione to estrone, estradiol and testosterone in breast tissue. J Steroid Biochem 1980; 13:89-94.
61. Preschtel K. Benign disease of the female breast: histology, normal and abnormal. In: Castelazo-Ayala L, McGregor C. Proceedings of the VIIIth World Congress on Gynaecology and Obstetrics. Amsterdam: Excerpta Medica 1977:135-138.
62. O'Neill JS, Miller WR. Aromatase activity in adipose tissue from women with benign and malignant breast disease. Br J Cancer 1987; 56:601-604.
63. O'Neill JS, Elton RA, Miller WR. Aromatase activity in adipose tissue from breast quadrants: a link with tumour site. Br Med J 1988; 296:741-743.
64. Bulun SE, Simpson ER, Breast cancer and expression of aromatase in breast adipose tissue. Trends Endocrinol Metab 1994; 5:113-120.
65. Mahendroo MS, Mendelson CR, Simpson ER. Tissue-specific and hormonally controlled alternative promoters regulate aromatase cytochrome P450 gene expression in human adipose tissue. J Biol Chem 1993; 268:19463-19470.
66. Abul-Hajj YJ, Iverson R, Kiang DT. Aromatization of androgens by human breast cancer. Steroids 1979; 33:205-222.
67. Miller WR. Steroid metabolism in breast cancer. In: Stoll BA, ed. Breast cancer: treatment and progress. Blackwell Scientific Publications, 1986:156-172.
68. Esteban JM, Warsi Z, Haniu M et al. Detection of intratumoral aromatase in breast carcinomas. Am J Pathol 1992; 140:337-343.
69. Sasano H, Nagura H, Harada N et al. Immunolocalization of aromatase and other steroidogenic enzymes in human breast disorders. Hum Pathol 1994; 25:530-535.
70. Miller WR, Hawkins RA, Forrest APM. Steroid metabolism and oestrogen receptors in human breast carcinomas. Eur J Cancer Clin Oncol 1981; 17:913-917.

71. Miller WR, O'Neill J. Mammary steroidogenesis: therapeutic implications. Nuclear Med Biol 1987; 14:369-376.

72. Bezwoda WR, Mansoor N, Dansey, R. Correlation of breast tumour aromatase activity and response to aromatase inhibition with aminoglutethimide. Oncology 1987; 44:345-349.

73. Thijssen JH, Blankenstein MA, Donker GH et al. Endogenous steroid hormones and local aromatase activity in the breast. J Steroid Biochem Molec Biol 1991; 39:799-804.

74. Vermeulen A. Human mammary cancer as a site of sex steroid metabolism. Cancer Surveys 1986; 5:585-595.

75. Reed MJ, Owen AM, Lai LC et al. In situ oestrone synthesis in normal breast and breast tumour tissues: effect of treatment with 4-hydroxyandrostenedione. Int J Cancer 1989; 44:233-237.

76. Hawkins RA, Thomson ML, Killen E. Oestrogen sulphate, adipose tissue and breast cancer. Breast Cancer Res Treat 1985; 6:75-87.

77. Santen RJ. Novel methods of oestrogen deprivation for treatment of breast diseases. Proc Roy Soc Edin 1989; 95B:255-269.

78. Santer SJ, Feil PD, Santen RJ. In situ estrogen production via the estrone sulfatase pathway in breast tumors: relative importance versus the aromatase pathway. J Clin Endocrinol Metab 1984; 59:29-33.

79. MacIndoe JH, Woods G, Jeffries L. The hydrolysis of estrone sulfate and dehydro-epiandrosterone sulfate by MCF-7 human breast cancer cells. Endocrinol 1988; 123:1281-1287.

80. Dao TL, Libby PR. Steroid sulfate formation in human breast tumors and hormone dependency. In: Dao TL, ed. Estrogen target tissue and neoplasia. Chicago University Press 1972:181-200.

81. Adams JB, Pewnim T, Chandra DP et al. A correlation between estrogen sulfotransferase levels and estrogen receptor status in human primary breast carcinoma. Cancer Res 1979; 39:5124-5126.

82. Adams JB, Phillips NS, Hall R. Metabolic fate of estradiol in human mammary cancer cells in culture: estrogen sulfate formation and cooperativity exhibited by estrogen sulfotransferase. Mol Cell Endocrinol 1988; 58:231-242.

83. Adams JB, Phillips NS, Pewnim T. Expression of hydroxysteroid sulphotransferase is related to estrogen receptor status in human mammary cancer. J Steroid Biochem 1989; 33:637-642.

84. Adams JB, Vrahimis R, Phillips N. Regulation of estrogen sulfotransferase by estrogen in MCF-7 human mammary cancer cells. Breast Cancer Res Treat 1992; 22:157-161.

85. Purohit A, Howarth NM, Potter BVL et al. Inhibition of steroid sulfatase activity by steroidal methylthiophosphonates—potential therapeutic agents in breast cancer. J Steroid Biochem 1994; 48:523-527.

86. Pollow K, Buquoi E, Baumann J et al. Comparison of the in vitro conversion of estradiol to estrone in normal and neoplastic human breast tissue. Mol Cell Endocrinol 1977; 6:333-348.

87. Santner SJ, Leszozynski D, Wright C et al. Estrone sulphate: a potential source of estradiol in human breast cancer tissues. Breast Cancer Res Treat 1986; 7:35-44.

88. Bonney RC, Reed MJ, Davidson K et al. The relationship between 17β-hydroxy-steroid dehydrogenase activity and oestrogen concentration in human breast tumours and in normal breast. Clin Endocrinol 1983; 19:727-739.

89. McNeil JM, Reed MJ, Beranek PA et al. A comparison of the in vivo uptake and metabolism of ^{3}H-oestradiol by normal breast and breast tumour tissue in postmenopausal women. Int J Cancer 1986a; 38:193-196.

90. Abul-Hajj YJ, Iverson R, Kiang DT. Estradiol 17β-dehydrogenase and estradiol binding in human mammary tumors. Steroids 1979; 33:477-484.

91. Adams EF, Newton CJ, Braunsberg H et al. Effects of human breast fibroblasts on growth and 17β-oestradiol dehydrogenase activity of MCF-7 cells in culture. Breast Cancer Res Treat 1988a; 11:165-172.

92. Adams EF, Newton CJ, Tait GH et al. Paracrine influence of human breast stromal fibroblasts on breast epithelial cells: secretion of a polypeptide which stimulates reductive 17β-oestradiol dehydrogenase activity. Int J Cancer 1988; 42:119-122.

93. Fournier S, Brihmat F, Durand JC et al. Estradiol 17β-hydroxysteroid dehydrogenase, a marker of breast cancer hormone dependency. Cancer Res 1985; 45:2895-2899.

94. Schatz F, Hochberg RB. Lipoidal derivatives of estradiol: the biosynthesis of a nonpolar estrogen metabolite. Endocrinol 1981; 109:697-703.

95. Abul-Hajj YL. Formation of estradiol-17β fatty acyl 17-esters in mammary tumors. Steroids 1982; 40:149-156.

96. Adams JB, Hall RT. Nott S. Esterification-deesterification of estradiol by human mammary cancer cells in culture. J Steroid Biochem 1986; 24:1159-1162.

97. Larner JM, Eisenfeld AJ, Hochberg RB. Synthesis of estradiol fatty acid esters by human breast tumors: fatty acid composition and comparison to estrogen and progesterone receptor content. J Steroid Biochem 1985; 23:637-641.

98. Martyn P, Smith DL, Adams JB. Selective turnover of the essential fatty acid ester components of estradiol-17β lipoidal derivatives formed by human mammary cancer cells in culture. J Steroid Biochem 1987; 28:393-395.

99. Janocko L, Larner JM, Hochberg RB. The interaction of C_{17} esters of estradiol with the oestrogen receptors. Endocrinol 1984; 114:1180-1186.

100. Larner JM, MacLusky NJ, Hochberg RB. The naturally occurring C-17 fatty acid esters of estradiol are long-acting estrogens. J Steroid Biochem 1985; 22:407-413.

101. Vazquez-Alcantara MA, Menjivar M, Garcia GA et al. Long-acting estrogenic responses of estradiol fatty acid esters. J Steroid Biochem 1989; 33:1111-1118.

102. Adams JB. Enzymatic regulation of estradiol-17β concentrations in human breast cancer cells. Breast Cancer Res Treat 1991; 20:145-154.

CHAPTER 6

LEVELS AND PATTERNS OF ESTROGEN WITHIN THE BREAST, ITS FLUIDS AND TISSUES

INTRODUCTION

Given the links between estrogens and the development of both normal and malignant breast it is surprising that comparatively little is known about the levels and profiles of estrogens within the breast. In part this stems from the difficulties of obtaining material from the breast in sufficient quantities to measure hormones. Milk is the most readily available fluid and is physiological but its production during lactation is at a time when estrogen levels within the breast may have little relevance to those found in the resting state. Small amounts of fluid may also be aspirated from the nipple of breasts of non-lactating women. Although small in volume these can be analysed for estrogen. Such nipple aspirates may however possess concentrations of constituents which are different to those of secretions formed deeper within the breast. Measurements have also been performed in breast tissue taken during surgical procedures but, in general, such surgery is necessary because of the presence of breast abnormalities and hormone levels may be primarily influenced by pathological changes. However, these analyses do allow an insight into the estrogenic environment which may exist within the breast. Such studies indicate that levels and profiles of estrogen within breast fluids and tissues differ substantially from those in the circulation. It is thus of interest to summarize the findings emanating from assays of breast-derived tissues and fluids.

MILK

Early measurements of estrogens employed relatively insensitive and non-specific methodology and, while these assays pointed to the presence of substantial quantities of estrogen in human milk, the suspicion remained that these were artifactual. However, studies using more specific methodology have confirmed high concentrations of estrogen in human milk and colostrum.[1,2] For example, the study of McGarrigle and Lachelin[1] indicated that both conjugated and unconjugated estrone, estradiol and estriol were present in nM amounts in milk obtained during the post-partum period. However, conjugated estrogens comprised more than 90% of the total estrogen content. The single major estrogen was estrone glucosiduronate with levels being significantly higher than those in plasma. Concentrations of unconjugated estrone, estradiol and estriol in milk were similar or somewhat lower compared with those in plasma. The mechanism whereby conjugated estrogen accumulates in milk is undetermined but presumably it involves some form of active uptake from the circulation; the high degree of correlation between levels in plasma and milk suggests that direct transfer is likely.[3] A similar process would account for the levels of oral contraceptive steroids such as ethinyl estradiol which may also be found in the milk of women taking such steroids.[4] The presence of steroids in human milk could also be responsible for the occasional cases of precocious puberty induced in breast-feeding infants.[5]

NIPPLE ASPIRATES

The breast is unusual in that in the non-lactating state its secretions are retained for varying times within the alveolar-duct system.[6] There, they may be metabolized or absorbed into blood and lymphatics. In a high proportion of adult premenopausal women samples of breast fluid can be obtained by nipple aspiration with a breast pump.[7] These fluids have a distinctive profile of constituents and appear to accumulate a variety of exogenous and endogenous materials.[6-15] Elevated levels of breast-derived proteins suggest that such fluids reflect the environment within the breast.[7,8,10] It is thus interesting that steroids and other hormones are present within breast fluids.[6,11-15] Estrogen is not only detectable within nipple aspirates but may also be found at levels which are higher than those in the circulation.[9,12] The most informative study is probably that of Petrakis and colleagues who undertook a large clinical and epidemiological study of breast disease in women at the University of California in San Francisco.[12,13] Levels of estrogens were determined in nipple aspirates and serum and then related to menstrual, reproductive and risk factors in healthy women and in women with breast disease. Estrone and estradiol were detectable in nipple aspirates from both pre- and postmenopausal women in levels five to 45 times higher than in serum (see also Table 6.1) but concentrations were not correlated with those in serum. Although there were substantial variations in estrogen levels in nipple aspirates, in contrast to circulating estrogens these did not relate to phases of the menstrual cycle in premenopausal women or differ between pre- and postmenopausal women—the mean concentration of estrogens in postmenopausal women were 40 times higher than those in serum despite the absence

Table 6.1. Estrogen levels (pmol/l) in nipple aspirates and serum

	Premenopausal		Postmenopausal	
	Estradiol	**Estrone**	**Estradiol**	**Estrone**
Nipple aspirates	3,000	4,558	2,930	4,200
Serum	330	270	50	115
Relative Excess	9	23	56	36

of ovarian function. These findings indicate that the estrogenic milieu of the normal breast as monitored by nipple aspirates is not directly related to circulating estrogens. Interestingly, concentrations of estradiol and estrone were highly correlated between right and left breast in women from whom secretions were obtained from both breasts suggesting that in individual women a common factor influences levels. Another striking feature was that mean levels of estradiol and estrone in nipple aspirates were lower in parous women as compared with nulliparous women and in parous women levels were related to time since last full-term birth. This is perhaps not surprising since levels of unconjugated estrogen are lower in milk compared with nipple aspirates from non-lactating women. It would seem that following parturition or discontinuance of nursing, estrogen levels remain low for up to two to three years. After pregnancy, therefore, the breast appears not to be exposed to high levels of estrogen for a substantial time (this might account for the protective effects of parity against breast cancer). However no significant differences were found in estrogen levels in nipple aspirates obtained from either women with breast cancer, benign breast disease or healthy control individuals (although when data were adjusted for the covariate of time since last full time birth, significantly elevated mean levels of estradiol and estrone were found in nipple aspirates of women who had been biopsied for benign breast disease [see Table 6.2]). Interestingly, mean levels of estradiol in nipple aspirates from the seven cancer patients studied were lower than those of control women although this finding was not statistically significant. The only other reported study[14] which has compared concentrations of estrogens in breast fluids from normal women and patients with benign breast disease also failed to detect significant differences.

Nipple aspirates may also contain exceptionally high levels of androgen conjugates such as dehydroepiandrosterone sulfate[15] (see Fig. 6.1). Such androgens may serve as precursors for the synthesis of other more potent hormones including estrogens and estrogenic steroids.

The mechanism whereby such high levels of steroid conjugates accumulate in nipple aspirates and are maintained is as yet unknown. Whatever the mechanism, the high concentrations indicate that breast tissue is potentially exposed to far greater levels of estrogenic hormones than might be expected from the levels in serum.

Table 6.2. Estrogen levels (pmol/l) in nipple aspirates from women with either benign or malignant breast disease and controls

	Controls	Benign	Malignant
Estradiol	2,580	4,220	1,440
Estrone	3,880	6,665	4,890

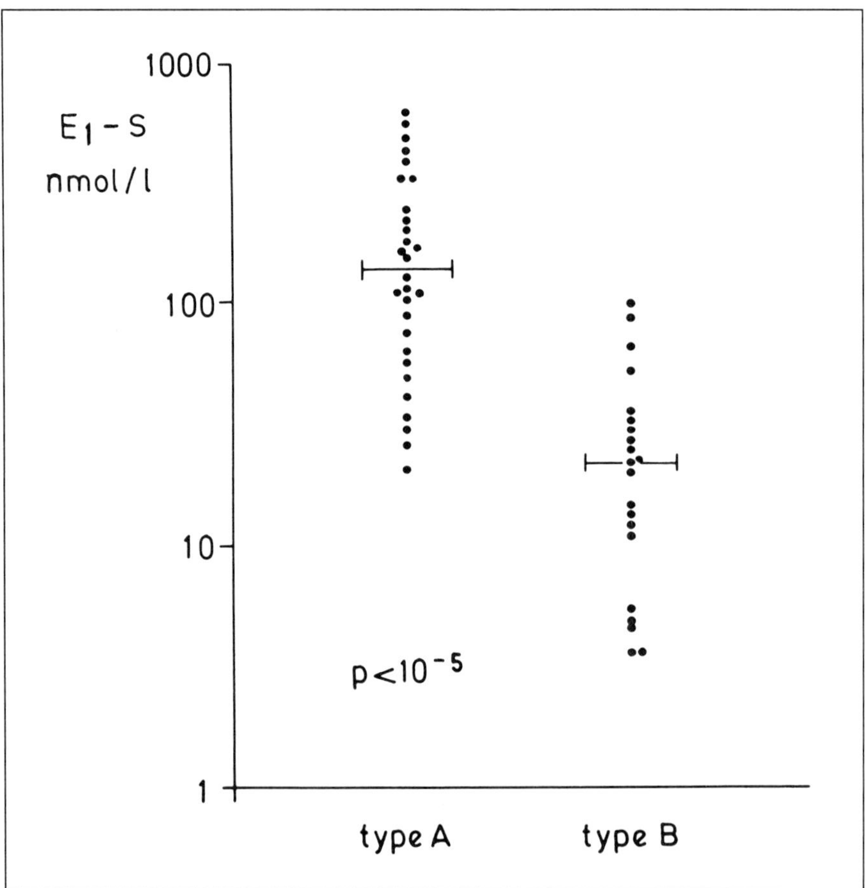

Fig. 6.1. Levels of DHA sulfate in nipple aspirates.

BREAST CYST FLUIDS

Breast cysts are a benign condition. They are routinely managed by needle aspiration of their fluid contents. Volumes of fluid in excess of several mls may be normally obtained. These may be analyzed and their constituents characterized.

Table 6.3. Estrogen levels (pg/ml) in breast cyst fluids and plasma

	Cyst Fluid	Plasma	Cyst Fluid Plasma
Estrone	28-715	100-1,000	< 1
Estradiol	130-835	125-2,500	1
Estrone Sulfate	6,135-57,500	1,300-2,450	30
Estradiol Sulfate	2,900-12,500	negligible	α

As with nipple aspirates, it has been possible to show breast cyst fluids contain a variety of estrogens.[16-23] (Table 6.3) Conjugated estrogens tend to predominate and both patterns and levels differ from those in the circulation. For example estradiol-3 sulfate is present in cyst fluids in concentrations ranging between 0.5 and >100 nM[16] but this conjugate has never been reported to be present in plasma in substantial amounts. Similarly, among estriol conjugates the sulfate predominates in cyst fluids whereas the glucuronide is the major form in plasma.[17] Estrone sulfate is also found in cyst fluids in concentrations which may be markedly in excess of those within the circulation. Thus, our own studies indicated that estrone sulfate was present in cyst fluids at concentrations ranging between 1.5 and 750 nM;[18] these levels being on average 30-fold higher than in the circulation. Furthermore no relationship was evident between concentrations of estrone sulfate in the circulation and those in cyst fluids. Cyst fluids may be subdivided into distinct groups according to their electrolyte composition.[24] It is thus interesting that fluids with low [Na$^+$]:[K$^+$]ratios (type I or A, which are derived from cysts having apocrine epithelium[25]) have significantly higher estrone sulfate levels than those with high [Na$^+$]:[K$^+$] ratios (type II or B, which have flattened lining epithelium[25]) (Fig. 6.2, Table 6.4).[17] A highly significant correlation also exists between levels of estrone sulfate and those of DHA sulfate in cyst fluids (although this is not apparent in plasma obtained from the same patients).

There is less agreement regarding levels of unconjugated estrogens. Schon and colleagues indicated that concentrations of estradiol in cyst fluids were significantly higher than those in blood[19] while Bradlow and co-workers found levels of estrone and estradiol in cyst fluids to be comparable with those in plasma.[16] Furthermore, in contrast to estrone sulfate, levels of estrone do not appear to be significantly different in fluids derived from cyst groups classified according to electrolyte composition.[20] Conflicting results have been presented for estradiol.[20-22]

The mechanism by which such high concentrations of estrogen conjugates accumulate in breast cyst fluids has also been the subject of investigation. Administration of radioactively labelled estriol or estriol sulfate indicated that only small amounts of radioactivity accumulate in cyst fluids aspirated hours later.[23] While this may result from the rapid clearance of these steroids from the circulation, the results of these isotope studies argue against the transfer of estriol sulfate from blood to

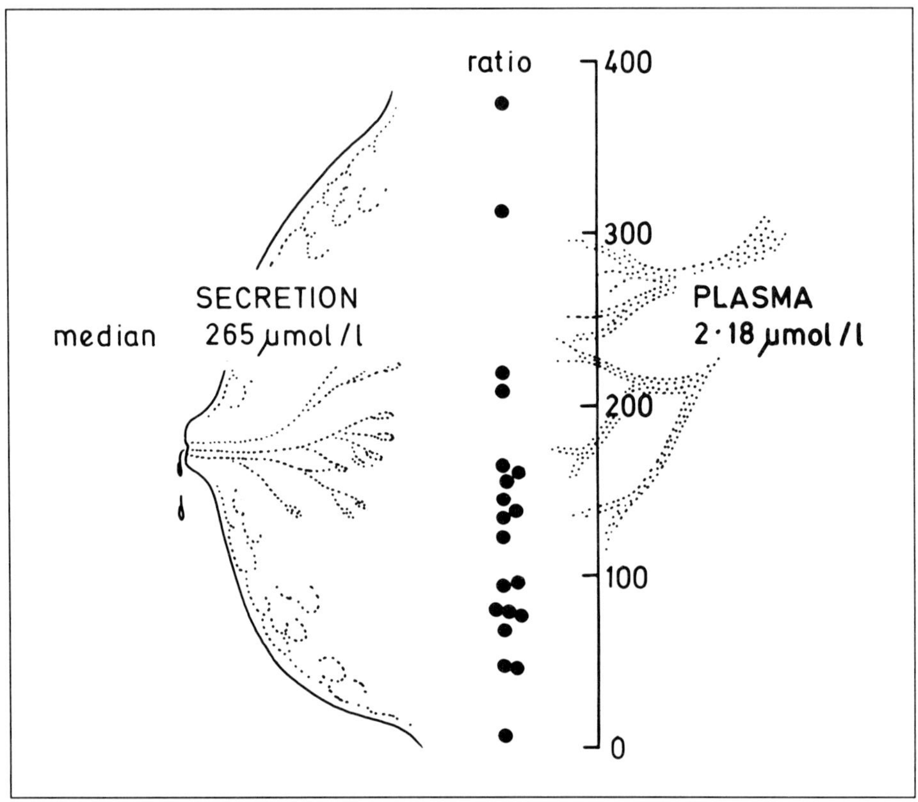

Fig. 6.2. Estrone sulfate in different subtypes of breast cyst fluids.

cyst fluid. It also appears unlikely that blood-borne estriol is the precursor of estriol sulfate found in the cyst fluid since endogenous plasma and cyst fluid concentrations of estriol are much lower than those of estriol sulfate in cyst fluid. However the possibility of a slow transfer of estriol sulfate from blood to cyst against a concentration gradient and the entrapment of the steroid conjugate in cyst fluid cannot be ruled out.

While there is no evidence that estrogens may be concentrated from plasma into cyst fluids, the data for the androgen conjugate, DHA sulfate, are much more convincing. Thus, our own studies in which radioactively labelled DHA sulfate has been infused into patients with multiple cysts show that at 48 hours many cysts contain levels of radioactivity markedly higher than those in the circulation (Fig. 6.3). Interestingly the highest levels of radioactively labelled DHA sulfate have been found in the subgroup of cyst fluids which have low [Na+]:[K+] ratios. While there is no definitive evidence that androgens such as DHA sulfate may be transformed into estrogens within breast cysts, the inter-relationship between DHA sulfate and estrone sulfate suggests some commonality of accumulation.[17]

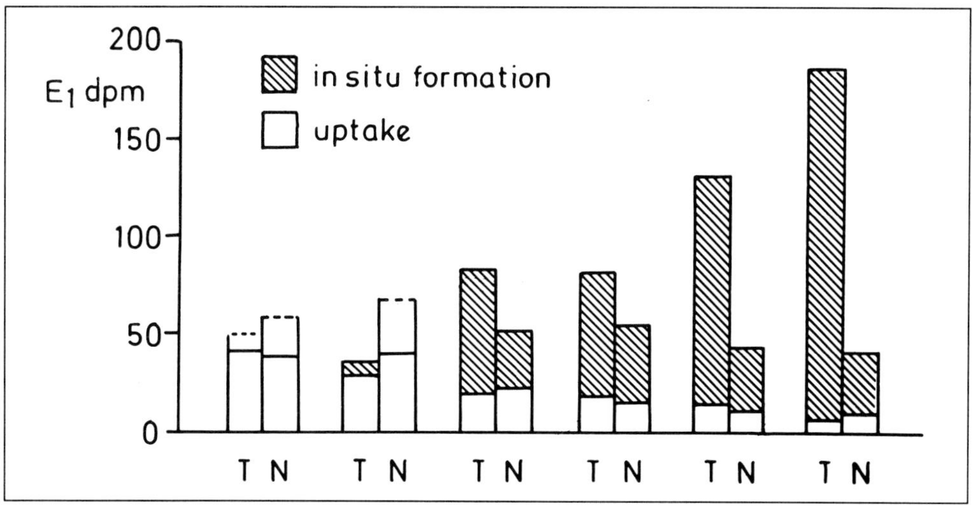

Fig. 6.3. Uptake of ³H DHA sulfate in breast cyst fluids.

Table 6.4. Estrogen levels (nmol/l) in different classes of cyst fluids

	Type I		Type II	
	Median	**(Range)**	**Median**	**(Range)**
Estradiol	17	(4-43)	2.7	(0.6-10.3)
Estrone sulfate	175	(25-750)	18	(1.5-300)

Irrespective of the mechanism by which steroid hormones accumulate in cyst fluids, these studies illustrate that no simple relationship exists between the levels of steroid hormones in cyst fluids and plasma. As a result it is not possible to predict concentrations of steroid hormones in cyst fluids from circulating levels. These observations may explain the difficulties encountered in relating endocrine activity as determined by circulating hormones to events occurring within the breast.

Measurements in cyst fluids of proteins induced by estrogen are also potentially informative since they may reflect biological activity. It is thus of interest that concentrations of cathepsin D and estradiol are inter-related in cyst fluids,[23] being significantly higher in low [Na⁺]:[K⁺] fluids as compared with those possessing high ratios. It may be that cathepsin D in human breast cyst fluid is regulated by estrogens, as has already been shown to be the case in breast cancer cell lines.[26] Equally the findings may merely reflect a common mode of accumulation between cathepsin D and estradiol, especially as pS2 concentrations (which are normally regulated by estrogen) are not closely correlated with those of estrogen and are not significantly different between two sub-groups of cysts.[23]

BREAST TISSUES

The availability of surgically dissected material from the breasts of women presenting with breast disease has provided a source of tissues for the assay of endogenous estrogens. These measurements have provided interesting results and will be reviewed. However, it ought to be emphasized that the assay of estrogens in breast tissues is beset with potential problems and limitations. These include the heterogeneity of tissue assayed; the specificity of the assays for estrogen and the problems of blanks, and the general inability to determine whether estrogens as assayed are located within cells or are simply found in extracellular fluids. Nevertheless the observations have provided an interesting perspective on the levels and profiles of estrogen within the breast. It is therefore proposed to summarize the general findings before presenting specific details of the levels and correlations which have been made within both malignant and non-malignant compartments of the breast.

GENERAL FINDINGS

Concentrations and patterns of estrogen differ markedly between the circulation and breast tissues, particularly in postmenopausal women.[27,28] Among the most striking disparities are the observations that tissue concentrations of estrogen are similar in pre- and postmenopausal women despite the marked fall in peripheral plasma levels after the menopause, that in postmenopausal women levels of estrogen are significantly higher in the breast compared with the circulation, and that while estrone and its sulfate predominate over estradiol in the circulation, levels of estradiol are similar to or higher than estrone in breast tissue.

In general these observations apply to both cancerous and non-malignant components of the breast but there is a trend for differences to be more marked in malignant tumors. Thus estradiol levels tend to be higher in cancers compared with normal or benign breast tissue.[29] Breast adipose tissue also displays levels of estrogen markedly in excess of those in peripheral plasma but these consist mainly of estrone.[30] These considerations indicate that endogenous concentrations of estrogen within the breast do not necessarily reflect those in the circulation.

Table 6.5. Estrogen levels in breast cancers

	pmol/g		pmol/mg cytosol protein		
	Estradiol	**Estrone**	**Estradiol**	**Estrone**	**Estrone Sulfate**
Premenopausal	0.70 (0.25 - 4.0)	1.00 (0.1 - 3.2)	– –	– –	– –
Postmenopausal	0.75 (0.15 - 4.0)	0.65 (0.01-2.25)	8.9 (0.4 -69.1)	6.8 (0.1 -67.0)	5.1 (0.1- 34.1)

Values are medians (range)

SPECIFIC DETAILS

BREAST CANCERS

Both estrone and estradiol are present in breast cancers in concentrations of pmol/g (Table 6.5). In premenopausal women, estrone levels exceed those of estradiol. While levels of estrone fall after the menopause, those of estradiol remain constant, so that values of estradiol are similar or greater than those of estrone. However it can be seen from the range of values that considerable variations exist between different tumors. This is particularly evident in tumors from postmenopausal women. Because expressing results as grams of tumor may hide differences caused by cellularity, it is appropriate to examine concentrations expressed per milligram of cytosol protein. These data are also presented in Table 6.5 and again it is evident that a wide range of values may be present between different tumors.

In terms of sub-cellular distribution, unlike in uterine tissues in which concentrations of estrogens appear to be higher in the nuclear fraction as compared with cytosols,[31] the reverse seems to hold in breast tissues.[27,31] Furthermore, while the mean estrogen receptor content in tumors from postmenopausal women is about twice that in tumors from premenopausal women, no significant differences have been found in the distribution of estradiol in subcellular fractions obtained from tumors derived from pre- and postmenopausal women.[27,32] Although the nuclear:cytosol ratio for estradiol does appears to be higher in the receptor-positive as compared with receptor-negative tumors, these observations also apply to concentrations of estrone[27] which has a lower affinity for the estrogen receptor than estradiol. Thus, it can be seen that estrogen receptor proteins cannot solely explain high concentrations of estrogen in breast cancer. It is also interesting that estradiol concentrations in human endometrium and myometrium is about 10-fold higher than those in breast tumors,[31] yet receptor concentrations are similar.[33]

Regardless of premenopausal status, levels of estrogen in tumors are not a simple reflection of those in plasma. This is particularly so for concentrations of estradiol in postmenopausal women. The relative ratio in breast cancer as compared with plasma is such that while levels of estradiol can exceed those in the circulation, the excess can vary enormously up to over 100-fold (Fig. 6.4).[29] A similar phenomenon exists for estrone which on average displays a 5-fold higher concentration in tumor than in plasma although not all tumors show this excess. In terms of estrone sulfate, levels are similar in tumors and the circulation and there is no evidence for preferential concentration except in a small number of tissues.[29] Consequently, whereas estrone is quantitatively the most important estrogen in plasma, in breast tissue estradiol concentrations are comparable or even higher than those of estrone.[27] Tissue: plasma gradients for estrone are greater than those in both pre- and postmenopausal women and are most pronounced in

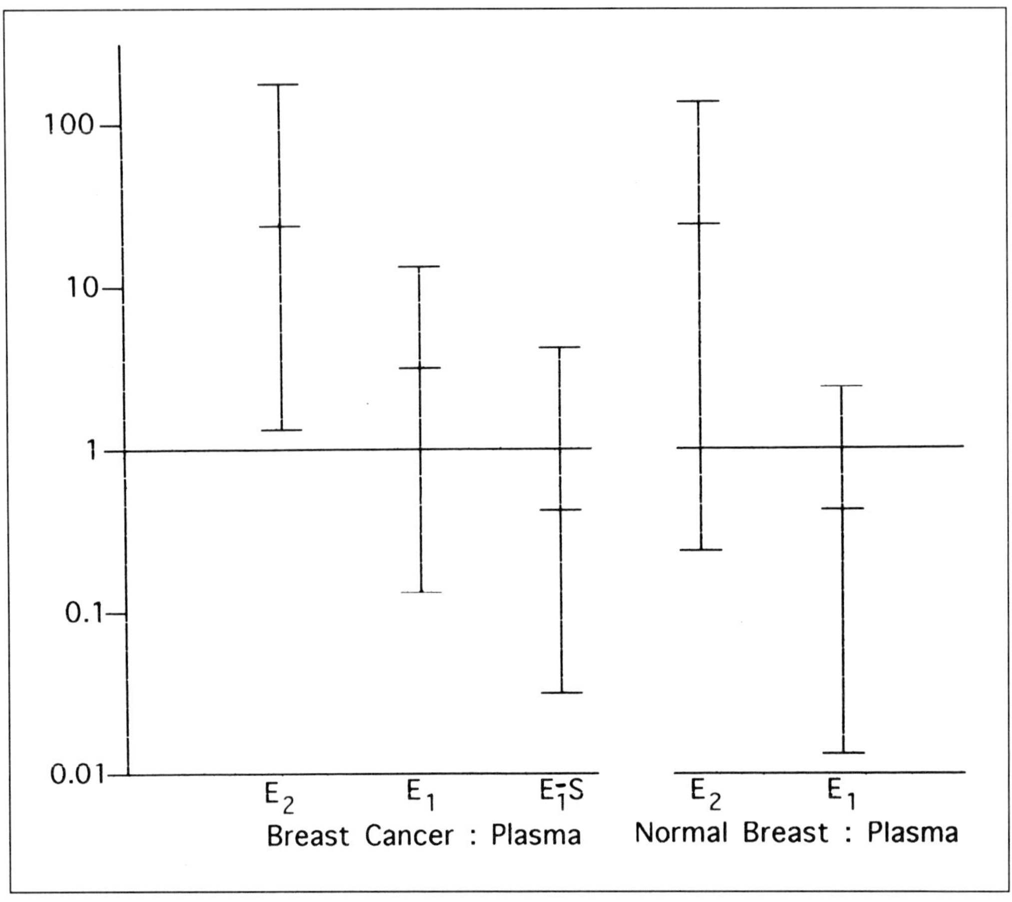

Fig. 6.4. Relative excess of estrogen in breast tissues compared with plasma.

Table 6.6 Estrogen levels in normal breast

	pmol/g Estradiol	Estrone	Estradiol	pmol/mg Estrone	protein Estrone Sulfate
	0.4	1.2	–	–	–
premenopausal	(0.2 - 1.7)	(0.2 - 2.3)	–	–	–
	0.3	0.4	5.7	3.9	0.6
postmenopausal	(0.2 - 0.5)	(0.3 - 0.6)	(0.8 - 15)	(0.1 - 20)	(0.1 - 1.2)

Values are median (range).

tumor extracts from postmenopausal patients. In contrast a distinct tumor: plasma gradient for estradiol is present only in postmenopausal patients in whom the gradient is much higher for estradiol than for estrone. Major variations in the ratio of estrone to estradiol between individual tumors clearly demonstrate that peripheral plasma levels are not reflective of endogenous tissue concentrations.

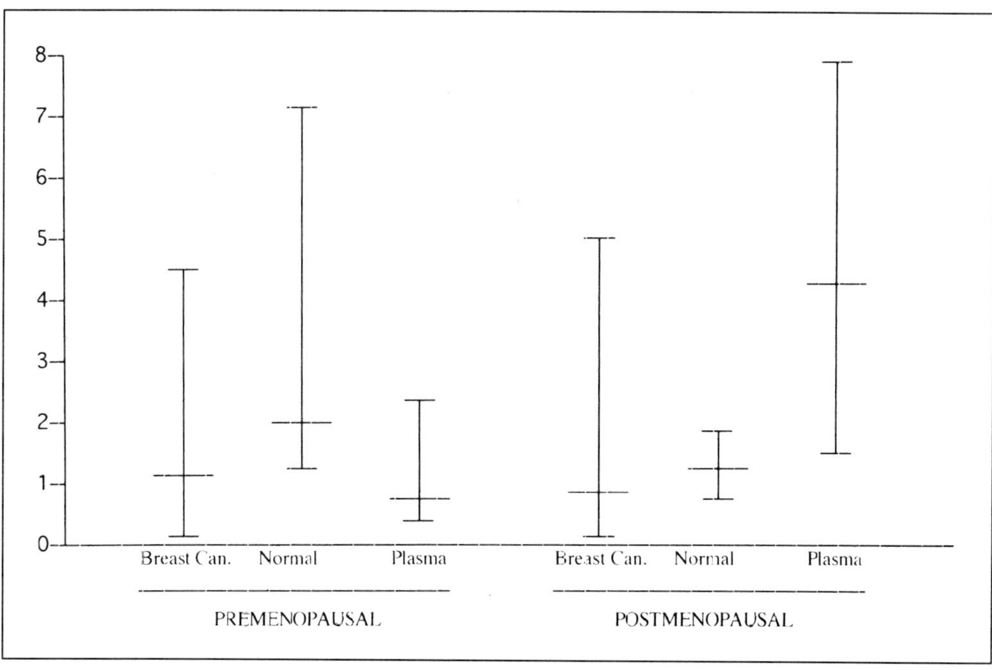

Fig. 6.5. *Relative ratio of estrone to estradiol in breast tissues and plasma of pre- and postmenopausal women.*

"NORMAL BREAST"

Levels of estrogens have also been measured in the so-called 'normal breast' and, more particularly, the glandular compartments of mastectomy specimens. These also display picomolar concentrations of estrone, estrone sulfate and estradiol (Table 6.6) although levels tend to be somewhat lower than those found in breast cancer.[29] There is also a large range of individual estrogens between different specimens. In terms of tissue:plasma ratio, many samples have values greater than unity. The differential is more pronounced for estradiol than estrone (Fig. 6.4). Consequently, the ratio of estrone to estradiol is different between normal and cancerous tissue; cancers tend to have lower ratios (Fig. 6.5). This is largely explained by the high concentrations of estradiol in tumor tissues rather than lower concentrations of estrone.

The striking and enormous variation in concentrations of estrogens between different specimens of breast relates only in part to menopausal status and the differences between normal and cancer. Other factors remain largely undefined although a study in which estrogen levels were determined in tumor specimens obtained from Poland and the Netherlands (countries with relatively low and high incidence of breast cancer) showed significantly lower concentrations of estrone and estradiol in the Polish samples.[34] Levels were about half those found in the Dutch tissues. The differences were particularly evident in the estradiol fractions extracted from fat tissue.

MECHANISM OF ACCUMULATION

The reason for such high concentrations of estrogen in breast tissue has been subject to substantial investigation. Clearly some form of active process must be responsible—either an active uptake of steroid hormones from the circulation against a concentration gradient or active biosynthesis within the breast. Evidence in support of both processes has been obtained.

In terms of uptake a positive arterial-venous gradient in the blood irrigating mammary tissues has been reported for estradiol.[35] Uptake of estrogens into breast tissues have been confirmed by infusing radioactive steroids into volunteer patients.[36,37] These studies have shown that both estradiol and estrone are taken up and concentrated within the breast. The accumulation is selective and can be variable. In particular, the process is more marked in breast cancer than normal breast and is especially associated with estradiol.

The mechanism by which this selective uptake occurs is unknown, but it is not unreasonable to postulate the presence of intracellular high affinity binding proteins capable of maintaining tissue levels of estrogen. However, no binding protein has been identified whose quantitative presence correlates with tumor concentrations of estrogen. Thus, while estradiol levels tend to be higher in estrogen receptor-positive tumors,[37] no correlation exists between levels of receptor and estradiol.[38] Levels of both estrone and estradiol in receptor-negative tumors are also markedly in excess of those in plasma.[39] Involvement of proteins with lower affinity and higher capacity for estrogen cannot be excluded.[40]

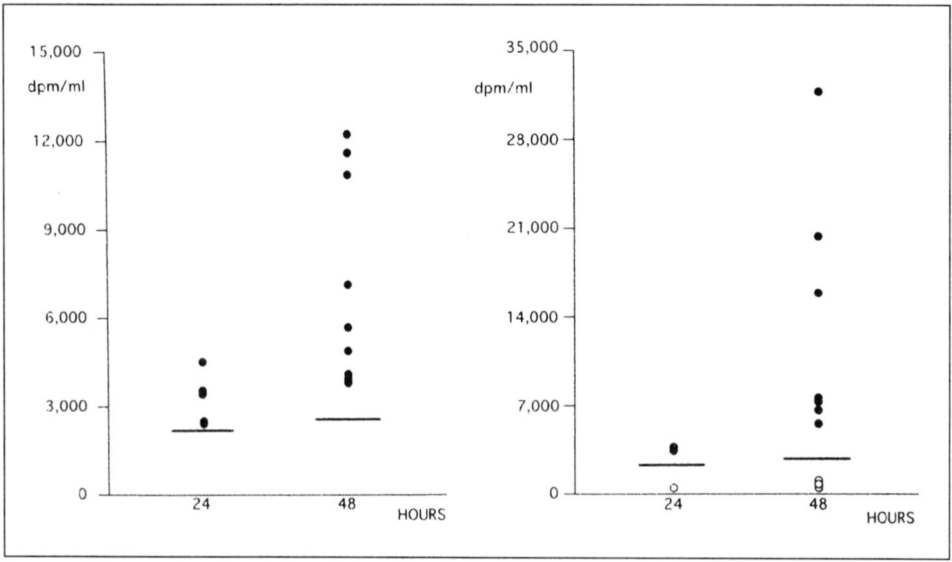

Fig. 6.6. Relative contribution of uptake and local biosynthesis to estrogen levels in breast cancers from postmenopausal women. (T = tumor, N = normal breast)

Both in vivo and in vitro studies show that breast tissues have the capacity for estrogen biosynthesis and inter-conversions.[41-44] Local activity of two transformations could potentially account for endogenous tumor levels of estrogens; namely, the aromatization of androgens to estrogens and the interconversion of estrone to estradiol. However, although these activities have been shown to be present in breast tissues[41-44] and influenced by local factors,[45-46] no correlation has been reported between either aromatase or 17β-hydroxysteroid dehydrogenase and tumor levels of estrogens.[47,48]

Using dual isotope techniques it is possible to make an estimate of the proportion of endogenous estrogen produced from androgen in situ within the breast as opposed to that taken up directly from the circulation.[49] In postmenopausal women with breast cancer the extent to which endogenous estrogen is derived either from uptake or from in situ production seems to be variable between different individuals. Certain breast cancers appear to obtain all estrogen from uptake, others from in situ synthesis, whereas the majority show a contribution from both sources (Fig. 6.6).

SUMMARY

Measurements of estrogens in breast fluids and tissues clearly indicate that levels may dramatically exceed those in the systemic circulation and that the relative proportion of individual estrogens differ from those in the peripheral plasma (in particular estradiol is proportionately higher in the breast). Conjugated rather than parent steroids accumulate in breast fluids, whether they be nipple or cyst aspirates. By contrast the phenomenon is associated with non-conjugated estrogens in breast tissues. There are still major questions to be resolved such as the mechanism whereby these high concentrations are maintained in breast tissues and whether these levels are of physiological significance and have biological activity within the breast. It might be expected that such high concentrations of estrogen would maintain a highly proliferative environment, yet after the menopause the breast atrophies as if deprived of estrogen. However it is possible that the normal parenchymal elements derived from postmenopausal breast are indeed maintained by local estrogens and breast cancers may display an abnormal response on account of their malignant phenotype.

REFERENCES

1. McGarrigle HHG, Lachelin GCL. Oestrone, oestradiol and oestriol glucosiduronates and sulphates in human puerperal plasma and milk. J Steroid Biochem 1983; 18:607-611.
2. Sahlberg BL, Axelson M. Identification and quantitation of free and conjugated steroids in milk from lactating women. J Steroid Biochem 1986; 25:379-391.
3. Nilsson S, Nygran KG, Johansson EDB. Transfer of estradiol to human milk. Am J Obstet Gynecol 1978; 132:643-657.

4. Nilsson S, Nygren KG, Johansson EDB. Ethinyl estradiol in human milk and plasma after oral administration. Contraception 1978; 17:131-139.

5. Tyson JE, Zacur HA. Diagnosis and treatment of abnormal lactation. Clin Obstet Gynecol 1975; 18:65-93.

6. Petrakis NL. Oestrogens and other biochemical and cytological components in nipple aspirates of breast fluid: relationship to risk factors for breast disease. Proc Roy Soc Edin 1989; 95B:169-181.

7. Petrakis NL. Physiologic, biochemical and cytologic aspects of nipple aspirate fluid. Breast Cancer Res Treat 1986; 8:7-19.

8. Yap PL, Miller WR, Humeniuk V et al. Milk protein concentrations in the mammary secretions of nonlactating women. J Reprod Immunol 1981; 3:49-58.

9. Wynder EL, Hill P, Laakso et al. Breast secretion in Finnish women. Cancer 1981; 47:1444-1450.

10. Williams CJ, Dion AS, Carten J et al. Epithelial membrane antigen expression in breast fluids and 'witch's milk.' Breast Cancer Res Treat 1992; 21:211-216.

11. Rose DP. Hormones in breast fluid. Breast Cancer Res Treat 1986; 8:25-28.

12. Ernster VL, Wrensch MR, Petrakis NL et al. Benign and malignant breast disease. Initial study results of serum and breast fluid analyses of endogenous estrogens. JNCI 1987; 79:949-960.

13. Petrakis NL, Wrensch MR, Ernster VL et al. Influence of pregnancy and lactation on serum and breast fluid estrogen levels: implications for breast cancer risk. Int J Cancer 1987c; 40:587-591.

14. Rose DP, Lahti H, Laakso K et al. Serum and breast duct prolactin and estrogen levels in healthy Finnish and American women and patients with fibrocystic disease. Cancer 1986a; 57:1550-1554.

15. Miller WR, Forrest APM. Factors affecting dehydroepiandrosterone sulfate levels in human breast secretions. Breast Cancer Res Treat 1981; 1267-272.

16. Bradlow HL, Rosenfeld RS, Kream J et al. Steroid hormone accumulation in human breast cyst fluid. Cancer Res 1981; 41:105-107.

17. Raju U, Ganguly M, Levitz M. Estriol conjugates in human breast cyst fluid and in serum of premenopausal women. J Clin Endocrinol Metab 1977; 45:429-434.

18. Scott WN, Hawkins RA, Killen E et al. Levels of androgen conjugates and oestrone sulphate in patients with breast cysts. J Steroid Biochem 1990; 35:399-402.

19. Schon HJ, Schurz B, Wenzl R et al. Beta endorphin, steroids and prolactin—immunoassay in breast cysts and blood. Arch Pathol Lab Med 1993; 117:248-253.

20. Bélanger A, Caron S, Labrie F et al. Levels of eighteen non-conjugated and conjugated steroids in human breast cyst fluid: relationships with cyst type. Eur J Cancer 1990; 26:277-281.

21. Lai LC, Cornell C, Lennard TWJ. Relationships between oestrogen-inducible proteins, oestradiol and electrolyte ratio in breast cyst fluid. Cancer Lett 1993; 69:21-25.

22. Boccardo F, Torrisi R, Zanardi S et al. EGF in breast cyst fluid: relationship with intracystic androgens, estradiol and progesterone. Int J Cancer 1991; 47:523-526.

23. Raju U, Noumoff J, Levitz M et al. On the occurrence and transport of estriol-3-sulfate in human breast cyst fluid: the metabolic disposition of blood estriol-3-sulfate in normal women. J Clin Endocrinol Metab 1981; 53:847-851.

24. Miller WR, Dixon JM, Scott WN et al. Classification of human breast cysts according to electrolyte and androgen conjugate composition. Clin Oncol 1983; 9:227-232.

25. Miller WR. Biochemistry of cyst fluids and its relevance. In: Steroid formation, degradation and action in peripheral tissues. Ann NY Acad Sci 1990; 595:459-463.

26. Vignon F, Capony F, Chambon M et al. Autocrine growth stimulation of the MCF-7 breast cancer cells by the estrogen regulated 52 kDa protein. Endocrinol 1986; 118:1537-1545.

27. van Landeghem AAJ, Poortman J, Nabuurs M et al. Endogenous concentration and subcellular distribution of estrogens in normal and malignant breast tissue. Cancer Res 1985; 45:2900-2904.

28. Vermeulen A, Deslypere JP, Paridaens R et al. Aromatase 17β hydroxysteroid dehydrogenase and intratissular sex hormone concentration in cancerous and normal glandular breast tissue in postmenopausal women. Eur J Cancer Clin Oncol 1986; 22:515-525.

29. Vermeulen A. Human mammary cancer as a site of sex steroid metabolism. Cancer Surveys 1986; 5:585-595.

30. Feher T, Bodrogi L, Valient K et al. Role of human adipose tissue in the production and metabolism of steroid hormones. Endocrinologie 1982; 80:173-180.

31. Poortman J, Thijssen JH, von Landeghem AA et al. Subcellular distribution of androgens and oestrogens in target tissues. J Steroid Biochem 1983; 19:939-945.

32. Thorsen T, Tangen M, Stoa KF. Concentration of endogenous oestradiol as related to oestradiol receptor sites in breast tumor cytosol. Eur J Cancer Clin Oncol 1982; 18:333-337.

33. Poortman J, Thijssen JHH, Schwarz F. Steroid receptors in human reproductive tissues. In: Wittliff JL, Dapunt O. Steroid receptors and hormone dependent neoplasia. New York: Masson Publishing Inc. 1980:45-58.

34. Thijssen JHH, Blankenstein MA, Miller WR et al. Estrogen in tissues: uptake from the peripheral circulation or local production. Steroids 1987; 50:297-306.

35. Duvivier J, Colin C, Hustin J et al. Comparison of levels of cytosol estrogen receptors with arterial and venous concentrations of gonadal steroids in mammary tumors. Clinica Chimica Acta 1981; 112:21-32.

36. McNeil JM, Reed MJ, Beranek PA et al. A comparison of the in vivo uptake and metabolism of ³H oestradiol by normal breast and breast tumour tissue in postmenopausal women. Int J Cancer 1986; 38:193-196.

37. James VHT, Reed MJ, Adams EF et al. Oestrogen uptake and metabolism in vivo. Proc Roy Soc Edin 1989; 95B:185-193.

38. Fishman J, Nisselbaum JS, Menendez-Botet CJ et al. Estrone and estradiol content in human breast tumours: relationship to estradiol receptors. J Steroid Biochem 1977; 8:893-896.

39. Thijssen JHH, Blankenstein MA. Oestrogens in breast tumours and fat. Proc Roy Soc Edin 1989; 95B:161-168.

40. Panko WB, Watson CS, Clark JH. The presence of a second steroid specific oestrogen binding site in human breast cancer. J Steroid Biochem 1981; 14:1311-1316.

41. Miller WR, Forrest APM. Oestradiol synthesis from C19 steroids by human breast cancer. Br J Cancer 1974; 33:16-18.

42. James VHT, McNeill JM, Lai LC et al. Aromatase activity in normal breast and breast tumour tissues: in vivo and in vitro studies. Steroids 1987; 50:269-279.

43. Perel E, Wilkin D, Killinger DW. The conversion of androstenedione to estrone, estradiol and testosterone in breast tissue. J Steroid Biochem 1980; 13:89-94.

44. Pollow K, Buquoi E, Baumann J et al. Comparison of the in vitro conversion of estradiol to estrone in normal and neoplastic human breast tissue. Molec Cell Endocr 1977; 6:333-348.

45. McNeill JM, Reed MJ, Newton CJ et al. The effect of epidermal growth factor, transforming growth factor, and breast tumour homogenates on the activity of oestradiol 17β-hydroxysteroid dehydrogenase in adipose tissue. Cancer Lett 1986; 31:213-219.

46. Miller WR, Mullen P. Factors influencing aromatase activity in the breast. J Steroid Biochem Molec Biol 1993; 44:597-604.

47. Bonney RC, Reed MJ, Davidson K et al. The relationship between 17-hydroxysteroid dehydrogenase activity and oestrogen concentration in human breast tumours and in normal breast. Clin Endocr 1983; 19:727-739.

48. Miller WR, O'Neill JS. The relevance of local oestrogen metabolism within the breast. Proc Roy Soc Edin 1989; 95B:203-217.

49. Reed MJ, Aherne GW, Ghilchik MW et al. Concentrations of oestrone and 4-hydroxyandrostenedione in malignant and normal breast tissues. Int J Cancer 1991; 49:562-565.

CHAPTER 7

MECHANISM OF ESTROGEN ACTION

ESTROGEN RECEPTORS

The major effects of estrogen in the breast appear to be mediated through specific intracellular receptors[1,2] by a mechanism depicted diagrammatically in Figure 7.1. These receptors are predominately located in the cell nucleus[3] and, although a fraction may shuttle between the cytoplasm and the nucleus,[4] the effect of estrogen binding to cytoplasmic receptors is to cause translocation to the nucleus.[4] Estrogen receptors also form transient complexes with heat shock proteins.[5] This interaction may ensure proper folding and the stability of the molecule. However, receptors cannot bind to DNA when complexed with heat shock proteins. Hormone binding causes in vitro disassociation from the complex.[6] Ligand binding also induces phosphorylation of receptors by kinases such as casein kinase II.[7] This may cause transactivation of the receptors, a process which allows a hinge region in the receptor to swing so that receptor dimerization can occur.[8] These conformational changes expose a cysteine-rich region which is capable of binding zinc in a manner which creates two peptide projections referred to as zinc fingers.[9] These zinc fingers promote the interaction of receptors with target enhancers known as estrogen response elements.[10] Interaction of dimerized receptor with its response element promotes initiation and transcription at nearby genes. The outcome of hormone receptor interactions with response elements is incompletely understood but it appears to be complicated and a variety of transcriptional events may result. In essence therefore, estrogen receptors act as nuclear transcription factors.[11] Estrogens may thus cause the accumulation of new species of RNAs which did not exist prior to stimulation.[12] As a result, a host of different types of proteins may be induced including enzymes involved in nucleic acid synthesis, known growth factors, proteolytic enzymes[13] and oncogene products.[14] These will be reviewed in more detail as they have been suggested to affect the development and progression of hormone-dependent breast cancers.

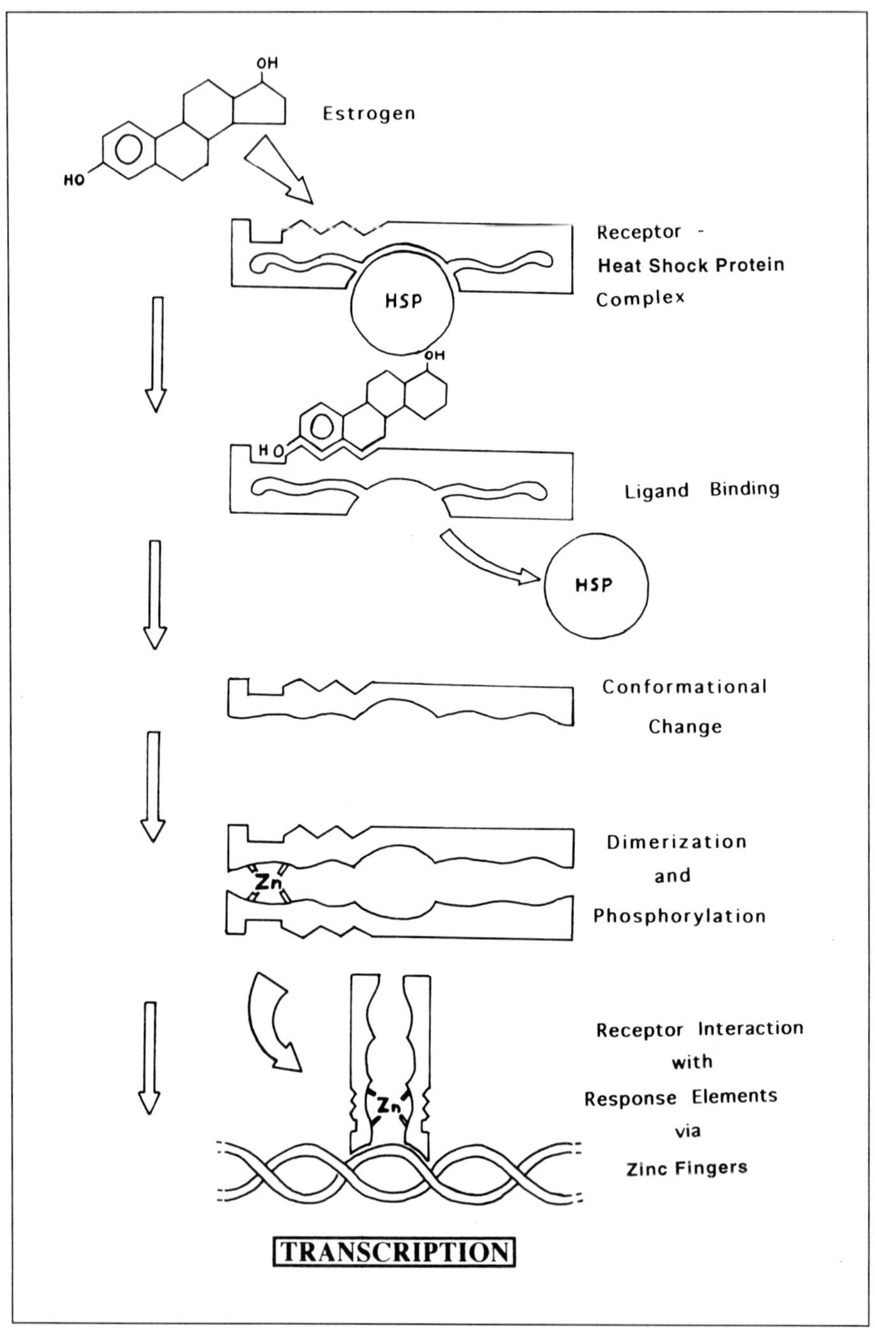

Fig. 7.1. Estrogen receptors as transducers of estrogen action.

NUCLEIC ACID SYNTHESIS

Estrogen induces a range of enzymes and other proteins involved in nucleic acid synthesis including DNA polymerase, thymidine and uridine kinases, thymidylate synthetase, carbamyl phosphate synthetase, aspartate transcarbamylase, dihydroorotase, glucose 6-phosphate dehydrogenase and dihydrofolate reductase.[15-19] Although increases in global transcription appear to be tightly coupled to estrogen action,[20] the most critically regulated genes have yet to be identified. However the effects are consistent with estrogen's effects on breast cancer proliferation.

SECRETION OF POLYPEPTIDE GROWTH FACTORS

Estrogen may induce polypeptides with growth regulatory properties.[13] These growth factors facilitate transition through restriction points in the cell cycle and it has been suggested that they act as mediators in the mitogenic control of breast cancer.[13] Such controls may be both distant and local. In terms of the former, estrogens are known to act on the pituitary to stimulate synthesis and secretion of growth factors such as prolactin and IGF-I.[21] These estromedin-like substances may act on the breast in an endocrine manner. Recently, however, the major interest has surrounded the possibility that growth factors are synthesized and secreted locally within the breast, thereby acting in either an autocrine or paracrine manner (Fig. 7.2).[22] The evidence for local regulation by growth factors has been facilitated by the availability of cell lines from breast tissue, particularly breast cancers. Although such lines have their limitations and have often been derived from pleural or ascitic fluid which represent advanced states of malignancy, nevertheless, if viewed with caution, the experimental findings can be illuminating. For example, many of the cell lines contain estrogen receptors and show direct proliferative responses to physiological doses of estradiol when grown both in vitro and in vivo as xenografts in immunocompromised animals.[23,24] Furthermore, media from estrogen receptor-positive cells grown in the presence of estrogen after the removal of estrogen may stimulate proliferation of other breast cancer cells in monolayer culture beyond that of media from cells cultured in the absence of estrogen,[25] as well as tumor formation in vivo in athymic nude mice.[24,26] These effects are at least partially specific since the media do not promote uterine growth in the same animals in which they induce tumor growth.[13] Such results suggest that estrogens induce the secretion of growth factors which specifically influence the proliferation of breast cells.

In terms of specific growth factors which may be involved, breast cancer cell lines may produce factors such as transforming growth factor (TGF)α,[15,27] insulin-like growth factors,[28] TGFβ[29] and fibroblast growth factors.[30] Secretion of many of these growth factors may be stimulated by estrogen in hormone-sensitive cell lines. For example,

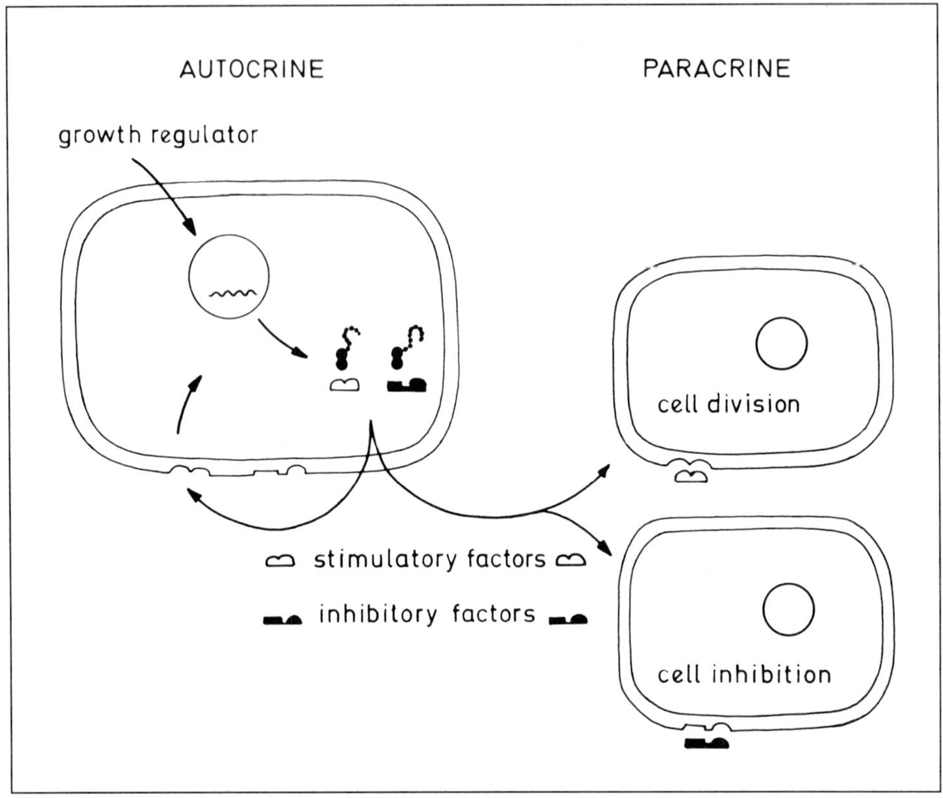

Fig. 7.2. Growth Factors acting as Autocrine/Paracrine Mediators of Estrogen Action.

TGFα-like material may be induced by estradiol in the estrogen receptor-positive MCF-7, T47D and ZR75-1 cell lines.[15,31] At least 70%
of primary breast carcinomas may express mRNA for TGFα[32] and the
peptide may be found in sufficient quantities to stimulate cell division.[33] However, no clear correlation has been reported with tumor
estrogen receptor status[32,34] although treatment with antiestrogens may
reduce tumor content of TGFα.[35]

Insulin-like growth factors I and II, as their names suggest, are
structurally similar to insulin. Although they are synthesized in many
body tissues, IGF I and II may also play an important role in breast
cancer. IGF-I is mitogenic for some breast cancer cells in culture[36,37]
and IGF-I-like material is secreted by breast cancer cells.[28] The nature
of this material is controversial as messenger RNA species corresponding to IGF-I have not been definitively identified in the cell lines.[38]
However, this IGF-like growth factor may be induced 3-to 6 fold following treatment of MCF-7 breast cancer cells with estrogen;[15] con-

versely secretion is inhibited by anti-estrogens.[39] Interestingly, growth hormone has negligible effect on the production of IGF-I-like growth factors by MCF-7 breast cancer cells,[40] whereas it is a strong stimulus for IGF-I production in liver, fibroblasts and other normal tissues.[41] However, the stromal component of breast tumors has been reported to be the major source of authentic IGF-I and IGF-II mRNA synthesis[38] and the production of IGF-I related polypeptides by fibroblasts in the stroma of breast tumors may, stimulate cancer cells by a paracrine mechanism.[38] Furthermore, there is evidence that insulin synergizes with estrogen in promoting growth of breast cancer cell lines both in vitro and in vivo[42] and it is possible that IGFs principally act by interacting with the estrogen to promote breast tumor growth.

It has also been reported that an IGF-II related gene product is produced by normal and malignant breast tissue.[43] IGF-II binds to multiple receptors (insulin, IGF-II and IGF-I) and these receptors have both been detected in human breast cancer.[44] In estrogen-dependent T47D human breast cancer cells, estradiol treatment increases IGF-II mRNA, whereas in the T61 human breast cancer xenograft (whose growth is inhibited by estrogen), estradiol down-regulates IGF-II.[45] These data support a role for IGF-II in estradiol-regulated breast cancer growth. It has also been hypothesized that IGF-II is involved in the progression of estrogen-dependence to estrogen-independence.[46]

Estradiol may also induce platelet derived growth factor (PDGF)[47] and while tumor cells do not express the PDGF receptors,[48] PDGF can stimulate IGF-I production in human fibroblasts.[49] Thus, an additional paracrine stimulation for breast cancer cells could operate through the effects of estrogen-induced tumor-derived growth factors stimulating stromal cells to secrete IGFs which could then stimulate adjacent tumor cells.

Transforming growth factor betas comprise three major isoforms, β1, 2 and 3. As their name suggests, these polypeptides are capable of transforming fibroblasts.[50] However, in contrast to TGFα and other growth factors, TGFβs inhibit the growth of most epithelial cells.[50] They may also stimulate differentiation in normal breast epithelial cells.[51] Interestingly, TGFβ secretion in MCF-7 breast cancer cells is inhibited by treatment with estrogen[52] and growth-inhibitory antiestrogens strongly stimulate secretion.[53] Furthermore TGFβ and medium from antiestrogen-treated MCF-7 cells inhibit the growth of estrogen receptor-negative cells such as the MDA-MB-231 cancer cell line.[54] Since breast cancers can exist as mixtures of estrogen receptor-positive and -negative tumor cells this opens up the possibility that anti-estrogen may inhibit estrogen receptor-negative clones as a consequence of induction of TGFβ in estrogen receptor-positive cells.

Because of these observations, it is tempting to postulate the mitogenic effect of estrogen is indirect and mediated by changes in growth factor secretion. Growth factors may be present in breast tumors in quantities sufficient to stimulate cell division and antiestrogen treatment may reduce concentrations. The antiestrogen, tamoxifen, also blocks cell line growth in the early to mid-GI phase of the cell cycle,[55] an effect which would be consistent with reduced availability of progression factors such as TGFα and IGF-I. However, studies with MCF-7-derived or transplantable solid human breast tumors in nude mice have failed to show an accumulation of cells in GI in tamoxifen-treated animals.[56] Furthermore, despite strong circumstantial evidence that TGFα may be an autocrine growth factor in breast tumors, other studies have failed to show that the blockade of TGFα action inhibits the growth of estrogen-sensitive breast cancer cell lines[57] or that overexpression of TGFα does not by-pass the need for exogenous estrogen for growth of MCF-7 tumors in nude mice.[58] TGFα and estradiol also induce different and distinctive profiles of intracellular peptides. These studies argue against an obligate intermediary role of TGFα in estrogen-dependent growth of human breast cancer.

However, estrogen may also sensitize estrogen responsive breast cancer cells to the mitogenic influences of insulin and insulin-like growth factors.[42,59] Such sensitization appears specific for estrogen and occurs at physiological levels of estradiol and is mediated by the Type I IGF receptor.[59] This may be an important mechanism by which estrogen stimulates the proliferation of hormone-dependent cells.[60] The regulation of the type I IGF receptor has a magnitude of sensitivity which is greater than that simple addition of growth factors.[61] Consequently it has been suggested that sensitization to IGFs is more important than the regulation of growth factors such as IGF-I, TGFα and TGFβ in the stimulation of breast cancer growth by estrogen.

PRODUCTION OF PROTEOLYTIC ENZYMES

In the same cell line systems as those studied for classical growth factors, estrogen may induce secretion of proteases such as plasminogen activator[63] and precursors of lysozymal cathepsins.[63] These are able to degrade extracellular matrix and may therefore facilitate tumor invasion (Fig. 7.3). Rochefort and his colleagues have made a detailed study of a glycoprotein with a molecular weight of 52 kD whose estrogen induction may be blocked by antiestrogens.[64] This protein has been subsequently shown to have a strong homology with the lysozymalenzyme, cathepsin D,[64,65] and to be able both to stimulate the proliferation of estrogen deprived MCF-7 cells[66] and to degrade extracellular matrix.[67] The secreted protein is partially taken up by cells through its interaction with the mannose 6-phosphate receptor,[68] which has been identified as the IGF-II receptor. This provides a possible explanation for the paradoxical mitogenic activity of a lysozymal protease. Interestingly some studies have shown that cathepsin D has prognostic significance in patients with breast cancer in that high concentrations in breast cancer cytosols are associated with a poor outlook.[69,70]

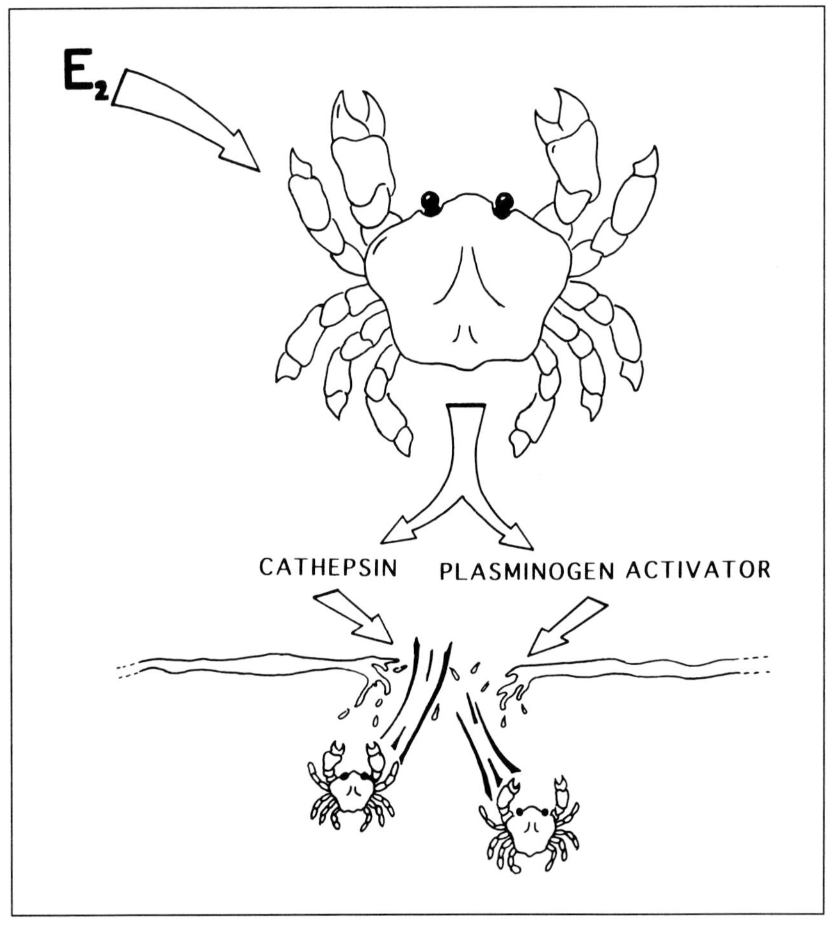

Fig. 7.3. Estrogen-induced secretion of proteolytic enzymes causing degradation of basement matrix and facilitating tumor invasion.

ONCOGENES

Estrogen may also stimulate the expression of oncogenes such as c-*myc* in breast cancers grown in vitro[14] or as xenografts.[71] Similarly, the tumor suppressor gene, p53, which when mutated may be oncogenic,[72] is increased in xenografts of breast cancer cells as a result of exposure to estrogen.[71] While these genes are involved in carcinogenesis, it is also clear that they are implicated[73,74] in the regulation of the cell cycle and may therefore influence proliferation rates. Paradoxically, however estradiol inhibits the expression in MCF-7 breast cancers of another oncogene, c-*erb*B$_2$[75] whose product is a putative growth factor receptor[76] and when overexpressed is associated with high proliferative capacity.[77]

SUMMARY

The major effects of estrogens are mediated through estrogen receptor proteins which act as nuclear transcription factors. As a result, estrogen may induce a variety of gene products which include enzymes connected with nucleic acid synthesis, growth factors, proteolutic enzymes and oncogene products. All these may influence and/or be components of the biosynthetic machinery associated with proliferation and spread which are ultimately associated with malignant transformation and progression.

REFERENCES

1. Jensen EV. In: Parker MG, ed. Nuclear hormone receptors. London: Academic Press 1991:1-13.
2. Korach KS. Insights from the study of animals lacking functional estrogen receptor. Science 1994; 266:1524-1526.
3. King WJ, Greene GL. Monoclonal antibodies localize oestrogen receptor in the nuclei of target cells. Nature 1984; 307:745-747.
4. Dauvois S, White R, Parker MG. The antiestrogen ICI 182780 disrupts estrogen receptor nucleocytoplasmic shuttling. J Cell Sci 1993; 106:1377-1388.
5. Schuh S, Yamemoto W, Brugge J et al. A 90,000 dalton binding protein common to both steroid receptors and the Rous sarcoma virus transforming protein pp60v-src. J Biol Chem 1985; 260:14292-14296.
6. Catelli MG, Binart N, Vourc'h C et al. Possible functional interaction between steroid hormone receptors and heat shock protein $M_r 90.00$ (hsp 90). In: Alexis MN, Sekeris CE, eds. Activation of hormone and growth factor receptors. The Netherlands: Kluwer Academic Publishers 1990:239-256.
7. Arnold SF, Obourn JD, Jaffe H et al. Serine 167 is the major estradiol-induced phosphorylation site on the human estrogen receptor. Mol Endocrinol 1994; 8:1208-1214.
8. Kumar V, Chambon P. The estrogen receptor binds tightly to its responsive element as a ligand-induced homodimer. Cell 1988; 55:154-156.
9. Parker MG. Structure and function of nuclear hormone receptors. Cancer Biol 1990; 1:81-87.
10. Parker MG, Bakker O. Nuclear hormone receptors: concluding remarks. In: Parker MG, ed. Nuclear Hormone Receptors. London: Academic Press 1991; 377-396.
11. Webster NJG, Green S, Jin JR et al. The hormone-binding domains of the estrogen and glucocorticoid receptors contain an inducible transcription activation function. Cell 1988; 54:199-207.
12. May FE, Westley BR. Identification and characterisation of oestrogen regulated RNAs in human breast cancer cells. J Biol Chem 1988; 263:12901-12908.
13. Dixon RB, Lippman ME. Estrogen regulation of growth and polypeptide growth factor secretion in human breast carcinoma. End Rev 1986; 8:29-43.

14. Dubik D, Dembinski TC, Shiu RP. Stimulation of c-myc oncogene expression associated with estrogen-induced proliferation of human breast cancer cells. Cancer Res 1987; 47:6517-6521.

15. Lippman ME, Dickson RB. Growth control of normal and malignant breast epithelium. Proc Roy Soc Edin 1989; 95B:89-106.

16. Edwards DP, Murphy SR, McGuire WL. Effect of estrogen and antiestrogen on DNA polymerase in human breast cancer. Cancer Res 1980; 40:1722-1726

17. Aitken SC, Lippman ME. Hormonal regulation of de novo pyrimidine synthesis and utilization in human breast cancer cells in tissue culture. Cancer Res 1983; 43:4681-4690.

18. Aitken SC, Lippman ME. Effect of estrogens and antiestrogens on growth-regulatory enzymes in human breast cancer cells in tissue culture. Cancer Res 1985; 45:1611-1620.

19. Dickson RB, Aitken S, Lippman ME. Assay of mitogen-induced effects on cellular thymidine incorporation. In: Barnes D, Sirbasku DA, eds. Methods in Enzymology 46, Hormone Action, Part II = Peptide growth factors. New York: Academic Press 1987:327-340.

20. Aitken SC, Lippman ME, Kasid A et al. Relationship between the expression of estrogen regulated genes and estrogens-stimulated proliferation of MCF-7 mammary tumor cells. Cancer Res 1985; 45:2608-2615.

21. Sirbasku DA. Estrogen-induction of growth factors specific for hormone responsive mammary, pituitary and kidney tumor cells. Proc Nat Acad Sci USA 1978; 75:3786-3790.

22. Lippman ME, Dickson RB, Bates S et al. Autocrine and paracrine growth regulation of human breast cancer. Breast Cancer Res Treat 1986; 7:59-70.

23. Engle LW, Young NW. Human breast carcinoma cells in continuous culture: a review. Cancer Res 1978; 38:4327-4339.

24. Soule HD, McGrath CM. Estrogen responsive proliferation of clonal human breast carcinoma cells in athymic mice. Cancer Lett 1980; 10:177-189.

25. Ikeda T, Danielpour D, Sirbasku DA. Isolation and properties of endocrine and autocrine type mammary tumor cell growth factors (estromedins). In: Bresciani F, King RJB, Lippman ME et al, eds. Progress in cancer research and therapy, Vol. 31. New York: Raven Press 1983:171-186.

26. Benz CC, Scott GK, Sarup JC et al. Estrogen-dependent, tamoxifen-resistant tumorigenic growth of MCF-7 cells transfected with HER2/neu. Breast Cancer Res Treat 1992; 24:85-89.

27. Bates SE, McManaway ME, Lippman ME et al. Characterization of estrogen responsive transforming activity in human breast cancer cell lines. Cancer Res 1986; 46:1707-1713.

28. Baxter RC, Maitland JE, Raisur RL et al. High molecular weight somatomedin-C (IGF-I) from T47D human mammary carcinoma cells: immunoreactivity and bioactivity. In: Spencer EM, ed. Insulin-like growth factors/somatomedins. Berlin: Walter de Gruyter Co. 1983:615-618.

29. Knabbe C, Zugmaier G, Dickson RB et al. Transforming growth factor beta and other growth inhibitory polypeptide in human breast cancer. In: Proceedings of the 3rd International Congress on Hormones and Cancer Hamburg. New York: Raven Press. 1988:258-262.
30. Swain S. Lippman M. Anchorage independent epithelial colony stimulating activity in human breast cancer cell lines. Proc Annual Mtg Am Assoc Cancer Res 1986; 27:Abstract 844.
31. Salomon DS, Kidwell WR, Kim N et al. Modulation by estrogen and growth factor of transforming growth factor alpha (TGFα) expression in normal and malignant human mammary epithelial cells. Cancer Res 1989; 113:57-69.
32. Bates SE, Davidson NE, Valverius E et al. Expression of transforming growth factor alpha and its messenger ribonucleic acid in human breast cancer: its regulation by estrogen and its possible functional significance. Mol Endocrinol 1988; 2:543-545.
33. Perroteau I, Salomon D, DeBortoli M et al. Immunological detection and quantitation of alpha transforming growth factors in human breast carcinoma cells. Breast Cancer Res Treat 1986; 7:201-210.
34. Nicholson RI, McClelland RA, Gee JM et al. Transforming growth factor-a and endocrine sensitivity in breast cancer. Cancer Res 1994; 54:1684-1689.
35. Gregory H, Thomas CE, Willshire IR et al. Epidermal and transforming growth factor a in patients with breast tumors. Br J Cancer 1989; 59:605-609.
36. Huff HK, McManaway M, Paik S et al. In vivo effects of insulin-like growth factor-I (IGF-I) on tumor formation by MCF-7 human breast cancer cells in athymic mic. Proc 70th Annual Mtg Endocrine Soc 1988a: Abstract 878.
37. Furlanetto RW, DiCarlo JN. Somatomedin C receptors and growth effects in human breast cells maintained in long-term culture. Cancer Res 1984; 44:2122-2128.
38. Yee D, Paik S, Lebovic GS et al. Analysis of insulin-like growth factor-I gene expression in malignancy: evidence for a paracrine role in human breast cancer. Mol Endocrinol 1989; 3:509-517.
39. Huff KK, Knabbe C, Lindsay R et al. Multihormonal regulation of insulin-like growth factor-I-related protein in MCF-7 human breast cancer cells. Molec Endocrinol 1988b; 2:200-208.
40. Clemmons DR, van Wyk JJ. Evidence for a functional role of endogenously produced somatomedin-like peptides in the regulation of DNA synthesis in cultured human fibroblasts and porcine smooth muscle cells. J Clin Invest 1986; 75:1914-1918.
41. Rechler MM, Bruni CB, Yang YWH et al. Regulation of insulin-like growth factor gene expression. In: Puett D, Ahmad F, Black S et al, eds. ICSU short reports, vol 4. Cambridge University Press, 1986:79-82.
42. Stewart AJ, Johnson MD, May FEB et al. Role of insulin like growth factors and the Type I insulin-like growth factor receptor in the estrogen-stimulated proliferation of human breast cancer cells. J Biol Chem 1990; 265:21172-21178.

43. Cullen KY, Yee D, Paik S et al. Insulin-like growth factor II expression and activity in human breast cancer. Proc 79th Annual Mtg Am Assoc Cancer Res 1988:Abstract 947.

44. DeLeon DD, Bakker B, Wilson DM et al. Demonstration of insulin-like growth factor (IGF-I and -II) receptors and binding protein in human breast cancer cell lines. Biochem Biophys Res Comm 1988; 152:398-405.

45. Brunner N, Yee D, Kern FG. Effect of endocrine therapy on growth of T61 human breast-cancer xenografts is directly correlated to a specific down-regulation of insulin-like growth factor-ii (igf-ii). Eur J Cancer 1993; 29:562-569.

46. Westley BR, May FEB. In vitro development of tamoxifen resistance. Endocrine-Rel Cancer 1995; 2:37-44.

47. Bronzert DA, Pantazis P, Antoniades HN et al. Synthesis and secretion of PDGF-like growth factor by human breast cancer cell lines. Proc Natl Acad Sci USA 1987; 84:5763-5767.

48. Yarden Y, Escobedo JA, Kwang WJ et al. Structure of the receptor for platelet-derived growth factor helps define a family of closely related growth factors. Nature 1986; 323:226-232.

49. Clemmons DR, Shaw DS. Variables controlling somatomedin production by cultured human fibroblasts. J Cell Physiol 1983; 115:137-143.

50. Roberts AB, Sporn MB. The transforming growth factor-βs. In: Spom MB, Roberts AB, eds. Handbook of experimental pharmacology, vol. 95. Heidelberg: Springer-Verlag 1990:419-472.

51. Roberts AB, Anzano MA, Wakefield LM et al. Type B transforming growth factor: a bifunctional regulator of cellular growth. Proc Natl Acad Sci USA 1985; 82:119-123.

52. Walker-Jones D, Valverius EM, Stampfer MS et al. Transforming growth factor beta (TGFβ) stimulates expression of milk fat globule protein in normal and oncogene transformed human mammary epithelial cells. Proc Am Assoc Cancer Res, New Orleans, LA 1988.

53. Knabbe C, Lippman ME, Wakefield LM. Evidence that TGF-beta is a hormonally regulated growth factor in human breast cancer cells. Cell 1987; 48:417-428.

54. Arteaga CL, Tandon AK, Von Hoff DD et al. Transforming growth factor β: potential autocrine growth inhibitor of estrogen receptor-negative human breast cancer cells. Cancer Res 1988; 48:3898-3904.

55. Sutherland RL, Green MD, Hall RE et al. Tamoxifen induces accumulation of MCF-7 human mammary carcinoma cells in the G_0/G_1 phase of the cell cycle. Eur J Cancer Clin Oncol 1983a; 19:615-621.

56. Brunner N, Bronzert D, Vindelov LL et al. Effect on growth and cell cycle kinetics of estradiol and tamoxifen on MCF-7 human breast cancer cells grown in vitro and in nude mice. Cancer Res 1989; 49:1515-1520.

57. Arteaga CL, Coronado E, Osborne CK. Blockade of epidermal growth factor receptor inhibits transforming growth factor α-induced but not estrogen induced growth of hormone dependent human breast cancer. Mol Endocrinol 1988; 2:1064-1069.

58. Clark R, Brunner N, Katz D et al. The effects of a constitutive expression of TGF-α on the growth of MCF-7 human breast cancer cells in vitro and in vivo. Molec Endocr 1989; 4:372-380.

59. van der Burg B, Rutteman GR, Blankenstein MA et al. Mitogenic stimulation of human breast cancer cells in a growth factor-defined medium: synergistic action of insulin and estrogen. J Cell Physiol 1988; 134:101-108.

60. Wiseman LR, Johnson MO, Wakeling AE et al. Type I IGF receptor and acquired tamoxifen resistance in oestrogen responsive human breast cancer cells. Eur J Cancer 1993; 29A:2256-2264.

61. Stewart AJ, Westley BR, May FE. Modulation of the proliferative response of breast cancer cells to growth factors by oestrogen. Br J Cancer 1992; 66:640-648.

62. Huff KK, Lippman ME. Hormonal control of plasminogen activator secretion in ZR-75-1 human breast cancer cells in culture. Endocrinol 1984; 114:1702-1710.

63. Morisset M, Capony F, Rochefort H. Processing and estrogen regulation of the 52-kDa protein inside MCF7 breast cancer cells. Endocrinol 1986; 119:2773-2783.

64. Rochefort H, Augereau P, Briozzo P et al. Oestrogen-induced pro-cathepsin D in breast cancer: from biology to clinical application. Proc Roy Soc Edin 1989; 95B:107-118.

65. Barrett AJ. Cathepsin D: purification of isoenzymes from human and chicken liver. Biochem J 1970; 117:601-607.

66. Vignon F, Capony F, Chambon M et al. Autocrine growth stimulation of the MCF-7 breast cancer cells by the estrogen-regulated 52K protein. Endocrinol 1986; 118:1537-1545.

67. Briozzo P, Morisset M. Capony F et al. In vitro degradation of extracellular matrix with Mr 52,000 cathepsin D secreted by breast cancer cells. Cancer Res 1988; 48:3688-3692.

68. Von Figura K, Hasilik A. Lysosomal enzymes and their receptors. Annu Rev Biochem 1986; 55:167-193.

69. Tandon A, Clark G, Chirgwin J et al. Cathepsin D and prognosis in breast cancer. New Eng J Med 1990; 322:297-302.

70. Thorpe SM, Rochefort H, Garcia M et al. Association between high concentrations of 52K cathepsin-D and poor prognosis in primary breast cancer. Cancer Res 1989; 49:6008-6014.

71. Thompson AM, Steel CM, Foster ME et al. Gene expression in oestrogen-dependent human breast cancer xenograft tumours. Br J Cancer 1990; 62:78-84.

72. Lane DP, Benchimol S. p53: oncogene or anti-oncogene? Genes Devel 1990; 4:1-8.

73. Musgrove EA, Sutherland RL. Cell cycle control by steroid hormones. Semin Cancer Biol 1994; 5: 381-389.

74. Allred DC, Clark GM, Elledge R et al. Association of p53 protein expression with tumor cell proliferation rate and clinical outcome in node-negative breast cancer. J Natl Cancer Inst 1993; 85:200-206.

75. Dati C, Antoniotti S, Taverna et al. Inhibition of c-erbB-2 oncogene expression by estrogens in human breast cancer cells. Oncogene 1990; 5:1001-1006.
76. Walker RA, Varley JM. The molecular pathology of human breast cancer. Cancer Surveys 1993; 16:31-57.
77. Tommasi S, Paradiso A, Mangia A et al. Biological correlation between HER-2/neu and proliferative activity in human breast cancer. Anticancer Res 1991; 11:1395-1400.

ESTROGENS AND ENDOCRINE THERAPY FOR BREAST CANCER

HISTORICAL BACKGROUND

It is remarkable not only that the first indication that the breast and its tumors were subject to endocrine control was put forward over 100 years ago but also that it was put forward without the knowledge of the nature of hormones. In 1889, the German surgeon Schinzenier, observed atrophy of the breast following cessation of ovarian function and suggested that removal of the ovaries might lead to regression of breast cancer.[1] However, he never followed through his observation and it was left to Sir George Beatson to show that surgical castration in premenopausal women with beast cancer had beneficial effects on the disease.[2] It is now clear that ovariectomy results in tumor regression in about one third of premenopausal patients with advanced breast cancer.[3] With the advent of synthetic glucocorticoids such as cortisone, which could be given as replacement corticosteroid therapy, operations such as adrenalectomy and hypophysectomy became practical propositions. Endocrine deprivation could then be applied to postmenopausal women. It then became apparent that removal of either the adrenals or pituitary could produce benefits in about 30-40% in postmenopausal patients with advanced breast cancer.[4,5] Paradoxically, pharmacological doses of estrogens also elicit meaningful responses in a similar percentage of patients.[6]

These observations illustrate the dilemma associated with endocrine therapy for breast cancer, i.e., objective remissions occur but only in the minority of patients. Furthermore, most women still die of cancer but with a disease which is evidently hormone-unresponsive.[7] If, therefore, hormone manipulations are not curative, their acceptability depends largely on the relative lack of toxicity in comparison with other major therapeutic modalities such as chemotherapy. There has, therefore, been a drive to develop reversible and less toxic forms of hormone treatment (Table 8.1). Agents such as LHRH agonists, antiestrogens and

Table 8.1. Comparative characteristics of "old" and "new" estrogen deprivation therapies

	Old	New
Method	surgery irradiation	drugs
Action	remove or destroy hormone-producing organ	inhibition of hormone synthesis/release/action
Properties	irreversible side effects	reversible minimal side effects

aromatase inhibitors are now widely used as endocrine therapies.[8] These developments have stemmed from a general understanding of the mechanisms by which estrogens are synthesized and exert their action within the breast (Fig. 8.1). This chapter will therefore consider the rationale behind the use of individual forms of estrogen deprivation and their place in the management of breast cancer.

OVARIAN ABLATION

Although ovarian ablation was the earliest form of endocrine therapy for breast cancer,[2] it still remains a major treatment option for patients who are premenopausal and who have advanced breast cancer. Ovariectomy is effective in between 30 and 40% of patients[3] and in patients with advanced breast cancer it produces a median duration of remission of about 9 months (although the length of response can be very variable).[9] Functional destruction of the ovary is generally been achieved either by surgery or radiation. However, whereas the effects of surgery are immediate, radiological ablation may require several weeks to become effective and the incomplete destruction of estrogen-producing follicles is more likely.[10] Benefits following ovarian ablation have also been reported in perimenopausal and postmenopausal patients, but response rates are markedly less than in women with regular ovarian function.[11] Oophorectomy has also been used as an adjuvant to local regional management of the breast in premenopausal patients with earlier stages of the disease.[12] Clear benefits in terms of both increased disease-free interval and survival have been demonstrated and it is calculated that ovariectomy reduces odds of death by an average of 28% compared with women not receiving therapy.[13] As a result, ovarian ablation represents a major treatment option for premenopausal patients with early breast cancer, particularly those who have invaded lymph nodes and estrogen receptor-positive tumors. Because of the benefits of oophorectomy as treatment in premenopausal women and the protective effects of such procedures in reducing the risk of developing

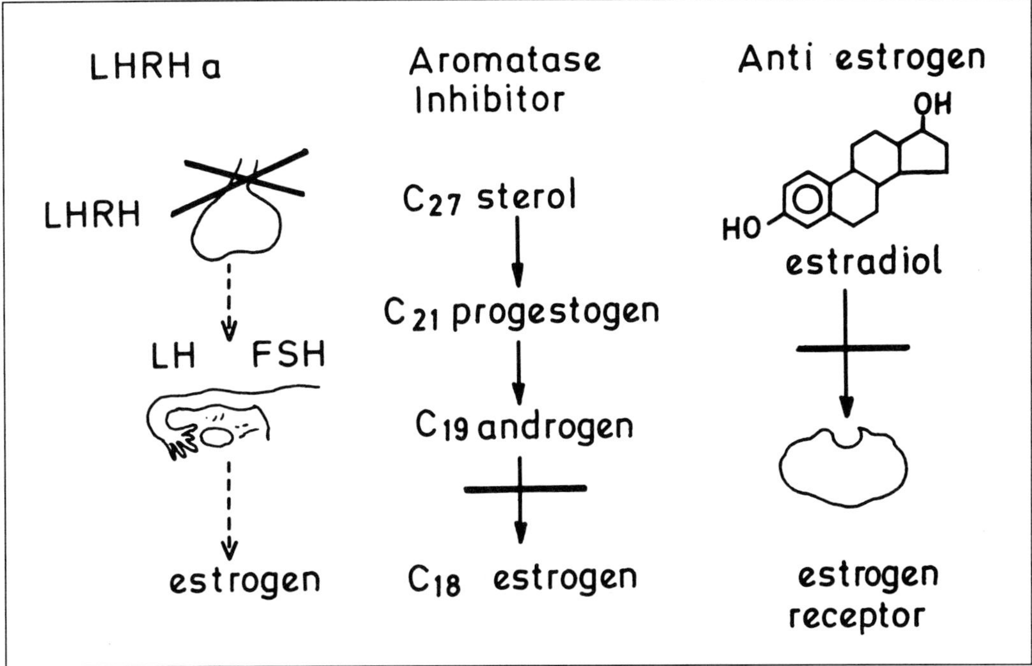

Fig. 8.1. Strategies underlying the development of drugs designed for estrogen-deprivation therapy.

breast cancer, it has been suggested that women with a genetic predisposition for breast disease should be offered oophorectomy prophylactically.[14] This, however, is still a matter of some controversy.

ADRENAL AND PITUITARY ABLATION

While adrenalectomy and hypophysectomy may affect the level and action of many hormones, their ability to reduce circulating levels of estrogens in postmenopausal women appears central to their anti-tumor effects. This is because, although benefits of these procedures are restricted to one third of postmenopausal women, they are particularly effective in tumors with estrogen receptors.[15] Further indirect evidence for the involvement of estrogen comes from the observation that patients who have previously received benefit from ovarian ablation are more likely to respond subsequently to either adrenalectomy or hypophysectomy.[16] As with other endocrine therapies a long disease-free interval, non-visceral metastasis and a good performance status also increases the likelihood of response.[16,17] A direct comparison of rates and length of response to adrenalectomy and hypophysectomy is difficult but hypophysectomy seems at least equal to or somewhat better than adrenalectomy. For example in one particular study, the duration of response with hypophysectomy was 15 months as compared with eight months with adrenalectomy.[18] The major drawbacks

associated with both adrenalectomy and pituitary ablation in postmenopausal women are the high incidence of morbidity and the long-term
management of adrenal/pituitary insufficiency.[19] Because of these considerations the procedures, although popular decades ago, are now rarely
performed.

LHRH AGONIST ANALOGUES

Surgical and radiological ablations of the ovaries are invasive and
irreversible procedures which produce benefits in the minority of patients. There has therefore been a desire to devise medical alternatives
which might be less traumatic and reversible. LHRH agonist analogues
have such characteristics, providing a means of suppressing ovarian
estrogen production in premenopausal women and effecting a "medical castration."[20] The basis for the development of these analogues has
come from a greater understanding of how gonadal synthesis of estrogen is regulated (Fig. 8.2). As was indicated in chapter 5, the production of steroid hormones in the ovary is under the control of pituitary
gonadotrophins whose secretion is in turn regulated by the hypothalamic releasing factor, LHRH.[21] Native LHRH is a decapeptide which
is intermittently secreted by the hypothalamus in regular pulses.[21,22]

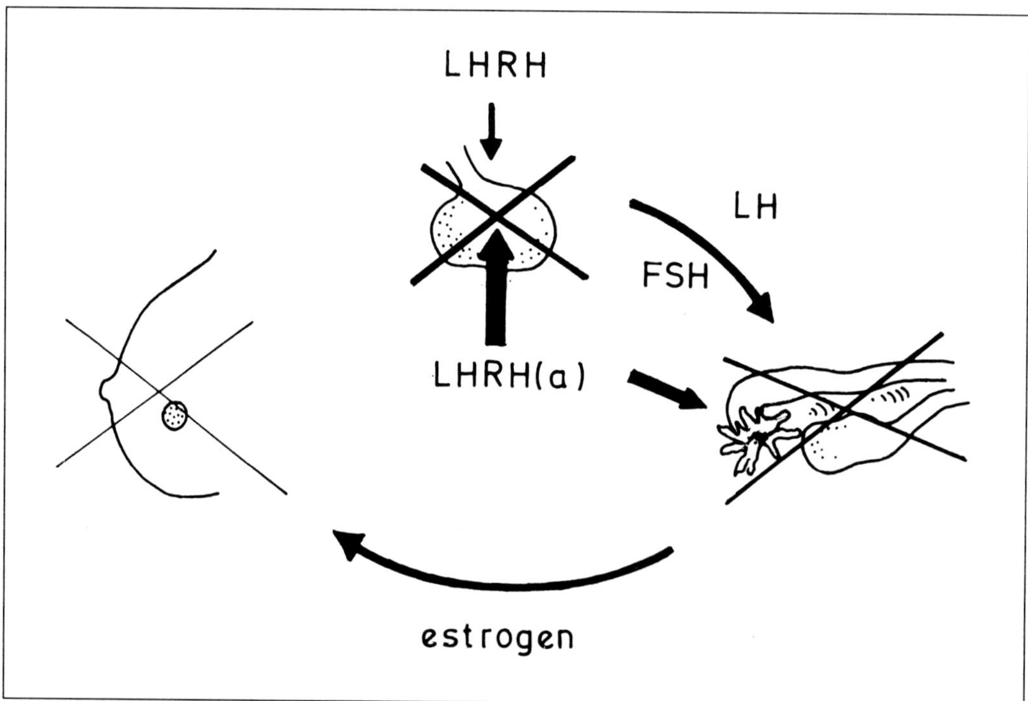

Fig. 8.2. Basis for the use of LHRH agonists as a form of medical castration.

LHRH travels via the portal circulation to the pituitary where it binds to specific receptors and stimulates the pulsatile release of gonadotrophins.[23] Recently, several highly potent LHRH analogues have been synthesized by introducing substituents of unusual amino acids within the molecule (particularly at position 6 and 10, Fig. 8.3).[24] When administered acutely, LHRH agonist analogues cause a rapid release of gonadotrophins into the circulation; in contrast when given chronically they produce paradoxical effects in that gonadotrophins fall.[25] This parallels responses to native LHRH which differ according to mode of presentation to the pituitary-pulsatile patterns producing stimulation of gonadotrophins whereas continuous infusion produces suppressive effects.[26] It seems likely therefore that potent analogues, even when given intermittently, maintain continuous receptor occupancy and simulate the suppressive effects of LHRH continuous infusion.[27] The fall in gonadotrophins following the administration of LHRH agonists results in a decreased drive to the ovaries and circulating levels of estrogen fall to castrate levels (Fig. 8.4)[25,28]—hence the term "medical ovariectomy."[19]

Initially LHRH agonist preparations required administration either by daily subcutaneous injection or by intra-nasal inhalation. More recently, however, depot formulations have become available.[29] In some, the peptide is linked to small rods of biodegradable polymers and the preparation can be injected once monthly and still maintain therapeutic levels of the analogue in the blood over 28 days. Hormone measurements confirm that this form of chronic treatment evokes an effective medical castration with reduced estrogen levels (Fig. 8.4) and induced amenorrhea.[30] These effects have led to the use of LHRH analogues treatment for premenopausal women with advanced breast cancer. The results of several studies using different types and regimes of LHRH agonists have confirmed the validity of such an approach and demonstrated therapeutic benefits similar to those produced either by radiation-induced or surgical castration (Fig. 8.5) i.e., about a

	1	2	3	4	5	6	7	8	9	10
LH-RH	pGlu	His	Trp	Ser	Tyr	Gly	Leu	Arg	Pro	Gly-NH
Zoladex						D-Ser(Bu^t)				Azygly-NH (ICI)
Buserelin						D-Ser(Bu^t)				Ethylamide (Hoechst)
Leuprolide						D-Leu				Ethylamide (Abbott)
—						D-Trp				Gly-NH (Debiopharm)

Fig. 8.3. Structure of LHRH agonists used in therapy.

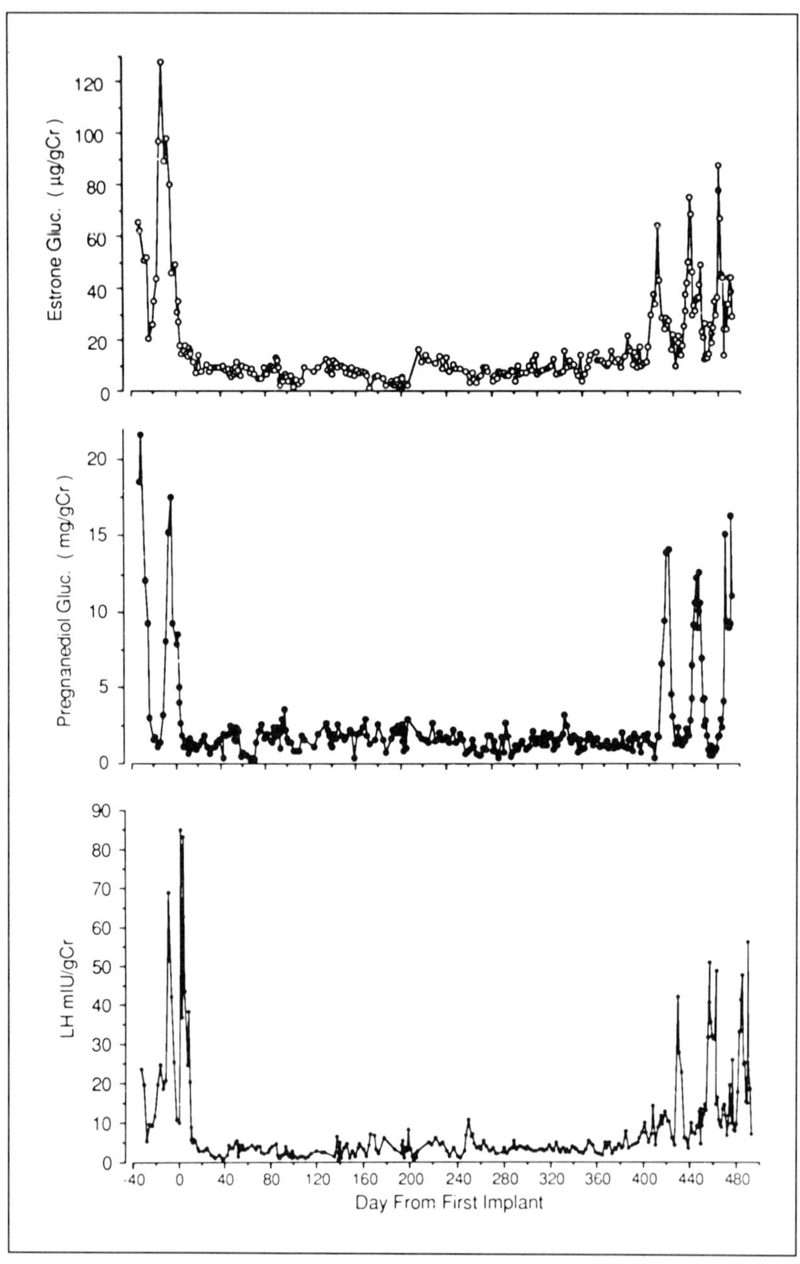

Fig. 8.4. *Estrogen levels following treatment with a depot preparation of LHRH agonist.*

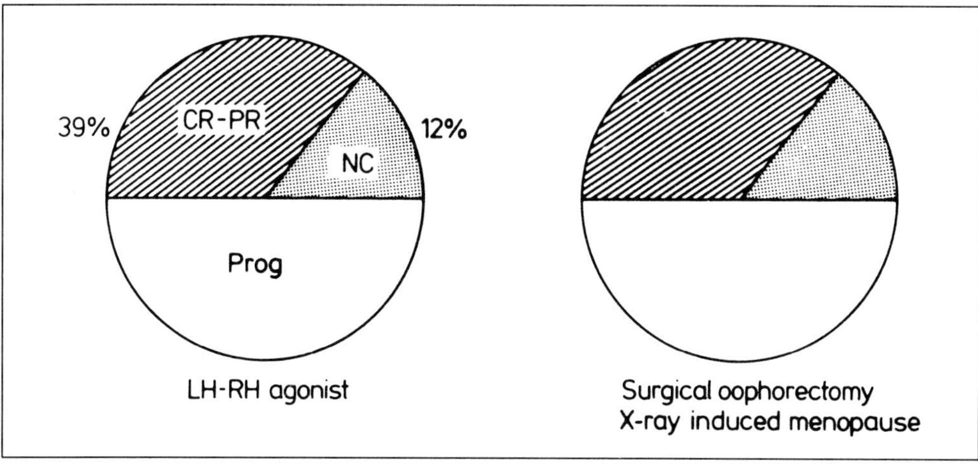

Fig. 8.5. Comparative effects of LHRH agonists and ovariectomy on clinical response of premenopausal patients with advanced breast cancer.

40% objective response rate in unselected patients and about a 50% benefit in patients with estrogen receptor-positive tumors.[31,32] There is a general lack of significant clinical toxicity although, as might be expected, patients report hot flushes and other menopausal symptoms. The immediate advantage of LHRH agonists over other forms of castration is that they alone are reversible and ovarian function returns on discontinuation of drug administration.[33] While, logically, the major clinical investigations of LHRH analogues have been performed in premenopausal women, small numbers of postmenopausal patients have also been treated. Interestingly about 10% of such patients with advanced breast cancer appear to gain some meaningful benefit.[30,34] The mechanism by which these are achieved is not immediately obvious. Thus it may be mediated through inhibiting residual ovarian function but effects on circulating estrogen are relatively small[34] (more substantial falls have been observed in androgen levels[35]). Direct effects on tumors are also possible, since inhibitory influences of LHRH and its analogues have been reported on breast cancer cells in culture[36] and certain breast tumors possess specific binding sites for LHRH agonists.[37]

The LHRH analogues which are currently clinically available are agonists rather than antagonists.[24] The reason for this is the toxicity associated with prototype drugs with antagonist activity.[38] It may be, however, that more rationally designed drugs have an improved clinical utility. The combination of LHRH agonists with antiestrogens may also provide a more complete estrogen blockade. In this respect the combination of LHRH agonists and tamoxifen produces a significantly greater decrease in serum levels of estradiol and FSH than does either agent alone.[39] Trials of LHRH analogues as adjuvant endocrine therapy for breast cancer are also in progress.[30,40] Because of their castration-like effects, LHRH agonists have also been proposed as preventative agents for breast cancer. It is postulated that reversible medical ovariectomy performed at critical risk periods may substantially reduce the incidence of breast cancer.[41] The calculation is that LHRH agonists plus low dose estrogen replacement therapy given to premenopausal women for 10 years will reduce lifetime risk of breast cancer by 50% while at the same time providing an effective contraceptive regime.[42]

ADDITIVE THERAPY WITH ESTROGENS

For reasons that still remain unclear (possibly down regulation of estrogen receptors), pharmacological concentrations of estrogen may induce remission in 30-35% of patients with advanced breast cancer when used as first-line therapy.[6,43] Response rates seem to increase with years after the menopause[9,18,44] and in estrogen receptor-positive tumors.[15,45] These characteristics suggest that, like other forms of endocrine therapy, additional estrogen therapy is mediated through the estrogen receptor. The most commonly used estrogen preparations are diethylstilbestrol, ethinyl estradiol and conjugated estrogens. No large randomized trials of the different estrogen preparations have been performed but it seems unlikely that the type or dose of estrogen markedly influences outcome.[46] However, up to 30% patients given estrogen therapy display substantial side effects[43] and it is because of these that estrogen therapy has largely been replaced (paradoxically) by antiestrogen treatment.

ANTIESTROGENS

If, as has been suggested in chapter 7, major effects of estrogen are mediated through its receptor then therapies based on using drugs which block the interaction of estrogen and receptor might be expected to produce beneficial anti-tumor effects. There has therefore been a major impetus to design drugs which might have these properties. In the forefront of such antiestrogens is the drug tamoxifen (Fig. 8.6). Tamoxifen can be shown to bind effectively to estrogen receptors and block the effects of endogenous estrogens, although weak estrogen agonist actions may be observed, particularly in the context of low endogenous estrogen levels.[47] The use of tamoxifen has been a major advance in the treatment of breast cancer. Since its first use as a palliative regime in advanced breast cancer,[48] results from almost 4000 women have shown that about one third of patients will obtain some form of clinical response to the drug.[49] Comparisons of tamoxifen with other drug-induced endocrine therapies in postmenopausal women are shown in Table 8.2. Because of its efficacy and general lack of toxicity, tamoxifen is now established as first-line endocrine therapy in postmenopausal women with breast cancer. As might be expected from a drug whose

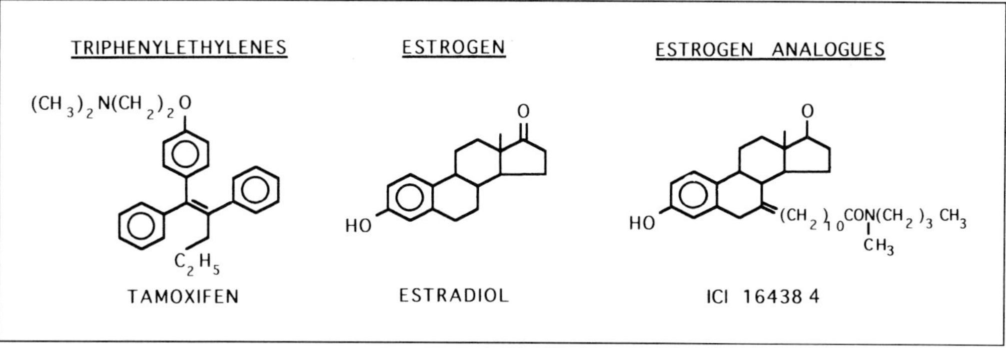

Fig. 8.6. Structure of antiestrogens.

Table 8.2. Clinical response to tamoxifen in patients with breast cancer

	Response CR+PR/Total	Response %
Nolvadex	63/205	31
Estrogen	67/203	33
Nolvadex	39/123	32
Androgen	30/139	22
Nolvadex	59/176	34
Progestin	67/173	39
Nolvadex	106/293	36
Aminoglutethimide	66/186	35

Data derived from ref. 49.

major mechanism of action is to interfere with estrogen receptor function, responses are much more likely to occur in tumors which are estrogen receptor-positive.[15] Insofar as the percentage of breast tumors which are estrogen receptor-positive increases with age,[50] it is perhaps not surprising that elderly women tend to have a relatively high response rate to tamoxifen.[31,51] This, together with lack of toxicity, has led to the suggestion that tamoxifen therapy be used as an alternative to surgery in patients who are elderly and may not find surgery an acceptable option. A large overview incorporating 30,000 patients has evaluated tamoxifen therapy as an adjuvant to surgical procedures in patients with early breast cancer. These studies have shown that adjuvant tamoxifen not only retards the appearance of recurrent disease but significantly reduces mortality in women aged 50 years or older (Table 8.3).[13] Effects were again more pronounced in patients having tumors possessing estrogen receptors. Because of this profile it has been

***Table 8.3. Clinical experience from using tamoxifen
therapy as an adjuvant in early breast cancer***

Patient age	Reduction in annual odds	
	Relapse	Death
<50 premenopausal	12%	6%
50-59 postmenopausal	28%	19%
60-69	29%	17%
> 70	28%	21%
Overall	25%	16%

suggested that tamoxifen represents a promising drug to use in preventative trials in women at high risk of developing breast cancer.[41,52]
Indeed such trials have now been embarked upon and initial data suggest that there may be hidden benefits to tamoxifen in terms of its
estrogenic agonist effects which may prevent bone loss and have a beneficial effect on blood profile lipids (this may account for the reduced
incidence of cardiovascular-related deaths in certain trials of tamoxifen[54]).[53]
Potential drawbacks have appeared in terms of induction of endometrial and hepatic cancers[47,55] and these are the subject of fierce debate.
Results from these prevention trials are eagerly awaited as extended
use and follow-up becomes available.

Other answers are still required for certain questions such as: what
is the optimal length of time for which antiestrogen is required to be
given in the adjuvant situation? Can antiestrogens have benefits in
estrogen receptor negative tumors? Is there a role for more potent and
specific antiestrogens?

The mechanism of action of antiestrogens is all important in terms
of the optimal time for which antiestrogens require to be given—if
tumorcidal, administration need only be given for the period covering
maximum cell kill; on the other hand, if antiestrogens are tumorstatic,
they potentially require to be given over an indefinite period. Experimental evidence points to tamoxifen being a cytostatic agent—the drug
retards the growth of hormone-sensitive breast cancer xenografts in
immunosuppressed animals but its effects are related to the time of
administration.[56] If tamoxifen is withdrawn and estrogens are present,
tumors will invariably resume growth. This suggests that tamoxifen
does not destroy all cancer cells and disease can be reactivated by exposure to an estrogen stimulus. Clinical trials in which different dura-
tions of therapy are directly compared also support this concept, suggesting that prolonged administration is more efficacious.[57,58]

Although there is almost total agreement that the major benefits
of tamoxifen in postmenopausal patients with advanced breast cancer
are achieved in estrogen receptor-positive tumors, a small but consistent proportion of estrogen receptor-negative tumors (about 10%) also

respond.[58] Similarly, trials of adjuvant therapy suggest that while major benefits are associated with tumors having high levels of estrogen receptors, increased disease-free interval and survival time can be spread throughout all groups, irrespective of estrogen receptor status.[58,59] Whether these minority effects are caused by tamoxifen having other actions in addition to those on the estrogen receptor still needs to be resolved. Equally it has been suggested that effects on estrogen receptor-negative tumors may be indirectly modulated through an estrogen receptor mechanism.[59] Thus, if other cells within the breast have estrogen receptors, they may be stimulated by tamoxifen to produce paracrine factors. Such a scenario has been put forward regarding tamoxifen induction of TGFβ in cells such as stromal fibroblasts,[59] the TGFβ acting in a paracrine manner to inhibit the growth of estrogen receptor-negative tumor cells.[60]

Antiestrogens such as tamoxifen may incompletely block the trophic actions of estrogen and also have partial estrogen agonist activity of their own. There is thus good reason to develop more potent antiestrogens devoid of intrinsic estrogen activity. Such drugs would be expected to produce more profound effects and have larger populations of target cells. Clinically, the proportion of complete tumor remissions might increase beyond that produced by the antiestrogens currently available. It is thus pertinent that 7α-alkyl amide analogues of estradiol (Fig. 8.6) have the pharmacological characteristics of pure antiestrogens, appear to be without estrogenic activity and block the trophic effects of exogenous and endogenous estrogens and partial agonists such as tamoxifen. In estrogen-responsive human breast cancer cells these pure antiestrogens are more effective inhibitors of cell growth than tamoxifen.[61] For example, the pure antiestrogen ICI164383 is a more potent inhibitor of the growth of MCF-7 estrogen-responsive breast cancer cells than tamoxifen, differences in efficacy being reflected in both the lower concentration of drug required for effect and the greater reduction in the proportion of cells continuing DNA synthesis (Fig. 8.7). These observations imply that pure antiestrogens will provide a more effective therapy of breast cancer. Indeed, preliminary clinical studies employing the pure antiestrogen ICI182780 have revealed responses in patients with tumors which had either acquired or inherent resistance to tamoxifen.[62] It remains to determine in more extensive studies whether these treatment benefits translate into increased survival. However a word of caution needs to be sounded with regard to pure antiestrogens in that they may produce accelerated bone loss and cardiovascular symptoms. In this respect some of the estrogenic effects of partial estrogen agonists are beneficial, and an ideal antiestrogen would have sufficient antiestrogenic potential to inhibit cancer growth effectively as well as by virtue of estrogenic properties protect against bone loss and other symptoms associated with estrogen deprivation. This profile corresponds closely to that of tamoxifen.

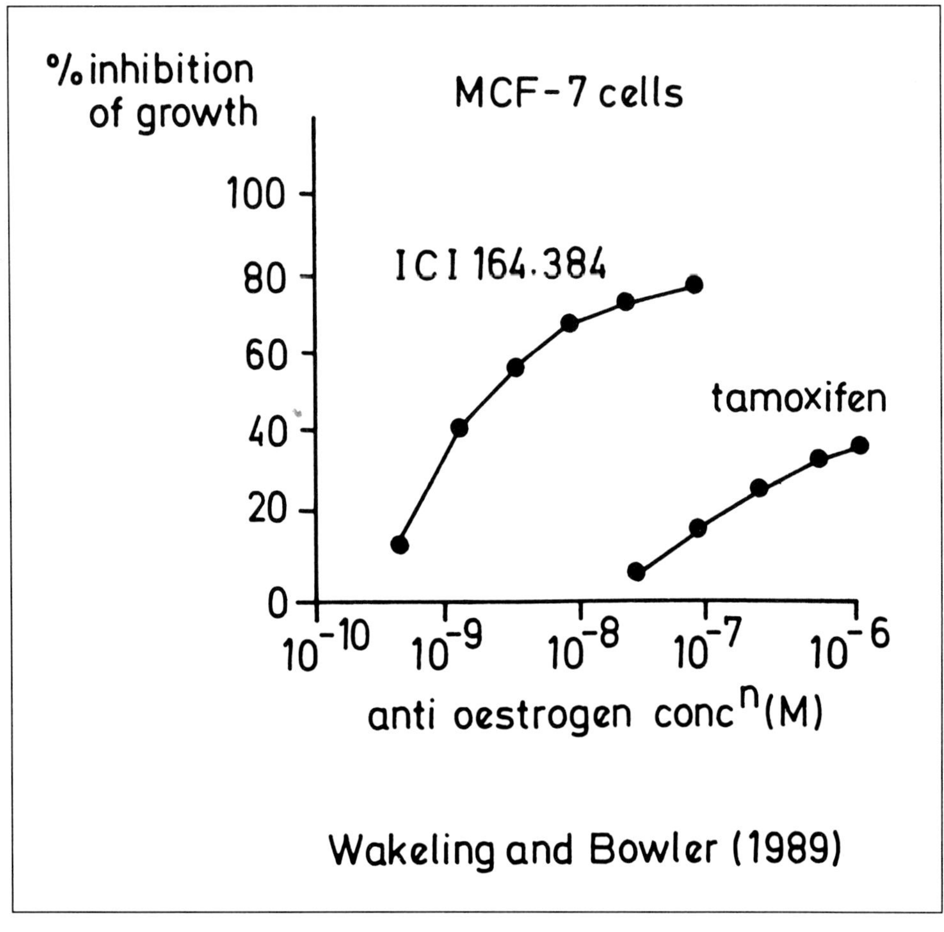

Fig. 8.7. Comparative effects of the pure antiestrogen and tamoxifen on the proliferation of the MCF-7 breast cancer cell line.

The use of antiestrogens in premenopausal women with breast cancer and the relative merits in comparison with oophorectomy are also the subject of controversy. Compared with postmenopausal women in which effects of tamoxifen on circulating estrogen levels are modest (indicating that the anti-tumor effects of tamoxifen are not directly mediated through alterations in glandular hormone secretion but rather a consequence of direct inhibition of estrogen actions at the tumor level), tamoxifen treatment in premenopausal women can be associated with marked elevations of gonadotrophin and estrogen levels.[31,63] These endocrine effects are likely to be counter-productive in terms of blocking estrogenic effects. Nevertheless it is clear that even in premenopausal women tamoxifen is capable of producing tumor regression.[31,59,64] Amenorrhea occurs in approximately one third of patients receiving tamoxifen and it may be that the drug's effects are comparable to castration in these particular patients although anti-tumor effects can also be seen in the absence of overt menstrual abnormalities.[65] These considerations need to be taken into account in assessing the potential value of tamoxifen as a preventative agent in high risk women, most of whom will be premenopausal. The main rationale for using tamoxifen in breast cancer prevention is the observed 35% reduction in contralateral breast cancer when the drug is used in the adjuvant setting. However, it should be noted that while the adjuvant use of tamoxifen in premenopausal breast cancer patients reduces the odds of death overall by a mean of 17%, premenopausal women with estrogen receptor-poor tumors appear to experience no benefit from tamoxifen.[13,66] This compares with the more dramatic effect of prophylactic oophorectomy which reduces the odds of death by 28% compared with women receiving no ablative treatment.[13]

AROMATASE INHIBITORS

The use of drugs which inhibit estrogen biosynthesis is an attractive strategy by which to treat estrogen-dependent cancers. In common with antiestrogen therapy this approach has several potential advantages over endocrine ablative therapy: the action of aromatase inhibitors may be reversible and self limiting—if therefore therapy proves ineffective, withdrawal of the drug should allow estrogen levels to return to normal; specific inhibition should affect estrogens alone and minimize side effects not associated with estrogen deprivation; as the aromatase enzyme seems similar in all tissues,[67] therapy should reduce estrogen levels irrespective of the site of biosynthesis—consequently, aromatase inhibitors have the potential to suppress estrogen levels beyond those achievable by surgical ablation of classical endocrine organs.[68]

As estrogens lie at the end of a sequence of steroid transformations, blockade of any conversion in the pathway will potentially cause a decrease in estrogen synthesis but more specific suppression will result from inhibition of the final step which is unique to estrogen biosynthesis. This, as indicated in chapter 1, comprises the aromatase reaction converting androgens into estrogen. The key role of aromatase enzymes in estrogen biosynthesis has generated considerable interest in the development of drugs to use as potential inhibitors.

Because the aromatase reaction is complex and involves multiple hydroxylation of the androgen substrate, employing NADPH as electron donor[69] and utilizing a specific cytochrome p450 as an electron transfer agent,[70] there are several potential mechanisms by which inhibition may be achieved (Fig. 8.8). In general, however, two major types of aromatase inhibitors have been developed (Fig. 8.9)—type I inhibitors, which interfere with the attachment of the androgen substrate to catalytic site and which are invariably substrate analogues and type II

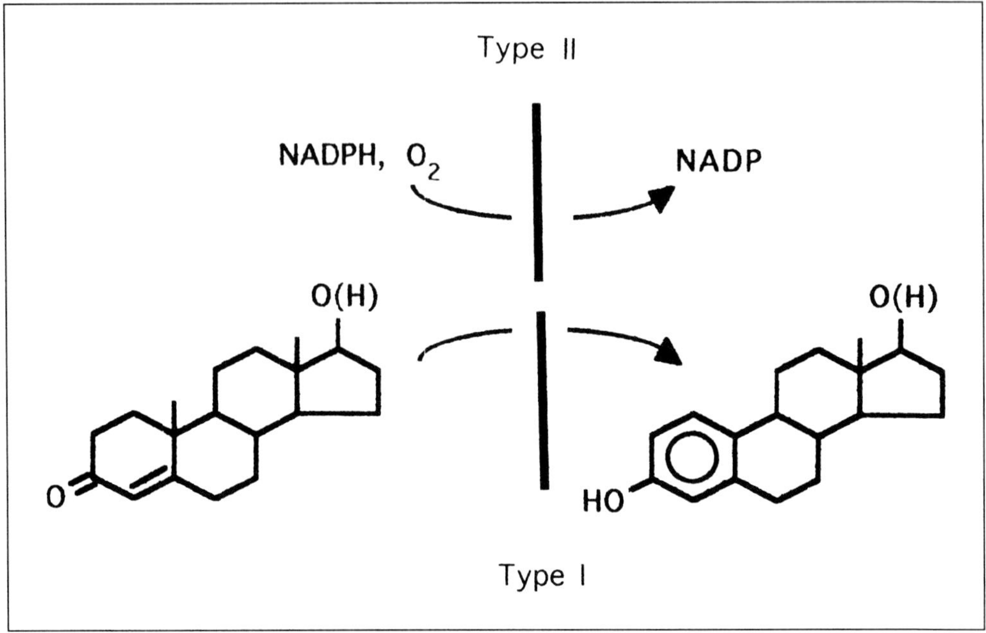

Fig. 8.8. Mechanisms by which to inhibit the aromatase enzyme.

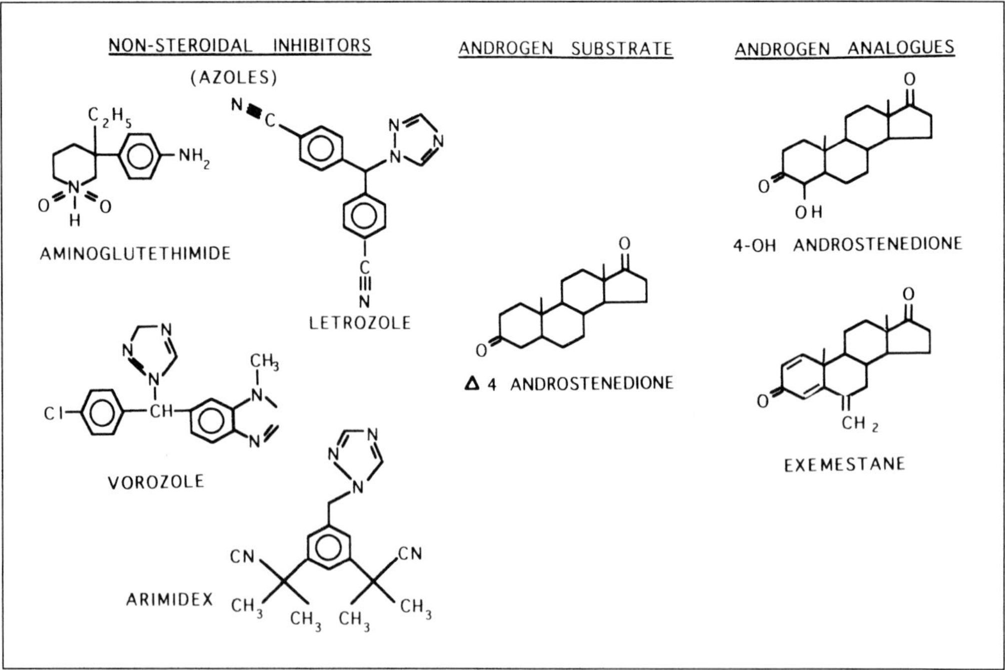

Fig. 8.9. Structure of some aromatase inhibitors.

inhibitors which interfere with the cytochrome p450 moiety of the enzyme.[71] Theoretically, type I inhibitors should be more specific although in designing substrate analogues it is important that the compounds themselves are not aromatized into metabolites with estrogenic characteristics. A subset of type I inhibitors known as "suicide inhibitors" are particularly interesting.[72] These compounds have little inherent inhibitory activity but once bound to the catalytic site of the aromatase enzyme are transformed into reactive intermediates which bind covalently to the active site causing loss of enzyme activity. The term "suicide" is particularly pertinent since the enzyme is only activated as a consequence of its own mechanism of action. An inhibitor acting in this way can be expected to have particular specificity since it should only inactivate enzymes for which it is substrate. Prolonged effects can also be predicted in vivo as the aromatase enzyme is not only inhibited but inactivated even after the unbound inhibitor has disappeared. Resumption of estrogen synthesis depends on the production of new aromatase molecules. These properties are to be contrasted with type II inhibitors which do not destroy the enzyme and whose actions are usually reversible and therefore dependent upon continued presence of inhibitors. Type II inhibitors often have the disadvantage of lack of specificity in that, in addition to aromatase, many other enzymes also have cytochrome p450 prosthetic groups and may therefore also be inhibited.[73] However, drugs are being developed which have a differential affinity towards cytochrome p450s in different enzymes and selective inhibition of aromatase may be achieved.[73,74]

The first and most widely used aromatase inhibitor was the drug, aminoglutethimide.[75] This was initially used as treatment for advanced breast cancer without the realization that it had anti-aromatase properties. Thus, aminoglutethimide was originally used as a form of "medical adrenalectomy."[76,77] Doses were given at concentrations sufficient to inhibit cholesterol side-chain cleavage in the adrenal and, as a result, the secretion of adrenal-derived steroids were markedly reduced. Administration of replacement corticoid steroids was required and this also prevented the reflex rise in ACTH.[78] Subsequently, it was shown that aminoglutethimide-hydrocortisone regimes blocked peripheral conversion of androgens to estrogens in vivo and profoundly reduced circulating estrogens in postmenopausal women.[79] These effects seem to mediate the anti-tumor effects of aminoglutethimide in that doses of the drug which inhibit aromatase and are ineffective against cholesterol side-chain cleavage are still capable of producing remissions in patients with breast cancer.[80-82] The rate, duration and sites of response to aminoglutethimide-hydrocortisone treatment in postmenopausal women with advanced breast cancer are similar to those reported for other endocrine therapies.[71,83] Thus, objective responses can be expected in about one third of patients and a further 15% may benefit from disease stabilization (Table 8.4). Patients with a previous response to other

Table 8.4. Clinical response of breast cancer to aromatase inhibitor

Inhibitor	Complete & Partial Responses (%)	Progressive Disease (%)
Aminoglutethimide	30	45
4-Hydroxyandrostenedione	30	45
Atamestane	20	30
Fadrozole	20	45

Modified from Hoffman. Cancer Treat Rev 1993; 19 Suppl B:37-44.

hormone therapies are twice as likely to respond compared with those who have failed such a treatment.[84] The median duration of response to aminoglutethimide is about 14 months.[84,85] In general, soft tissue and lymph nodes respond better than visceral sites.[86] The presence of estrogen receptors in tumors also predicts response to aminoglutethimide, with estrogen receptor-negative tumors having a response rate less than 10% whereas estrogen receptor-positive tumors show a rate between 50-60%.[86-88] These latter observations would substantiate that the major effects of aminoglutethimide are mediated through estrogen deprivation. This also explains why the drug is less successful in premenopausal women in whom therapy does not effectively reduce circulating estrogen levels.[89] As a second line endocrine therapy, aminoglutethimide is capable of producing responses in up to one half of patients previously treated with either tamoxifen, adrenal-ectomy or hypophysectomy.[86] The latter may result from the ability of the drug to decrease circulating estrogens in both adrenalectomized and hypophysectomized patients.[68] The interrelationship between amino-glutethimide and tamoxifen is interesting. Thus, while aminoglutethimide is effective in about 30% of patients when given after tamoxifen, the antiestrogen less frequently causes remission when given after amino-glutethimide.[83,90] Furthermore, the combination of tamoxifen and aminoglutethimide is not substantially more effective than the two drugs given singly or sequentially.[91,92] The reasons for these interactions are not completely clear and, indeed, it is not known whether they are specific for aminoglutethimide and tamoxifen or more general for aromatase inhibitors and antiestrogens. However, in terms of amino-glutethimide and tamoxifen it is clear that the sequence of treatment should be tamoxifen before amino-glutethimide.

As an aromatase inhibitor, aminoglutethimide has several drawbacks in that it is not particularly potent, lacks specificity and has side effects not associated with its anti-aromatase properties and it requires concomitant administration of corticoids. As a consequence there has been an interest in developing other aromatase inhibitors which might avoid these disadvantages. In terms of other type II inhibitors, drugs have been developed which have selective affinity towards the cytochrome p450 in the aromatase enzyme.[74] This characteristic is exploited in the imidazole derivative of aminoglutethimide (CGS16949) which is about 1000-fold more potent as an aromatase inhibitor than aminoglutethimide[74] and, at concentrations which maximally inhibit aromatase, the drug has minimal effects on other cytochrome p450 containing enzymes.[75,93] CGS16949 may therefore be given without the need for corticoid replacement and preliminary results in postmenopausal women with advanced breast cancer show that it can effectively suppress circulating estrogens[94] and produce anti-tumor effects even in patients who have been heavily treated with other endocrine therapies.[95]

Among type I inhibitors the substrate analogue, 4-hydroxy-androstenedione, was specifically designed as an aromatase inhibitor.[96,97] It produces a time-dependent inactivation of the aromatase enzyme and is about 60-fold more potent than aminoglutethimide in inhibiting aromatase activity.[72,97] The drug has been used to treat advanced breast cancer in postmenopausal women and produces tumor remissions in about 33% of patients and disease stabilization in a further 15% (Table 8.4);[31,95,98] responses have also been observed in tumors which appear resistant to aminoglutethimide.[95] The drug also offers the advantage of comparatively low toxicity. Again there appears to be no requirement for corticoid replacement therapy.

The development of the second generation aromatase inhibitors has offered the promise of reduced toxicity and enhanced efficacy over traditional drugs. However, it would seem that even the more potent of these inhibitors, while having the potential to exert total inhibition of aromatase activity,[79] do not completely reduce circulating estrogen levels.[87] It is therefore of interest that third generation inhibitors such as vorazole and CGS20267 have even greater potency and seem to be able to reduce levels of circulating estrogen to values which are almost undetectable by current assay procedures.[100-104] Preliminary clinical results suggest that these drugs are able to induce tumor remissions in patients who are resistant to less powerful aromatase inhibitors.[95,101] It is also possible that these highly potent aromatase inhibitors may extend the use to premenopausal women. To date, aromatase inhibitors have not been effective in premenopausal women because, even when large doses have been given, the higher levels of aromatase in the ovary and the compensatory regulation produced by feedback loops have resulted in secondary increases in both androgen substrate and aromatase in the ovary (Fig. 8.10).[89,105]

Finally it is worth maintaining some additional perspective about the use of aromatase inhibitors. For example, while passage of time has seen the evolution of aromatase inhibitors move from agents whose properties coincidentally included suppression of estrogen biosynthesis

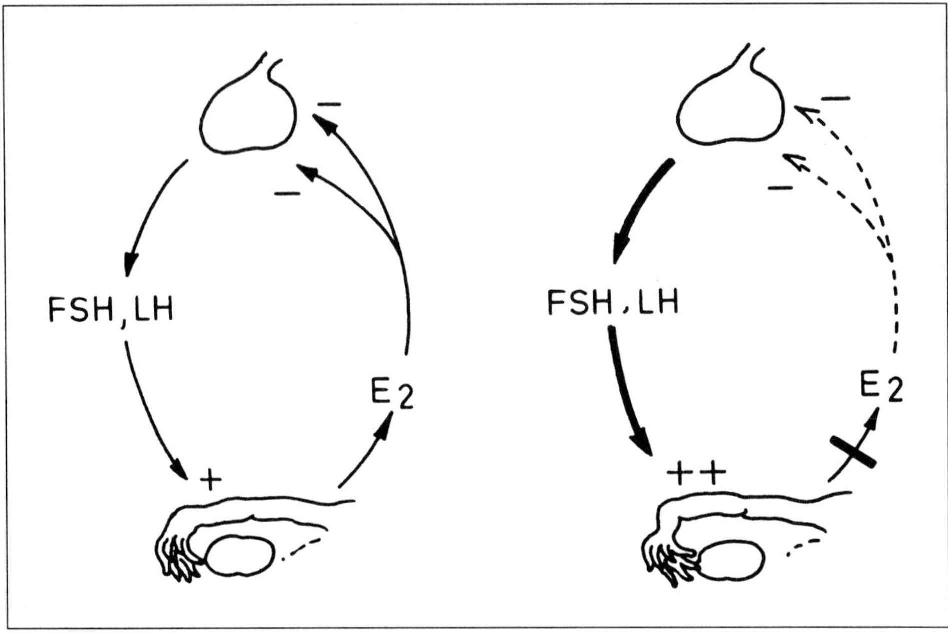

Fig. 8.10 Rationale for the inefficient effects of current aromatase inhibitors in premenopausal women.

to drugs purposely designed to inhibit the aromatase enzyme, it has to be asked if there is a good rational for developing even more potent inhibitors. This is because current aromatase inhibitors already inhibit peripheral estrogen biosynthesis almost completely. If endogenous estrogen production is totally suppressed, can exogenous sources of estrogens (such as those in the diet[106] and adrenal androgens with estrogenic activity[107]) still maintain hormone-dependent growth? These are sources which specific aromatase inhibitors will not directly affect. Theoretically, the use of antiestrogens which block the mechanism of action of estrogenic steroids irrespective of their structure and source would seem to have greater utility.

NOVEL METHODS OF ESTROGEN DEPRIVATION

By their nature, these methods are more speculative. For example, inhibition of the C17-20 lyase enzyme which is responsible for the conversion of progestogens to androgens would block the estrogen biosynthetic pathway at a higher point. This has advantages insofar as it would theoretically reduce both androgen and estrogen biosynthesis which has potential merits as certain androgens, particularly those produced by the adrenals, are capable of eliciting estrogenic responses.[107] Ketoconazole is such a drug but it needs to be given in high doses which also affect corticoid biosynthesis.[108] The evolution of more specific drugs would allow inhibition of sex steroids alone. Other inhibitors of steroid metabolism which may have potential include drugs which block the sulfatase activity involved in converting estrone sulfate into unconjugated steroids and thereby decrease estrogenic activity.[109] Such inhibitors are about to enter clinical practice but it seems likely that maximum benefits will be obtained by using the drugs in combination with aromatase inhibitors.

It is also possible that specific antiestrogen effects may be obtained by using antigenic or molecular biological approaches. Antibodies against estrogen and its receptor are available and have some therapeutic potential,[110] especially if these could be coupled to cytotoxic agents or radionucleotides.[111] There are however problems to overcome such as tumor targeting, permeability of cells to antibodies and potential uncoupling of antibodies at non-target sites. Antisense messenger-RNA against the estrogen receptor or estrogen-induced products may also potentially block estrogen action, especially as the latter may give growth advantage to and aid metastatic spread of tumors.[112] However more work needs to be performed in order to determine the physiological effects of such approaches, the doses required and an optimal mode of delivery of messenger-RNA into tissues. Additionally, since many of these factors induced by estrogen appear to be similar to those required by normal tissue, problems of specificity will probably need to be overcome if side effects, particularly in tissues containing dividing cells, are to be avoided.

FUTURE PERSPECTIVES

Recent years have seen major changes in the nature of endocrine deprivation therapy of breast cancer. Endocrine surgery, which was irreversible and held substantial risk of morbidity, has been largely superseded by drugs which either diminish the availability of estrogen or block its action within breast cancer. Because these agents are effective and specific, side-effects not associated with hormone deprivation have been greatly reduced. Novel drugs are also about to enter the clinic including pure antiestrogens, potent and specific aromatase inhibitors and long acting preparations of LHRH analogues. These agents offer the promise of non-toxic sustained estrogen deprivation which can be expected to simplify treatment and reduce the discomfort to patients. While these new drugs will first be administered to those with overt metastatic disease, a wider application can be considered if the characteristics of minimal side effects are realized. Most women present with cancer evidently confined to the breast. The natural history of the disease suggests that the majority already have occult distant metastasis and would benefit from systemic therapy. The advent of non-toxic hormone therapy will make such adjuvant treatment acceptable to women who can see no evidence of residual tumor following breast surgery. However, if survival rates are to be markedly improved with hormone therapy it will be necessary to kill more tumor cells while they are held in antiestrogen-induced quiescence and also prevent the emergence of clones of estrogen-resistant cells. Increased knowledge of molecular mechanisms underlying such events should help identify processes which are under the control of estrogens in endocrine-sensitive tumors and regulated by other factors in more autonomous cancers. The final perspective must be that the knowledge derived from treating patients with cancer may also be applied to earlier stages in the disease process such as the transformation of high-risk normal breast epithelium into cancer cells and the transition from non-invasive to invasive cancer.

REFERENCES

1. Schinzengier. In: Verh ditsch Ges Chir 1889; 18:28. Cited by Halberstaeder L & Hochman A. The artificial menopause and cancer of the breast. JAMA 1946; 131:810-816.
2. Beatson GT. On the treatment of inoperable cases of carcinoma of the mammary. Suggestions for a new method of treatment with illustrative cases. Lancet 1986; 2:104-107, 162-165.
3. Thomson A. Analysis of cases in which oophorectomy was performed for inoperable carcinoma of the breast. Br Med J 1902; 2:1538-1541.
4. West CD, Hollander VP, Whitmore WF et al. The effect of bilateral adrenalectomy upon neoplastic disease in man. Cancer 1952; 5:1109-1018.
5. Luft R, Olivercrona H, Sjorgen BJ. Hypophysektomie pa manniska. Nordisk Med 1952; 47:351-354.
6. Haddow A, Watkinson JM, Paterson E. Influence of synthetic oestrogens upon advanced malignant disease. Br Med J 1944; 2:393-398.
7. Dowsett M. Rationale for the endocrine treatment of breast cancer. In: Dowsett M, ed. Endocrine aspects of breast cancer. UK: The Parthenon Pub Group 1992:11-24.
8. Miller WR. Endocrine treatment for breast cancers: biological rationale and current progress. J Steroid Biochem Molec Biol 1990; 37:467-480.
9. Kennedy BJ. Hormonal therapies in breast cancer. Semin Oncol 1974; 5:119-130.
10. Nissen-Meyer R. Castration as part of the primary treatment for operable female breast cancer. Acta Radiologica. Supplementum 1984:249.
11. Vernonesi U, Pizzocaro G Rpsso A. Oophorectomy for advanced carcinoma of the breast. Surg Gynecol Obstet 1975; 141:569-570.
12. Baum M. Adjuvant systemic treatment of breast cancer. In: Dowsett M, ed. Endocrine aspects of breast cancer. UK: The Parthenon Pub Group 1992:25-36.
13. Early Breast Cancer Trialists' Collaborative Group. Systemic treatment of early breast cancer by hormonal, cytotoxic or immune therapy. Lancet 1992; 339:1-15.
14. Kelsey JL. A review of the epidemiology of human breast cancer. Epidemiol Rev 1979; 1:74-109.

15. Hawkins RA, Roberts MM. Oestrogen receptors and breast cancer: current status. Br J Surg 1980; 67:153-169.
16. Schmidt ML, Nemoto T, Dao T et al. Prognostic factors affecting adrenalectomy in patients with metastatic cancer of the breast. Cancer 1971; 27:1106-1111.
17. Moseley HS, Fletcher WS, Leung BS et al. Predictive criteria for the selection of breast cancer patients for adrenalectomy. Am J Surg 1974; 128:143-151.
18. Henderson IC, Canellos GP. Cancer of the breast—the past decade. New Eng J Med 1980; 302:17-30.
19. Lippman ME, Gellman EP. Endocrine management of malignant disease. In: DeGroot LJ. Endocrinology, Vol 3, Chapt 152. Philadelphia: WB Saunder & Co, 1995:2846-2869.
20. Harvey HA, Lipton A, Max DT et al. Medical castration produced by the GnRH analogue leuprolide to treat metastatic breast cancer. J Clin Oncol 1985; 3:1068-1072.
21. Schally AV, Arimura A, Kartin AJ et al. Gonadotropin releasing hormone: one polypeptide regulates secretion of luteinizing and follicle-stimulating hormones. Science 1971; 173:1036-1037.
22. Fraser HM, Baird DT, Clinical applications of LHRH analogues. In: Bailliere's Clin Endocrinol Metab 1987; 1:43-67.
23. Clayton RN. Gonadotrophin-releasing hormone: its actions and receptors. J Endocrinol 1989; 120:11-19.
24. Karten MJ, Rivier JE. Gonadotropin-releasing hormone analog design. Structure function studies toward the development of agonists and antagonists: rationale and perspective. Endocr Rev 1985; 7:44-66.
25. Nicholson RI, Walker KJ, Walker RF et al. Review of the endocrine actions of luteinizing hormone-releasing hormone analogues in premenopausal women with breast cancer. Horm Res 1989; 32 (Suppl 1):198-201.
26. Belchetz PE, Plant TM, Nakai Y et al. Hypophysial responses to continuous and intermittent delivery of hypothalamic gonadotropin releasing hormone. Science 1978; 202:631-633.
27. Clayton RN, Bailey LC, Cottam J et al. Radioimmunoassay for GnRH agonist analog in serum of patients with prostate cancer treated with D-ser(tBu)[6] AZA Gly[10]-GnRH. Clin Endocrinol 1985; 22:453-462.
28. Nicholson RI, Walker KJ, Turkes A et al. Therapeutic significance and mechanism of action of the LH-RH agonist ICI 118630 in breast and prostate cancer. J Steroid Biochem 1984; 20:129-135.
29. Kaufmann M, Jonat W, Kleebert U et al. Goserlin, a depot gonadotropin releasing hormone agonist in the treatment of premenopausal patients with metastatic breast cancer. J Clin Oncol 1989; 7:1113-1119.
30. Nicholson RI, Walker KJ. Use of LH-RH agonists in the treatment of breast disease. Proc Roy Soc Edin 1989; 95B:271-281.
31. Santen RJ, Manni A, Harvey H et al. Endocrine treatment of breast cancer in women. Endocr Rev 1990; 11:1-45.

32. Blamey RW, Dixon AR. LHRH analogues. In: Medical management of breast cancer. Eds TJ Powles, IE Smith. Dunitz, London 1991:109-114.
33. Lemay A. Clinical appreciation of LHRH analogue formulations. Horm Res 1989; 32 (Suppl 1):93-102.
34. Harris AL, Carmichael J, Cantwell BMJ et al. Zoladex: therapeutic effects in postmenopausal breast cancer. Horm Res 1989; 32 (Suppl 1):213-217.
35. Dowsett M, Cantwell B, Lal A et al. Suppression of postmenopausal ovarian steroidogenesis with the luteinizing hormone-releasing hormone agonist goserelin. J Clin Endocr Metab 1988; 66:672-677.
36. Miller WR, Scott WN, Morris R et al. Growth of human breast cancer cells inhibited by a luteinizing hormone-releasing hormone agonist. Nature 1985; 313:231-233.
37. Eidne LA, Flanagan CA, Millar RP. Gonadotropin-releasing hormone binding sites in human breast carcinoma. Science 1985; 229:989-991.
38. Asch RH, Balmaceda JP, Borghi M. LH-RH antagonists in rhesus and cynomologus monkeys. In: Vickery BH, Nestor JJ Jr, Hafesz ESE. LH-RH and its analogs. UK: MTP Press 1984:107.
39. Walker KJ, Turkes A, Robertson JFR et al. Endocrine effects of combination antioestrogen and LH-RH agonist therapy in premenopausal advanced breast cancer patients. Eur J Cancer Clin Oncol 1989; 25:651-654.
40. Jonat W. LHRH analogues in early breast cancer. Hormone Res 1989; 32 (Suppl 1):223-225.
41. Fentiman IS. Prevention of Breast Cancer. Austin: RG Landes Co 1993.
42. Pike MC, Ross RK, Lobo RA et al. LHRH agonists and the prevention of breast and ovarian cancer. Br J Cancer 1989; 60:142-148.
43. Muss HB. Endocrine therapy for advanced breast cancer: a review. Breast Cancer Res Treat 1992; 21:15-26.
44. Stoll BA. Palliation by castration or by hormone administration. In: Stoll BA, ed. Breast cancer—early and late. Chicago: Year Book, 1977:133-146.
45. Korsten CB, Englesman E, Persin JP. Clinical value of estrogen receptors in advanced breast cancer. In: McGuire WL, Carbone PP, Vollmer EP, eds. Estrogen receptors in human breast cancer. New York: Raven Press. 1975:93-105.
46. Carter AC, Sedransk N, Kelley RM et al. Diethylstilbestrol: recommended dosages for different categories of breast cancer patients. Report of the Cooperative Breast Cancer Group. JAMA 1977; 237:2079-2080.
47. Jordan VC, Murphy CS. Endocrine pharmacology of antiestrogens as antitumor agents. Endo Rev 1990; 11:49-81.
48. Cole MP, Jones CTA, Todd IDH. A new antioestrogenic agent in late breast cancer. Br J Cancer 1971; 25:270-275.
49. Jackson IM, Lowery C. Clinical uses of antioestrogens. In: Furr BJA, Wakeling AE. Pharmacology and clinical uses of inhibitors of hormone secretion and action. London: Bailliere Tindall 1987:87-105.
50. Thorpe SM, Rose C. Oestrogen and progesterone receptor determinations in breast cancer: technology and biology. Cancer Surveys 1986; 5:505-525.

51. Bradbeer JW, Kyngdon J. Primary treatment of breast cancer in elderly women with tamoxifen. Clin Oncol 1983; 9:31-34.

52. Jordan VC. Chemosuppression of breast cancer with long-term tamoxifen therapy. Prev Med 1991; 20:3-14.

53. Love RR, Mazess RB, Barden HS et al. Effects of tamoxifen therapy on lipid and lipoprotein levels in postmenopausal patients with node-negative breast cancer. J Natl Cancer Inst 1990; 82:1327-1332.

54. McDonald C, Stewart HJ. Fatal myocardial infarction in the Scottish adjuvant tamoxifen trial. BMJ. 1991; 303:435-7.

55. Jordan VC, Parker CJ, Morriw M. Update: breast cancer treatment and prevention with antiestrogens in the 1990s. Endo Rev 1993; 1:82-85.

56. Gottardis MM, Robinson SP, Jordan VC. Estradiol-stimulated growth of MCF-7 tumours implanted in athymic mice: a model to study the tumouristatic actions of tamoxifen. J Steroid Biochem 1988; 29:57-60.

57. Jordan VC. Optimisation of antioestrogen therapy: laboratory and clinical concepts. Proc Roy Acad Sci 1989; 95B:239-246.

58. Stewart HJ. Clinical experience in the use of the antioestrogen tamoxifen in the treatment of breast cancer. Proc Roy Soc Edin 1989; 95B:231-237.

59. Baum M, Fraser SCA, Colletta AA et al. Current controversies in the role of antioestrogens in the treatment of carcinoma of the breast. Proc Roy Soc Edin 1989; 95B:221-229.

60. Arteaga CL, Tandon AK, Von Hoff DD et al. Transforming growth factor β: potential autocrine growth inhibitor of estrogen receptor-negative human breast cancer cells. Cancer Res 1988; 48:3898-3904.

61. Wakeling AE, Bowler J. Novel antioestrogens. Proc Roy Soc Edin 1989; 95B:247-252.

62. De Friend DJ, Howell A, Nicholson RI et al. Investigations of a new pure antiestrogen (ICI-182780) in women with primary breast cancer. Cancer Res 1994; 54:408-414.

63. Sherman BM, Chapler FK, Crickard K et al. Endocrine consequences of continuous antiestrogen therapy with tamoxifen in premenopausal women. J Clin Invest 1979; 64:398-404.

64. Margreiter R, Wiegele J. Tamoxifen (Nolvadex) for premenopausal patients with advanced breast cancer. Breast Cancer Res Treat 1984; 4:45-48.

65. Sawka CA, Pritchard KI, Paterson AHG et al. Role and mechanism of action of tamoxifen in premenopausal women with metastatic breast carcinoma. Cancer Res 1986; 46:3152-3156.

66. Manni A, Santen RJ, Harvey HA. Endocrine treatment of breast cancer: Update 1993. Endo Rev 1993; 1:46-48.

67. Simmons DL, Lalley PA, Kasper CB. Chromosomal assignments of genes coding for components of the mixed function oxidase system in mice. J Biol Chem 1985; 260:515-521.

68. Samojlik E, Santen RJ, Worgul TJ. Suppression of residual oestrogen production with aminoglutethimide in women following surgical hypophysectomy or adrenalectomy. Clin Endocrinol 1984; 20:43-51.

69. Fishman J, Goto J. Mechanisms of oestrogen biosynthesis: participation of multiple enzyme sites in placental aromatase hydroxylations. J Biol Chem 1981; 256:4466-4471.

70. Thompson EA, Siiteri PK. Utilization of oxygen and reduced nicotinamide adenine dinucleotide phosphate by human placental microsomes during aromatization of androstenedione. J Biol Chem 1974; 249: 5364-5372.

71. Miller WR. Aromatase inhibitors in the treatment of advanced breast cancer. Cancer Treat Rev 1989; 16:83-93.

72. Johnston JO, Metcalf BW. Aromatase: a target enzyme in breast cancer. In: Sunkara PS, ed. Novel approaches to cancer chemotherapy. London: Academic Press 1984:307-328.

73. Santen RJ, Worgul TJ, Samojlik E et al. A randomised trial comparing surgical adrenalectomy with aminoglutethimide plus hydrocortisone in women with advanced breast cancer. N Eng J Med 1981; 305:545-551.

74. Steele RE, Mellor LB, Sawyer WK et al. In vitro and in vivo studies demonstrating potent and selective estrogen inhibition with the nonsteroidal aromatase inhibitor CGS16949A. Steroids 1987; 50:147-161.

75. Griffiths CT, Hall TC, Saba Z et al. Preliminary trial of aminoglutethimide in breast cancer. Cancer 1973; 32:31-37.

76. Lipton A, Santen RJ. Medical adrenalectomy using aminoglutethimide and dexamethasone in advanced breast cancer. Cancer 1974; 33:503-512.

77. Newsome HH, Brown PN, Terz JJ et al. Medical and surgical adrenalectomy in patients with advanced breast carcinoma. Cancer 1977; 39:542-546.

78. Santen RJ, Wells SA. The use of aminoglutethimide in the treatment of patients with metastatic carcinoma of the breast. Cancer 1980; 46:1066-1074.

79. Santen RJ, Santner S, Davis B et al. Aminoglutethimide inhibits extraglandular estrogen production in postmenopausal women with breast cancer. J Clin Endocrinol Metab 1978; 47:1257-1265.

80. Harris AL, Dowsett M, Cantwell BMJ et al. Endocrine effects of low dose aminoglutethimide with hydrocortisone—an optimal hormone suppressive regime. Breast Cancer Res Treat 1986; Suppl 7:68-72.

81. Harris AL, Cantwell BMJ, Sainsbury JR et al. Low dose aminoglutethimide (125 mg twice daily) with hydrocortisone for the treatment of advanced breast cancer. Breast Cancer Res Treat 1986; Suppl 7:41-44.

82. Stuart-Harris R, Dowsett M. Bozet T et al. Low dose aminoglutethimide in treatment of advanced breast cancer. Lancet 1984; 2:604-607.

83. Santen RJ, Samojlik E, Worgul TJ. Aminoglutethimide produce profile. In: Santen RJ, Henderson IC. Pharmanual: A comprehensive guide to the therapeutic use of aminoglutethimide. Basel: S Karger 1981:101-160.

84. Harris AL, Powles TJ, Smith IE et al. Aminoglutethimide for the treatment of advanced postmenopausal breast cancer. Eur J Cancer Clin Oncol 1983; 19:11-17.

85. Santen RJ, Worgul TJ, Harvey H et al. Aminoglutethimide as treatment of postmenopausal women with advanced breast cancer. Correlation of clinical and hormonal responses. Ann Intern Med 1982; 96:94-101.

86. Harris AL. Could aminoglutethimide replace adrenalectomy. Breast Cancer Res Treat 1985; 6:201-211.

87. Lawrence DV, Lipton A, Harvey HA et al. Influence of estrogen receptor status on response of metastatic breast cancer to aminoglutethimide. Cancer 1980; 45:786-791.

88. Santen RJ, Worgul TJ, Samojlik E et al. A randomised trial comparing surgical adrenalectomy with aminoglutethimide plus hydrocortisone in women with advanced breast cancer. N Eng J Med 1981; 305:545-551.

89. Harris AL, Dowsett M, Jeffcoate SL et al. Endocrine and therapeutic effects of aminoglutethimide in premenopausal patients with breast cancer. J Clin Endocrinol Metab 1982; 55:718-720.

90. Smith IE, Harris AL, Morgan M et al. Tamoxifen versus aminoglutethimide in the treatment of advanced breast carcinoma. A control randomised cross-over trial. Br Med J 1981; 283:1432-1434.

91. Smith IE, Harris AL, Morgan M et al. Tamoxifen versus aminoglutethimide versus combined tamoxifen and aminoglutethimide in the treatment of advanced breast carcinoma. Cancer Res 1982; Suppl 42:3430-3433.

92. Smith IE, Stuart-Harris R, Harris AL et al. Aminoglutethimide alone and in combination in the treatment of advanced breast cancer: clinical and endocrine aspects. In: Harvey HA, Lipton A, Michaels MA. Breast cancer: therapeutic modalities current and future. Canada: MES Medical Education Services, Mississauga 1984:145-149.

93. Bhatnager AS, Hausler A. Fortschritte in der Entwicklung neuer wirksamer und selektiver Aromatasehemmer. In: Possinger K, Miller WR, Zuchshverat W, eds. Aromatasehemmer Neue Perspektiven in der Behandlung des Mammakaranoms. Aktuelle Onkologie, 38. Verlag München 1987:23-28.

94. Santen RJ, Demers LM, Adlercreutz H et al. Inhibition of aromatase with CGS16949A in postmenopausal women. J Clin Endocrinol Metab 1989; 69:99-106.

95. Coombes RC, Stein RC, Dowsett M. Aromatase inhibitors in human breast cancer. Proc Roy Soc Edin 1989; 95B:283-291.

96. Brodie AMH, Schwarzel WC, Sheikh AA et al. The effect of an aromatase inhibitor, 4-hydroxyandrostenedione on estrogen-dependent processes in reproduction and breast cancer. Endocrinol 1977; 110:1684-1685.

97. Brodie AMH, Garnett WM, Henderson JR et al. Inactivation of aromatase in vitro by 4-hydroxyandrostenedione and 4-acetoxyandrostenedione and sustained effects in vitro. Steroids 1981; 38:693-702.

98. Hoffken K, Jonat W, Possinger K et al. Aromatase inhibition with 4-hydroxy-androstenedione in the treatment of postmenopausal patients with advanced breast cancer: a phase II study. J Clin Oncol 1990; 8:875-880.

99. Harris AL, Dowsett M, Jeffcoate SL et al. Endocrine and therapeutic effects of aminoglutethimide in premenopausal patients with breast cancer. J Clin Endocrinol Metab 1982; 55:718-720.

100. Demers LM, Lipton A, Harvey HA et al. The efficacy of CGS 20267 in suppressing estrogen biosynthesis in patients with advanced stage breast cancer. J Steroid Biochem 1993; 44:687-691.

101. Iveson TJ, Smith IE, Ahern J et al. Phase I study of the oral nonsteroidal aromatase inhibitor CGS 20267 in postmenopausal patients with advanced breast cancer. Cancer Res 1993; 53:166-270.

102. Plourde PV, Dyroff M, Dukes M. Arimedex (TM): a potent and selective fourth-generation aromatase inhibitor. Breast Cancer Res Treat 1994; 30:103-111.

103. Johnston SRD, Smith IE, Doody D et al. Clinical and endocrine effects of the oral aromatase inhibitor Vorozole in postmenopausal patients with advanced breast cancer. Cancer Res 1994; 54:5875-5881.

104. Goss PE, Gwyn KMEH. Current perspectives on aromatase inhibitors in breast cancer. J Clin Oncol 1994; 12:2460-2470.

105. Wander HE, Blossey H Ch, Nagel GA. Aminoglutethimide in the treatment of premenopausal patients with metastatic breast cancer. Eur J Cancer Clin Oncol 1986; 22:1371-1374.

106. Jordan VC. Antioestrogen action and breast cancer therapy. In: Santen RJ, Juhos E eds. Endocrine-dependent breast cancer: critical assessment of recent advances. Hans Hubert, Bern 1988:92-102.

107. Hackenberg R, Turgetto I, Filmer A et al. Estrogen and androgen receptor-mediated stimulation and inhibition of proliferation by androst-5-ene-3-beta, 17-beta-diol in human mammary cancer cells. J Steroid Biochem 1993; 46:597-603.

108. Harris AL, Cantwell BM, Dowsett M. High dose ketoconazole: endocrine and therapeutic effects in postmenopausal breast cancer. Br J Cancer 1988; 58:493-496.

109. Purohit A, Howarth NM, Potter BVL et al. Inhibition of steroid sulfatase activity by steroidal methylthiophosphonates—potential therapeutic agents in breast cancer. J Steroid Biochem 1994; 48:523-527.

110. Lorincz MA, Holt JA, Greene GL. Monoclonal antibody recognition of multiple forms of estrogen receptor tagged with [125] methoxy-iodovinyl estradiol in ovarian carcinomas. J Clin Endocrinol Metab 1985; 61:412-417.

111. Schlom J, Molinolo A, Simpson JF et al. Advantage of dose fractionation in monoclonal antibody-targeted radioimmunotherapy. JNCI 1990; 82:763-771.

112. Carter C, Lemoine NR. Antisense technology for cancer therapy: does it make sense? Br J Cancer 1993; 67:869-876.

CHAPTER 9

PREDICTION OF ESTROGEN SENSITIVITY/DEPENDENCE

Although estrogen deprivation therapies are generally better tolerated by patients than cytotoxic chemotherapy, estrogen dependence is a characteristic of only the minority of tumors. Indiscriminate application of estrogen deprivation therapy has therefore undesirable consequences in terms of the majority of patients being needlessly subjected to the morbidity associated with endocrine treatments and the implementation of potentially effective chemotherapy being delayed. This has stimulated the search for reliable predictive tests by which to select patients for endocrine treatment. The application of such assays represents a major route along which endocrine management of breast cancer has evolved. This chapter therefore considers the utility and practical application of assays by which to identify estrogen-sensitive tumors.

ESTROGEN RECEPTORS

As discussed in chapter 7, the initial step in estrogen action is the binding of the hormone to highly specific receptor proteins. The concept, therefore, developed that target organs for estrogens (including estrogen-sensitive breast cancer) possess receptors for estrogen whereas non-target organs (including estrogen-independent breast cancer) will be without such receptors. Based on this premise, Jensen[1] and Terrenius[2] independently demonstrated specific binding of radioactive estrogen to some human breast cancer specimens and correlated the presence of this binding to clinical responsiveness. Subsequently, numerous investigators have confirmed these pioneering investigations and assays for estrogen receptors have become routine. Between 60 and 75% of breast cancers possess receptors for estrogen in concentrations ranging up to 1000 fmol (10^{-15} mol) receptor sites per mg of cytosolic protein.[3-5] Within this range the distribution of tumors appears continuous with a progressive increase in proportion to lower values. The proportion of estrogen receptor-positive tumors may vary from study to study according to differences in method sensitivity and criteria used to define positivity. Subdivision according to presence or absence of receptors may be academic since physiological and clinical significance may depend on a critical level and it has become recent practice to subdivide tumors according to whether they are estrogen receptor-rich or -poor.[4,6] Receptor content may also be influenced by age, menopausal status of the patient, the histological grade of the tumor and source of tumor material;[5,7] additionally, but more controversially, the stage of the menstrual cycle[8] and the time of year[9] may also affect levels.

Tumors from premenopausal women are less frequently estrogen receptor-positive[7,10] and quantitatively contain lower concentrations of receptors.[3,7] This may be caused in part by occupation of receptor sites by the higher levels of circulating estrogens in premenopausal women,[5,11] but, equally, higher levels of circulating progesterone in the luteal phase of the cycle of premenopausal women may inhibit estrogen receptor synthesis.[12] Some support comes from this in that some but not all studies have found highest values of estrogen receptor in the early proliferative phase of the menstrual cycle and lower incidence of estrogen receptor-positive tumors during the secretory phase.[8]

Several studies have also concluded that estrogen receptor levels are related to age, particularly in elderly patients. Thus older women are more likely to be estrogen receptor-positive than younger women[13-15] and there is a steady rise in the proportion of estrogen receptor-positive tumors with advancing age.[15] It is possible that this reflects the appearance of more slow-growing cancers. Estrogen receptor status is more strongly correlated with age than menopausal status and is still significantly related to age after adjustment for menopausal status while the relationship between ER and menopausal status is no longer significant after adjusting for age.[10]

Several studies have also indicated that hormone receptor levels correlate with the histological grade of breast cancers.[16,17] Those tumors with a poor grade tend to be estrogen receptor-negative whereas highest receptor levels are found in more differentiated and more cellular tumors. A variety of different histological parameters, such as cellularity, elastosis, nuclear grade, and ultra-structural features have also been related to receptor status.[3,18,19]

Some evidence exists to suggest that with time the proportion of estrogen receptor-positive tumors in populations of patients with breast cancer is increasing. Thus, a recent study has reported that in the last two decades the median level of receptors has risen from 15 to 60 fmol per mg protein; in the same period the percentage of receptor-positive tumors rose from 73-78%.[20] Whether this is because of increased assay sensitivity and expertise in performing measurements, or is caused by a change in the inherent nature of tumors, is still to be resolved.

While lymph node metastasis may give substantially higher values than the primary tumor (perhaps because of increased tumor cellularity of lymph nodes),[3,21] differences in terms of qualitative presence or absence between primary and lymph nodes rarely occur.[22] Although some studies have found that receptor levels tend to be lower in metastatic disease as compared with primary tumors,[23] there is again a general concordance between receptor status performed in primary tumors and metastases taken at the same time.[24] This is of practical importance if one is to use assays in primary tumors (which are more accessible to biopsy) to predict the response of metastatic deposits to endocrine therapy. The incidence of detectable receptor activity is similar in most metastatic sites except for liver and adrenal gland which show a higher percentage of receptor-positive tissues (> 80%).[25]

RELATIONSHIP BETWEEN ESTROGEN RECEPTORS AND RESPONSE TO ENDOCRINE THERAPY OF ADVANCED BREAST CANCER

If 60-75% of breast cancers possess estrogen receptors, and yet only one third of tumors respond to estrogen deprivation therapy, it is clear that there cannot be an absolute correlation between estrogen receptor status and clinical response. However, considerable research has been invested in determining the role of estrogen receptors as a predictive indices of estrogen sensitivity. These results have been summarized in several overviews[3,5,25] and a typical cross-section is shown in Table 9.1. Overall, estrogen receptor-positive tumors are associated with a 50-60% objective response rate to ablative therapies whether ovariectomy in premenopausal women or adrenalectomy/hypophysectomy in postmenopausal patients. In contrast, less than 10% of estrogen receptor-negative tumors are associated with objective response rates to these ablative therapies. Estrogen additive therapy also produces similar

---

Table 9.1. Estrogen receptors and response to endocrine therapy

	ER-positive		ER-negative	
	% response	(No. responses/total)	% response	(No. responses/total)
Ovariectomy	58%	(53/91)	5%	(7/134)
Tamoxifen	49%	(150/306)	9%	(11/116)
Medroxyprogesterone-Acetate	56%	(31/55)	16%	(7/42)
Total	52%	(234/452)	9%	(25/292)

Derived from:
(i) Hawkins RA, Roberts MM, Forrest APM. Oestrogen receptors and breast cancer: current status. Br J Surg 1980; 67:153-169.
(ii) Paterson JS, Battersby LA, Edwards DG. In: Iacobelli S, Lippman ME et al. The Role of Tamoxifen in Breast Cancer. New York: Raven Press, 17.
(iii) C Bumma. In: Nagel GA, Robustellin Della Cuna G, Lanius P, eds. Medroxyprogesterone-Acetate in the therapy of hormone dependent tumors. 1983:93.

results, estrogen receptor-positive tumors experiencing a 60% response rate compared with less than 10% for estrogen receptor-negative tumors. Similarly, as has already been discussed in Chapter 8, drug induced estrogen deprivation whether by antiestrogens or aromatase inhibitors or LHRH agonists produce 50-60% response rates in estrogen receptor-positive tumors but beneficial effects in a only a small minority of estrogen receptor-negative tumors. If there is an exception to these general effects, it is in the response of tamoxifen in estrogen receptor-negative tumors, since several studies have shown response rates up to 27% in this cohort of patients.[26,27] The possibility is, however, that certain of these responses may be achieved by mechanisms other than through estrogen receptor. In general, therefore, about 50-70% of tumors that are estrogen receptor-positive can be expected to respond objectively to estrogen deprivation therapy whereas only about 5-10% of receptor-negative tumors will respond. Overall response to endocrine therapy can thus be predicted with an accuracy of about 75%.[28] While this is an improvement over random allocation of patients the issues of why some receptor-negative patients respond and a substantial proportion of receptor-positive patients fails to respond still need to be resolved (Table 9.2). One explanation for so-called false negative results is based on methodology. Estrogen receptors are thermo-labile proteins and sub-optimal sample storage and assay conditions may destroy binding activity leading to false negative results. Secondly, it is possible that the sample taken for analysis may inadvertently not contain tumor cells—the histological presence of tumor in material for analysis should be checked. It is also possible that a proportion of cells when resting or dormant displays an estrogen receptor-negative phenotype but when given an appropriate stimulus to enter the cell cycle will express levels of hormone receptors. Tumors composed of these resting cells might regress if exposed to reduced levels of estrogen. Estrogen receptor measurements would not distinguish between true endocrine autonomy and cellular dormancy in these tumors. Finally, the excised material may be truly estrogen receptor-negative and unresponsive, whereas other tumor deposits which will respond to endocrine therapy are estrogen receptor-positive. Positive results in non-responding tumors are common, occurring in about half

Table 9.2. Reason for estrogen receptors not correlating with endocrine response

Non-response of ER+ve tumours	Response of ER-ve tumors
1. Mixture of ER+ve and ER-ve cells in tumor	1. Methodological failure
2. Inefficient endocrine therapy	2. Tissue sample contains no tumor
3. ER variant and mutation	3. Dormant ER+ve cells display ER-ve phenotype
4. Defective processing distal to receptor	4. ER heterogeneity between tissue sample and disease being assessed

the cases. The most frequently invoked explanation for this is tumor heterogeneity—a sample may contain a sufficient number of tumor cells with estrogen receptors to provide a positive assay result but yet still represent only a minority of the total tumor cell population. As a result, following deprivation therapy only the proliferation of the subset of estrogen receptor-positive cells is affected—these may regress but are outgrown by estrogen receptor-negative cells. If this hypothesis is true, a quantitative relationship between receptor concentration and response rate might be expected. Certain studies support this with response rates of 75-85% in tumors containing the highest concentrations of estrogen receptors.[28] Furthermore, histochemical methods show that tumors are generally heterogeneous with regard to estrogen receptors[29,30] although this heterogeneity and receptor level do not appear generally to change with therapy.[31] This will be discussed later with regard to endocrine resistance. Certain endocrine therapies may also not be efficient at estrogen deprivation and as a result estrogen receptor-positive tumors can continue to grow. More effective therapy might be expected to produce responses and this might account for the 10-15% of patients who fail initial therapy yet respond to subsequent endocrine therapy.[28] It has also been suggested that clinical responsiveness to hormone therapy is related to the molecular species of estrogen receptors[32,33] and that those with the higher molecular form (8S) of receptors are more likely to show response and smaller molecular forms of receptor are not predictive. Other variants of estrogen receptor also exist which exhibit altered function, including changed responsiveness to hormone therapy—their differential measurement may yet prove to be a better predictor of tumor response. Finally, some receptor-containing tumors fail to respond to endocrine manipulation because some step distal to the initial binding of hormone to receptor is deranged. If this is the case it may be more logical to examine tumors for estrogen responsiveness rather than hormone binding. As will be discussed later these approaches are offering promise but at the moment estrogen receptor status represents the single best predictor by which to discriminate between estrogen-dependent and -independent tumors.

ESTROGEN RECEPTORS AND PROGNOSIS IN PATIENTS WITH EARLY BREAST CANCER

It is now established that patients with estrogen receptor-positive tumors have a better prognosis than those with estrogen receptor-negative cancers.[5,7,10,34] Given that many patients are offered some form of estrogen deprivation therapy as adjuvant treatment, the benefits associated with estrogen receptor-positive tumors may be related to increased likelihood of response to adjuvant treatment. There is evidence to support this. An informative study was performed by Howell et al[35] in which patients with "early breast cancer" were classified according to response to endocrine therapy given to treat recurrent disease. These results showed that those with estrogen receptor-positive tumors which did not respond to endocrine therapy had a similar survival to those who had estrogen receptor-negative tumors. This suggests that survival benefit in patients with estrogen receptor-positive tumors is achieved through increased likelihood of response to endocrine therapy. However, as a group, estrogen receptor-positive tumors may also display inherently better behavior. In patients never offered adjuvant endocrine therapy estrogen receptor-negative tumors are more likely to be associated with rapid recurrence than estrogen receptor-positive tumors;[36] conversely, survival benefits are associated with estrogen receptor-positive tumors although in many studies the early survival advantage is not maintained over long observation times.[7,34] The effect does not seem to be associated with lymph node involvement (which does not relate to estrogen receptor status) but, as indicated earlier, tumors with low grade differentiation are more likely to be estrogen receptor-positive and these have an inherently benign behavior. Since metastatic spread also differs between estrogen receptor-positive and -negative tumors (patients with estrogen receptor-positive tumors are more likely to metastasize to bone rather than other sites), site of metastatic spread might also be involved.[37] However, irrespective of the mechanism by which these benefits are achieved, it seems logical to determine the likelihood of early recurrence (and need for adjuvant therapy) and to select those proceeding to endocrine therapy according to tumor estrogen receptor status.

There is therefore a need for a robust reproducible routine assay for estrogen receptors—with the advent of monoclonal antibodies for the estrogen receptor this has been achieved. Assays may be performed either on tumor cytosols to determine the quantitative level of estrogen receptors (ELISA) or in histological sections (ERICA) to determine the distribution of receptors. There are advantages and disadvantages to these two approaches. The ELISA assays provide an absolute number but give no indication of the source or heterogeneity of estrogen receptor-positive cells within a tumor. Conversely, the immunochemical assay is only semi-quantitative but it can indicate the heterogeneity of estrogen receptor positivity across a tumor. Furthermore, the advent of immunochemical staining has allowed the application of estrogen receptor assays to small samples, including fine needle aspirates and holds the expectation of being able to estimate estrogen receptor levels co-incidentally in the same samples being used for histological confirmation of the presence of cancer. Several studies have confirmed the feasibility of this approach, indicating a strong correlation between biochemical and immunological assays for the estrogen receptor.[38,39] Furthermore, there is an excellent correlation between response to endocrine therapy of primary tumors and the estrogen receptor status of the tumor as determined immunohistochemically on fine needle aspirates of the tumor (Fig. 9.1).[40,41] Interestingly the predictor with most clinical utility is the

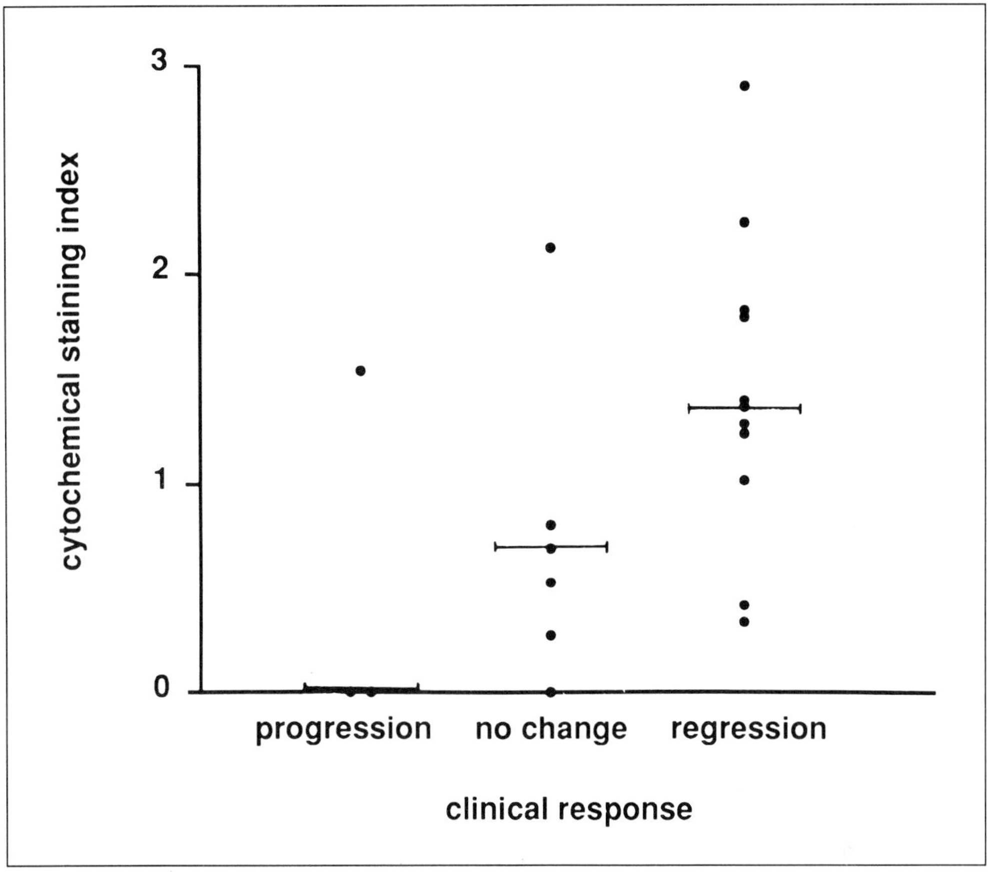

Fig. 9.1. Relationship between estrogen receptor status as determined on tumor fine needle aspirates and response to endocrine therapy.

proportion of cells taking up the stain rather than the intensity of stain within individual cells.[40] Thus, the proportion of estrogen receptor-positive and -negative cells within ERICA assays relates to hormone sensitivity and patients with tumors in which ERICA staining is not observed in any tumor cell show very few remissions following endocrine therapy.[41,42] The group of tumors which contain approximately equal proportions of estrogen receptor-positive and -negative cells shows an intermediate response rate whereas highly ERICA positive tumors are associated with a high degree of hormone sensitivity. These data support the notion that the proportion of tumor cells which are estrogen receptor-positive contribute to the endocrine sensitivity.

The knowledge that tumor estrogen receptor status relates both to prognosis and likelihood of response to endocrine therapy is now influencing management decisions for therapy—treatment of breast cancer is becoming rational rather than empirical.

PROGESTERONE RECEPTORS

Because the synthesis of progesterone receptors in target tissues depends upon the action of estrogens and requires intact estrogen receptor machinery,[43] it has been proposed that progesterone receptors may be a marker of estrogen action. This hypothesis is supported by the observation that the progesterone receptor is absent in almost all estrogen receptor-negative tumors but is present in about one half of the estrogen receptor-positive tumors;[44] a proportion close to response rates in patients having estrogen receptor-positive tumors. Accumulative experience confirms the importance of progesterone receptor in predicting response to hormone therapy (Table 9.3). Thus, the highest response rate (71%) is seen in patients whose tumors contain both estrogen receptors and progesterone receptors compared with only 9% women with tumors lacking both receptors.[5,44,45] If the hypothesis of the progesterone receptor indicating an intact estrogen receptor pathway is strictly true, no responses should be seen in estrogen receptor-positive progesterone receptor-negative tumors. Practical experience suggests that while estrogen receptor-positive progesterone receptor-negative tumors are much less likely to respond than those with both receptors, a substantial proportion appear to derive benefit from estrogen deprivation therapy.[15,44,45] There are several possible explanations— (i) in postmenopausal women progesterone receptors may be absent because of inadequate endogenous estrogen stimulation to cause the expression of progesterone receptors, despite a functional estrogen response mechanism, (ii) in premenopausal women high endogenous progesterone levels in the luteal phase may mask progesterone receptors and (iii) it is conceivable that the estrogen dependent properties of growth and progesterone receptor expression might be uncoupled in some tumors. Interestingly, the small sub-group of estrogen receptor-negative but progesterone receptor-positive tumors (2% of patients) consistently show about a 53% response rate[44-47] suggesting the possibility of false negative-estrogen receptor determination. The enigma surrounding responses in estrogen receptor-negative progesterone receptor-positive tumors has been the subject of molecular analysis. These studies suggest that estrogen receptor molecules defective in their steroid binding domain may exist.[48] This may result in constitutively active

---

Table 9.3. Estrogen receptor-progesterone receptor and response to endocrine therapy

Total patients	ER-positive		ER-negative	
	% response	(No. responses/total)	% response	(No. responses/total)
638	55	(249/452)	13	(241/186)
	ER+/PR+	**ER+/PR-**	**ER-/PR+**	**ER-/PR-**
	71% (188/263)	32% (61/189)	53% (8/15)	9% (16/171)

receptors which do not bind estrogen but nevertheless are capable of producing the progesterone receptor. One such receptor lacks exon 5 of the hormone-binding domain and interestingly is the predominant estrogen receptor RNA in estrogen receptor-negative progesterone receptor-positive tumors.[49] However it is not clear why, if the estrogen does not bind to these receptors, estrogen deprivation therapy should be successful.

Although highest response rates are found in tumors containing both estrogen and progesterone receptors, the substantial therapy failures in this group and the responses to endocrine therapy in estrogen receptor-positive progesterone receptor-negative groups limit the clinical utility of the progesterone receptor. Additionally the phenotypic expression of the progesterone receptor appears more variable than the estrogen receptor. For example, the rate of discordance in progesterone receptor status between primary metastatic deposits is 30-40% compared with 20-25% in equivalent samples for estrogen receptor.[6,50] Furthermore, in one study 44% of all initial progesterone receptor-positive tumors showed negative values on a second later biopsy,[51] and 56% of tumors which were progesterone receptor-positive prior to endocrine therapy, were subsequently progesterone receptor-negative. (This contrasts with only 9% of initially progesterone receptor -negative patients converting to progesterone receptor-positive status on re-biopsy.) Loss of progesterone receptor, however, parallels reduced response to hormone therapy—no more than 50% of patients who respond to initial endocrine treatment do so to a second hormonal manipulation after relapse.[52] Patients who are initially progesterone receptor-positive but later become progesterone receptor-negative have a worse prognosis than those who retain progesterone receptor-positive status.[51] Furthermore, as progesterone receptors are more frequently found in primary tumors compared with metastatic deposits (unlike estrogen receptors) it may be that progesterone receptors are lost during the metastatic process.[56] This may confound a prediction of hormone sensitivity of metastatic disease if measurements are being made on the primary lesion. Studies of cell lines also have produced data which suggests that progesterone receptor heterogeneity may be associated with a mixed and potentially unsustained response to antiestrogen treatment.[53] Given these variations in progesterone receptors and, the positive quantitative correlation between concentrations of estrogen receptor and presence of progesterone receptors, quantitative assays for the former may provide as much predictive accuracy for endocrine sensitivity as determination of presence of the latter.

However, findings in earlier stage disease suggest that the presence of estrogen receptor and progesterone receptor may correlate with different biological characteristics.[54-56] In patients who have not yet developed clinical evidence of malignant spread, i.e., stage I breast cancer, the ability to metastasize is reflected more by factors such as histology, high proliferative rate and lack of estrogen receptor. In those patients whose tumors have already shown evidence of malignant spread to axillary nodes, progesterone receptor expression may assume a more important role in determining the subsequent prognosis. Progesterone receptor status has also been shown in several studies to be an important factor in predicting the benefits of adjuvant tamoxifen treatment.[57]

pS2

pS2 (or pNR-2) is a 6.45 kD peptide which has strong homology with spasmolysins and pancreatic spasmolytic polypeptides.[58] Although similar molecules are expressed in normal stomach mucosa and inflammatory diseases of the digestive tract,[59-61] pS2 was first identified by virtue of being induced by estrogen in the breast cancer cell line, MCF-7, in which its synthesis is controlled at the transcriptional level by estrogens.[62] An association of pS2 mRNA with the expression of estrogen receptors in human breast cancers has been shown;[63] transcripts for pS2 found in 50% of breast tumors but largely restricted to estrogen receptor-positive tumors are present in about 40-50% compared with about 10% of estrogen receptor-negative tumors. The development of monoclonal antibodies against pS2 proteins means that immunocytochemical assays for use on histological sections and radioimmunometric assays for use on tumor cytosols are now available.[64-68] While results from such studies have shown considerable variation in terms of both the proportion of cells staining within histological sections and the incidence of pS2-positive tumors, most (but not all) have confirmed an association with estrogen receptor-positive tumors.

Several studies have suggested that pS2 mRNA transcripts were useful in predicting the outcome of endocrine therapy.[69-72] While the consensus is that little additional information is gained over using measurements of estrogen receptor or progesterone receptor status, pS2 expression may define a subset of estrogen receptor-positive tumors which on relapse are more likely to respond to tamoxifen.[68]

Certain reports have suggested that expression of the protein is associated with improved survival.[64,69,73-75] Indeed, in patients offered adjuvant hormone therapy, pS2 may have independent prognostic power[69,75] even beyond that of hormone receptor status.[69] However, for the overall population of breast cancers, most studies have not been able to demonstrate that pS2 adds to already established prognostic parameters such as tumor size, histological grade, hormone receptors and lymph node involvement.

ESTROGEN INDUCIBLE GENES

The approach of screening molecular libraries from estrogen responsive and resistant breast cancers or cell lines derived from such tumors before and after culture with estrogen for genes whose expression is differentially transcribed has been used to discover other directive markers[63,76] (see Fig. 9.2 for a diagrammatic representation of the strategy). For example, pLIVI is expressed in some, but not all, estrogen receptor-positive breast cancers in which it is regulated by estrogen. Interestingly the gene appears to be particularly associated with tumors metastasizing to lymph nodes.[77] In contrast pMGT1 is suppressed by estrogens and induced by antiestrogens.[78] The value of these markers in selecting patients for endocrine-based therapies and monitoring anti-tumor activities of antiestrogen therapy is still yet to be fully evaluated.

HSP27 (HEAT SHOCK PROTEIN 27,000)

HSP27 is an important small molecular weight heat shock protein which is found in both cancer and normal cells.[79] In addition to having a putative role in thermo-tolerance the protein may be influential in drug and endocrine resistance.[79] HSP27 is particularly found in cell types such as the breast, uterus, cervix, placenta, skin and platelets.[80]

In breast cancer, concentrations of HSP27 are qualitatively and quantitatively linked to the estrogen receptor.[81,82] HSP27 was initially identified in human breast cancer cell lines as an estrogen responsive protein[83] and subsequent work in other breast cancer cell lines have

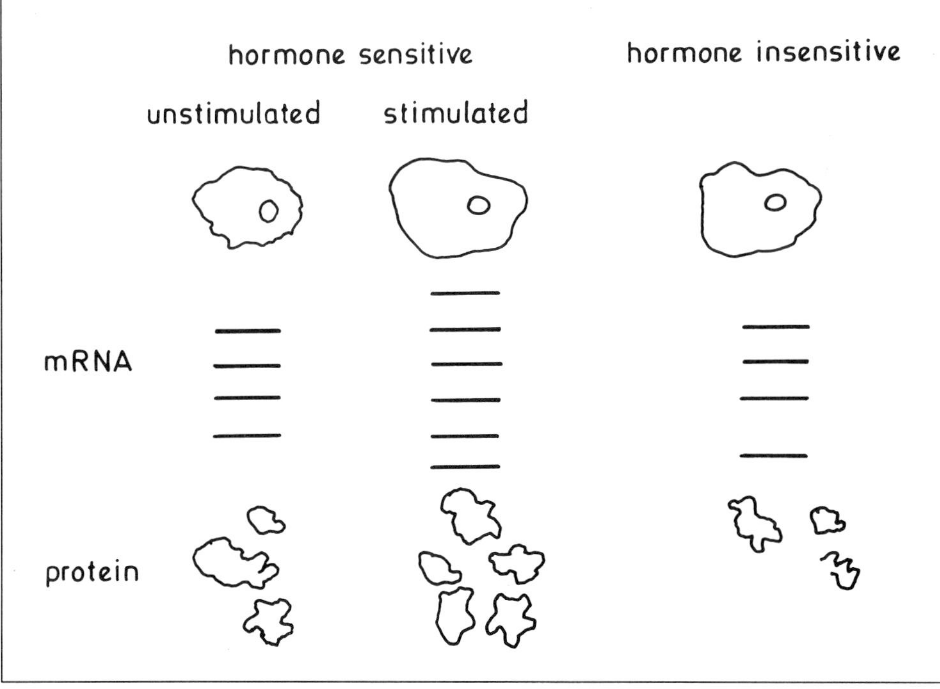

Fig. 9.2. Screening mRNA and protein for species induced by estrogen or expressed in estrogen-dependent tumor cells rather than estrogen-independent cells.

confirmed its presence as a marker of estrogen activity.[84,85] Although HSP may be a marker for estrogen stimulation, it only correlates weakly with progesterone receptors.[86] The utility of HSP27 as a predictor of response to hormone treatment in patients with breast cancer is still controversial. While it cannot be considered as a major determinant of hormone dependence, tumors co-expressing HSP27 and estrogen receptors have been reported to have an increased likelihood of clinical response to hormone therapy as compared with patients expressing estrogen receptors alone.[81,87]

Certain studies have also found that HSP27 overexpression in breast carcinomas is associated with more aggressive behavior[88-90] In contrast, other investigators have reported that HSP27-positive tumors were associated with a better outcome, having a higher rate of response to chemotherapy and relatively prolonged survival.[91]

TYPE I TYROSINE KINASE RECEPTORS

Epidermal growth factor receptor and the proto-oncogene, c-*erb*B-2, show substantial homology in that they are transmembrane receptors which have the function to phosphorylate tyrosine on their internal domains.[92] Interestingly, they are overexpressed in a proportion of breast cancers, these invariably being estrogen receptor-negative or -poor.[93,94] An inverse relationship between estrogen receptors and type 1 tyrosine kinase receptors has also been confirmed at a cellular level.[95] Tumor overexpression of both epidermal growth factor receptor and c-*erb*B-2 appears to be associated with aggressive phenotypes which lead to poor prognosis and resistance to treatment.[93,95,96] In the context of this particular chapter, it is relevant that the EGF receptor-positive tumors may be associated with lack of response to hormone therapy.[97] Similarly, although more controversially, several studies have reported that c-*erb*B-2 positive tumors have a poorer response to endocrine therapy than those which are c-*erb*B-2 negative.[98,99]

SUMMARY

The attraction of estrogen deprivation therapy for patients with breast cancer is founded upon relative lack of side effects and toxicity in comparison with chemotherapy. However, endocrine therapy is effective in only the minority of cases and if potentially beneficial chemotherapy is not to be unnecessarily delayed it is important to be able to predict likelihood of response to endocrine therapy before starting treatment. At this time there is no tumor marker which correlates absolute with endocrine dependence but it is clear that estrogen receptor-negative tumors rarely respond to estrogen deprivation therapy. Tumor estrogen receptor status should therefore be taken into account, especially when stratifying patients for trials of endocrine therapy. The value of other marker are less proven and more controversial. A case has been made for the progesterone receptor in that tumors which possess both progesterone receptors and estrogen receptors are more likely to respond to endocrine treatment than those with estrogen receptors alone but benefits are also seen in a substantial number of the latter tumors. However, molecular technology can be expected to uncover more genes whose products are likely to predict more accurately for hormone dependence. This should allow the realization of a totally rational approach to the use of estrogen deprivation in the management of patients with breast cancer.

REFERENCES

1. Jensen EV DeSombre ER, Jungblut PW. Estrogen raceptors in hormone-responsive tissue and tumors. In: Wissler RW, Dao TL, Wood S Jr., eds. Endogenous factors influencing host-tumor balance. Chicago: University of Chicago Press 1967:15-30.
2. Terenius L. Selective retention of estrogen isomers in estrogen-dependent breast tumors of rats demonstrated by in vitro methods. Cancer Res 1968; 28:328-337.
3. Hawkins RA, Roberts MM, Forrest APM. Oestrogen receptors and breast cancer: current status. Br J Surg 1980; 67:153-169.
4. Leclerq G, Heuson JC, Deboel MC et al. Estrogen and progesterone receptors in human breast cancer. In: McGuire WL et al. Progesterone receptors in normal and neoplastic tissues. New York: Raven Press 1977:141-153.
5. Jordan VC, Wolf MF, Mirecki DM et al. Hormone receptor assays: clinical usefulness in the management of carcinoma of the breast. CRC Crt Rev Clin Lab Sciences 1988; 26:97-151.
6. Merkel DE, Osborne CK. Steroid receptors in relation to response. In: Stoll BA, ed. Endocrine management of cancer; 1. Biological Bases. Basel: Karger 1988:84-99.
7. Thorpe SM, Rose C. Oestrogen and progesterone receptor determinations in breast cancer: technology and biology. Cancer Surveys 1986; 5:505-525.
8. Heise E, Garlich M. Estradiol receptor in human breast cancers throughout the menstrual cycle. Oncology 1982; 39:340-344.
9. Mason BH, Holdaway IM, Stewart AW et al. Season of initial discovery of tumour is an independent variable predicting survival in breast cancer. Br J Cancer 1990; 61:137-141.
10. Clark GM, McGuire WL. The clinical usefulness of oestrogen-receptor and other markers of hormone dependence. Proc Roy Soc Edin 1989; 95B:145-150.
11. Sakai F, Saez S. Existence of receptors bound to endogenous estradiol in breast cancer of premenopausal and postmenopausal women. Steroids 1976; 27:99-110.
12. Saez S, Martin PM, Chouvet CD. Estradiol and progesterone receptor levels in human breast adenocarcinoma in relation to plasma estrogen and progesterone levels. Cancer Res 1978; 38:3468-3473.

13. Elwood JM, Godolphin W. Oestrogen receptors in breast tumors: associations with age, menopausal status and epidemiological and clinical features in 735 patients. Br J Cancer 1980; 42:635-644.

14. McCarty KS Jr, Silva JS, Cox EB. Relationship of age and menopausal status to estrogen receptor content in primary carcinoma of the breast. Ann Surg 1983; 197:123-127.

15. Clark GM, Osborne CK, McGuire WL. Correlations between estrogen receptor, progesterone receptor, and patient characteristics in human breast cancer. J Clin Oncol 1984; 2:1102-1109.

16. Maynard PV, Davis CJ, Blamey RW et al. Relationship between oestrogen-receptor content and histological grade in human primary breast tumors. Br J Cancer 1978; 38:745-748.

17. McCarty KS Jr, Barton TK, Fetter BF et al. Correlation of estrogen and progesterone receptors with histological differentiation of mammary carcinoma. Cancer 1980; 46:2851-2858.

18. Masters JRW, Hawkins RA, Sangster K et al. Oestrogen receptors, cellularity, elastosis and menstrual status in human breast cancer. Eur J Cancer 1978; 14:303-307.

19. Fisher ER, Sass R, Fisher B. Pathological findings from the National Surgical Adjuvant Breast Project. Cancer 1987; 59:1554-1559.

20. Pujol P, Hilsenbeck SG, Chamness GC et al. Rising levels of estrogen-receptor in breast cancer over 2 decades. Cancer 1994; 74:1601-1606.

21. Hawkins RA, Roberts MM, Freedman B et al. Oestrogen receptors in human breast cancer: the Edinburgh experience. In: King RJB, ed. Steroid receptor assays in human breast tumours: methodological and clinical aspects. Cardiff: Alpha Omega Alpha 1979.

22. LeClercq G, Heuson J, Deboel M et al. Oestrogen receptors in breast cancer: a changing concept. Br Med J 1975; 1:185-189.

23. DeSombre ER, Jensen EV. Estrophilin assays in breast cancer: quantitative features and application to the mastectomy specimen. Cancer 1980; 46:2783-2788.

24. Brennan MJ, Donegan WL, Appleby DE. The variability of estrogen receptors in metastatic breast cancer. Am J Surg 1979; 137:260-262.

25. McGuire WL, Carbone PP, Sears ME et al. Estrogen receptors in human breast cancer: an overview. In: McGuire WL, Carbone PP, Vollmer EP. Estrogen receptors in human breast cancer. New York: Raven Press 1975:1.

26. Maas H, Trams G, Engel B. Clinical significance of receptor determinations in breast cancer patients. In: Vermeulen A, Jungblut P, Klopper A et al, eds. Research in steroids VII. Amsterdam: Elsevier North Holland 1977:387-391.

27. Barnes DM, Ribeiro CG, Skinner LG. Simultaneous estimation of oestrogen and progestin receptor activity in human breast tumours and correlation with response to treatment. In: King RJB, ed. Steroid receptor assays in human breast tumours: methodological and clinical aspects. Cardiff: Alpha Omega Alpha 1979.

28. Lippman ME, Allegra JC. Current concepts in cancer: estrogen receptor and endocrine therapy of breast cancer. New Eng J Med 1978; 299:930-933.

29. Nenci I. Receptor and centriole pathways of steroid action in normal and neoplastic cells. Cancer Res 1978; 38:4204-4211.

30. Mercer WD, Carlson CA, Wahl TM et al. Identification of estrogen receptors in human breast cancer cells by immunofluorescence. Am J Clin Pathol 1978; 70:330.

31. Hawkins RA, Tesdale AL, Anderson EDC et al. Does the oestrogen receptor concentration of a breast cancer change during systemic therapy? 1990; 61:877-880.

32. Kute TE, Heidemann P, Wittliff JL. Molecular heterogeneity of cytosolic forms of estrogen receptors from human breast tumors. Cancer Res 1978; 38:4307-4313.

33. Jozan S, Julia AM, Carretie A et al. 65 and 47kDa forms of estrogen receptor in human breast cancer: relation with estrogen responsiveness. Breast Cancer Res Treat 1991; 19:103-109.

34. McGuire WL. Prognostic factors in primary breast cancer. Cancer Surveys 1986; 5:527-536.

35. Howell A, Barnes DM, Harland RN et al. Steroid-hormone receptors and survival after first relapse in breast cancer. Lancet 1984; 1:588-591.

36. Crowe JP, Hubay CA, Pearson OH et al. Estrogen receptor status as a prognostic indicator for stage I breast cancer patients. Breast Cancer Res Treat 1982; 2:171-176.

37. Koenders PG, Beex LVAM, Langens R et al. Steroid hormone receptor activity of primary human breast cancer and pattern of first metastasis. Breast Cancer Res Treat 1991; 18:27-32.

38. Ryde CM, Smith D, King N et al. Comparison of 4-immunochemical methods for the measurement of estrogen-receptor levels in breast cancer. Cytopathol 1992; 3:155-160.

39. Marazzo A, Russo A, Bazan V et al. Immunocytochemical determination of estrogen and progesterone receptors and flow cytometric DNA analysis of breast cancer on fine-needle aspirates. Anticancer Res 1993; 13:2435-2440.

40. Gaskell DJ, Hawkins RA, Sangster K. Relationship between immunocytochemical estimation of oestrogen receptor in elderly patients with breast cancer and response to tamoxifen. Lancet 1989:1044-1046.

41. Gaskell DJ, Hawkins RA, de-Carteret S et al. Indications for primary tamoxifen therapy in elderly women with breast cancer. Br J Surg 1992; 79:1317-1320.

42. Nicholson RI, Bouzubar N, Walker KJ et al. Hormone sensitivity in breast cancer: Influence of heterogeneity of oestrogen receptor expression and cell proliferation. Eur J Cancer 1991; 27:908-913.

43. Horwitz KB, McGuire WL, Pearson OH et al. Predicting a response to endocrine therapy in human breast cancer: a hypothesis. Science 1975; 189:726-727.

44. Knight WA III, Osborne CK, Yochmowitz MG et al. Steroid hormone receptors in the management of human breast cancer. Annals Clin Res 1980; 12:202-207.
45. Clark GM, McGuire WL. Progesterone receptors and human breast cancer. Breast Cancer Res Treat 1983; 3:157-163.
46. McGuire WL. Steroid receptors in human breast cancer. Cancer Res 1978; 38:4289-4291.
47. Wittliff JL. Steroid-hormone receptors in breast cancer. Cancer 1984; 53:630-643.
48. McGuire WL, Chamness GC, Fuqua SA. Abnormal oestrogen receptors in clinical breast cancers. Eur J Cancer 1992; 28:309-310.
49. Fuqua SAW, Wiltschke C, Castles C et al. A role for estrogen-receptor variants in endocrine resistance. Endocrine Related Ca 1995; 1:19-25.
50. Osborne CK. Heterogeneity in hormone receptor status in primary and metastatic breast cancer. Semin Oncol 1985; 12:317-326.
51. Gross CE, Clark GM, Chamness GC. Multiple progesterone receptor assays in human breast cancer. Cancer Res 1984; 44:836-840.
52. Powles TJ, Ashley S, Ford HT et al. Treatment of disseminated breast cancer with tamoxifen, aminoglutethimide, hydrocortisone and danazol used in combination or sequentially. Lancet 1984; i:1369-1372.
53. Horowitz KB. How do breast cancers become hormone resistant? J Steroid Biochem Mol Biol 1994; 49:295-302.
54. Clark GM, McGuire WL, Hubay CA et al. Progesterone receptors as a prognostic factor in stage II breast cancer. N Eng J Med 1983; 309:1343-1347.
55. Clark GM, McGuire WL. High risk profile for recurrence and survival of 1647 node-negative breast cancer patients. Proc AACR 1986; 5:65.
56. McGuire WL, Clark GM. The prognostic role of progesterone receptors in human breast cancer. Semin Oncol 1983; Suppl 4:2-6.
57. Fisher B, Redmond C, Brown A et al. Influence of tumor estrogen and progesterone receptor levels on the response to tamoxifen and chemotherapy in primary breast cancer. J Clin Oncol 1983; 1:227-241.
58. Baker ME. Oestrogen induced pS2 protein is similar to pancreatic spasmoytic polypeptide and the kringle domain. Biochem J 1988; 253:307-309.
59. Wright NA, Poulsom, R, Stamp GW et al. Epidermal growth factor (EGF/URO) induces expression of regulatory peptides in damages human gastrointestinal tissues. J Pathol 1990; 162:279-284.
60. Theisinger B, Walter C, Seitz G et al. Expression of the breast cancer associated gene pS2 and the pancreatic spasmolytic polypeptide gene (hSP) in diffuse type of stomach carcinoma. Eur J Cancer 1991; 27:770-773.
61. Rio MC, Chennard MP, Wolf C et al. Induction of pS2 and hSP genes as markers of mucosal ulceration of the digestive tract. Gastroenter 1991; 100:375-379.
62. Masiakowski P, Breathnach R, Bloch J et al. Cloning of cDNA sequences of hormone regulated genes from MCF-7 human breast cancer cell line. Nucleic Acids Res 1982; 10:7895-7903.

63. Henry JA, Nicholson S, Hennessy C et al. Expression of the estrogen regulated pNR-2 mRNA in human breast cancer: relation to estrogen receptor mRNA levels and response to tamoxifen therapy. Br J Cancer 1990; 61:32-38.

64. Foekens JA, Rio MC, Seguin P et al. Prediction of relapse and survival in breast cancer patients by pS2 protein status. Cancer Res 1990; 50:2832-2837.

65. Henry JA, Piggott NH, Mallick UK et al. pNR-2/pS2 immunohistochemical staining in breast cancer: correlation with prognostic factors and endocrine response. Br J Cancer 1991; 63:615-622.

66. Koerner FC, Goldberg DE, Edgerton SM et al. pS2 protein and steroid hormone receptors in invasive breast carcinomas. Int J Cancer. 1992; 52:183-188.

67. Dookeran KA, Rye PD, Dearing SJ et al. Expression of the pS2 peptide in primary breast carcinomas: comparison of membrane and cytoplasmic staining patterns. J Pathol 1993; 171:123-129.

68. Pichon MF, Milgrom E. Clinical significance of the estrogen regulated pS2 protein in mammary tumors. Crit Revs Oncol/Hematology 1993; 15:13-21.

69. Predine J, Spyratos F, Prud'homme JF et al. Enzyme-linked immunosorbent assay of pS2 in breast cancers, benign tumors and normal breast tissues. Cancer 1992; 69:2116-2123.

70. Luqmani YA, Ricketts D, Ryall G et al. Prediction of response to endocrine therapy in breast cancer using immunocytochemical assays for pS2, oestrogen receptor and progesterone receptor. Int J Cancer 1993; 54:619-623.

71. Schwartz LH, Koerner FC, Edgerton SM et al. pS2 expression and response to hormonal therapy in patients with advanced breast cancer. Cancer Res 1991; 51:624-628.

72. Charpin, C, Devictor B, Bonnier P et al. Quantitative imaging of pS2 immuno-cytochemical assays in breast carcinoma. Int J Oncol 1993; 2:443-448.

73. Thor AD, Koerner FC, Edgerton SM et al. pS2 expression in primary breast carcinomas: relationship to clinical and histological features and survival. Breast Cancer Res Treat 1992:111-119.

74. Cappelletti V, Coradini D, Scanziani E et al. Prognostic relevance of pS2 status in association with steroid receptor status and proliferative activity in node-negative breast cancer. Eur J Cancer 1992; 28A:1315-1318.

75. Spyratos F, Anddrieu C, Hacene K et al. pS2 and response to adjuvant hormone therapy in primary breast cancer. Br J Cancer 1994; 69:394-397.

76. Skilton RA, Luqmani YA, McClelland RA et al. Characterisation of a messenger RNA selectively expressed in human breast cancer. Br J Cancer 1989; 60:168-175.

77. Manning DL, Robertson JFR, Ellis IO et al. Oestrogen regulated genes in breast cancer: Association of pLIVI with lymph node involvement. Eur J Cancer 1994; 30A:675-678.

78. Manning DL, Nicholson RI. Isolation of pMGT1: a gene that is repressed by oestrogen and increased by antioestrogens and antiprogestins. Eur J Cancer 1993; 29A:759-762.

79. Ciocca DR, Oesterreich S, Chamness GC et al. Biological and clinical implications of heat shock protein 27000 (Hsp27): a review. JNCI 1993; 85:1558-1570.

80. Ciocca DR, Adams DJ, Edwards DP et al. Distribution of an estrogen-induced protein with a molecular weight of 24,000 in normal and malignant human tissues and cells. Cancer Res 1983; 43:1204-1210.

81. King RJB, Coffer AI. The generation of antibodies against partially purified estradiol receptor from human myometrium. In: Jordan VC, ed. Estrogen/antiestrogen action and breast cancer therapy. Madison: Univ Winsconsin Press 1986:375-394.

82. Dunn DK, Whelan RDH, Hill B et al. Relationship of HSP27 and oestrogen receptor in hormone sensitive and insensitive cell lines. J Steroid Biochem Mol Biol 1993; 46:469-479.

83. Edwards DP, Adams DJ, Savage N. Estrogen induced synthesis of specific proteins in human breast cancer cells. Biochem Biophys Res Commun 1980; 93:804-812.

84. Ciocca DR, Fuqua SAW, Lock-Lim S et al. Response of human breast cancer cells to heat shock and chemotherapeutic drugs. Cancer Res 1992; 52:3648-3654.

85. Fucqua SAW, Blum-Salingaros M, McGuire WL. Induction of the estrogen-regulated "24K" protein by heat shock. Cancer Res 1989; 49:4126-4129.

86. Ciocca DR, Stato AO, Amprino de Castro MM. Colocalization of estrogen and progesterone receptors with an estrogen-regulated heat shock protein in paraffin sections of human breast and endometrial cancer tissue. Breast Cancer Res Treat 1990; 16:243-251.

87. Cano A, Coffer AI, Adatoa R et al. Histochemical studies with an estrogen receptor-related protein in human breast tumors. Cancer Res 1986; 46:6475-6480.

88. Chamness CG, Ruiz A, Fulcher L et al. Stress responsive protein srp27 predicts recurrence in node-negative breast cancer. Breast Cancer Res Treat 1988; 12:130.

89. Tandon AK, Clark GM, Chamness GC et al. Heat shock/stress responsive proteins: biological and clinical significance in breast cancer. Proc ASCO 1988; 9:84.

90. Thor A, Benz C, Moore II D et al. Stress response protein (srp-27) determination in primary human breast carcinomas: clinical, histological, and prognostic correlations. JNCI 1991; 83:170-178.

91. Seymour L, Bezwoda WR, Meyer K. Tumor factors predicting for prognosis in metastatic breast cancer. The presence of p24 predicts for response to treatment and duration of survival. Cancer 1990; 66:2390-2394.

92. Connelly PA, Stern DF. The epidermal growth factor receptor and the product of the neu protooncogene are members of a receptor tyrosine phosphorylation cascade. Proc Nat Acad Sci USA 1990; 87:6054-6057.

93. Slamon DJ, Clark GM, Wong SG et al. Human breast cancer: correlation of relapse and survival with amplification of the HER-2/neu oncogene. Science 1987; 235:177-182.

94. Nicholson RI, McClelland RA, Finlay P et al. Relationship between EGF-R, c-erbB-2 protein expression and Ki67 immunostaining in breast cancer and hormone sensitivity. Eur J Cancer 1993; 29A:1018-1023.

95. Sharma AK, Horgan K, Douglas-Jones A et al. Dual immunocytochemical analysis of oestrogen and epidermal growth factor receptors in human breast cancer. Br J Cancer 1994; 69:1032-1037.

96. Muss HB, Thor AD, Berry DA et al. c-erbB-2 expression of response to adjuvant therapy in women with node-positive early breast cancer. New Eng J Med 1994; 330:1308-1309.

97. Nicholson RI, McClelland RA, Gee JMW et al. Epidermal growth factor expression in breast cancer: association with response to endocrine therapy. Breast Cancer Res Treat 1994; 29:117-125.

98. Nicholson S, Wright C, Sainsbury JRC et al. Epidermal growth factor receptor (EGFr) as a market for poor prognosis in node-negative breast cancer patients: NEU and tamoxifen failure. J Steroid Biochem Mol Biol 1990; 6:811-814.

99. Borg A, Baldetorp B, Ferno M et al. ERBB2 amplification is associated with tamoxifen resistance in steroid-receptor positive breast cancer. Cancer Letts 1994; 81:137-144.

CHAPTER 10

ESTROGEN INDEPENDENCE

While strategies which deprive the breast of estrogen are associated with atrophy of normal structures and the regression of a minority of breast cancers, the growth of most breast cancers appears to be independent of hormonal restraints.[1] Whether at an early stage in their evolution these autonomous cancers have passed through a hormone-sensitive state is uncertain. However, the natural history of estrogen-dependent cancers suggests that under the selective pressure of estrogen deprivation most will acquire the phenotype of autonomy. Clinical experience shows that, even following successful endocrine treatment, most estrogen-dependent tumors resume growth and will subsequently kill.[2] Irrespective of whether resistance appears to be primary or acquired it is of importance to determine the causes of estrogen resistance and how they may occur (Table 10.1).

PRIMARY RESISTANCE

There appear to be two major underlying reasons for primary resistance (i) the tumor may be inherently autonomous and may not require estrogen for the maintenance of growth. Most estrogen receptor-negative tumors appear to fall into this category and, as has been discussed, estrogen receptor-negative tumors rarely respond to any form of endocrine deprivation,[3,4] and (ii) while tumor cells themselves may still require estrogen for growth, the therapy employed fails to reduce estrogens below a critical level required by the tumor. If this were the case, more efficient endocrine therapies should cause tumors to respond. Such a mechanism accounts for the second line responses seen after primary endocrine failure.[5] However, these are relatively infrequent and the following primary endocrine treatment, levels of estrogen tend to be similar in responding and non-responding patients.[6]

ACQUIRED RESISTANCE

There are several possible mechanisms for acquired resistance: the endocrine system may adapt to constraints put upon it and compensate by producing more estrogen, perhaps from an alternative source; pharmokinetic influences when drugs are used for estrogen deprivation; breast cancers like other malignancies display heterogeneity and

Table 10.1. Potential causes of endocrine resistance

Mechanisms of Estrogen Resistance	Characteristics
Inherent insensitivity	Estrogen receptor negativity
Clonal heterogeneity	Selection of ER+ve cells; outgrowth of ER-ve cells Changed phenotype with acquired resistance
Ineffective deprivation/Endocrine compensation	Estrogen levels in sufficiently reduced or raised second-line responses to more effective treatment
Drug metabolism/Efflux pump	Reduced levels of drugs in tumor cells
Variant/mutant ER	Reduced expression of induced markers in presence of estrogen Presence of transcriptional active ER in the absence of estrogen
Estrogen requirement by-passed	Overexpression of mitogenic growth factors and/or their receptors

following hormone deprivation clones of estrogen independent cells may selectively emerge from the hormone sensitive clones; during treatment hormone-dependent cells learn to by-pass the requirement for external sources of estrogen by means of phenotypic changes. It is worth considering each of these possibilities in more detail.

ENDOCRINE COMPENSATION

Relapse on treatment may be associated with hormone escape in patients in whom levels of circulating estrogens increase at time of relapse after successful endocrine treatment (Fig. 10.1). If hormone escape induces tumor regrowth, other measures which suppress estrogen levels more efficiently could be beneficial. It is thus pertinent that second line therapies which reduce estrogen levels, have produced responses after failed endocrine therapy.[8] This suggests that a proportion of tumors which are apparently resistant to treatment are still endocrine-sensitive. It should also be noted that increased estrogen at relapse might be the consequence rather than the cause of progressive disease (for example progressive metastatic disease might reduce the metabolic clearance of estrogens).[9] Finally it has to be emphasized that in most patients treatment failure is not associated with a change in circulating steroids.[10]

DRUG METABOLISM/EFFLUX PUMP

Experience from treatment of patients with chemotherapeutic drugs suggests that resistance to such agents may occur as a result of metabolism or the induction of cellular efflux pumps (such as P-glycoprotein); these effectively reduce levels of active drug within target

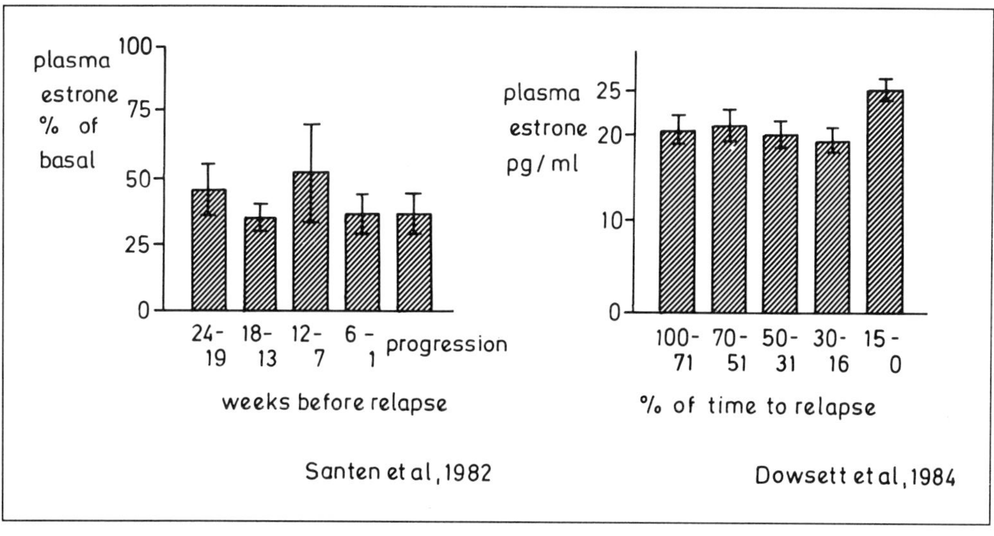

Fig. 10.1. Endocrine compensation as a mechanism of resistance (increased levels of circulating estrogens at relapse). Left hand side—lack of evidence.[10] Right hand side—supportive evidence.[5]

cells.[11] A similar mechanism has been postulated as a reason for resistance to drugs which affect the endocrine system, e.g., tamoxifen.[12] Furthermore, aromatase inhibitors such as aminoglutethimide are able to induce liver hydroxylase enzymes[13] which decrease the plasma half-life of the drug.[14] Additional consideration with regard to antiestrogens and aromatase inhibitors are presented in later sections.

Outgrowth of Hormone Independent Clones

It is also possible that the appearance of hormone resistance during therapy results from the outgrowth of sub-clones of independent cells which were present from the initiation of therapy (Fig. 10.2). Such cellular heterogeneity of breast cancers has been well documented both in regard to hormone sensitivity and hormone receptors.[2,11,12] Selective cell kill has also been demonstrated after successful hormone therapy.[13,14] Furthermore second-line responses to further endocrine manipulations are more likely in tumors responding to first line therapy.[15] These data would be compatible with a successive destruction of cellular populations with differing hormone sensitivity. However, clinical observations are not totally compatible with the clonal destruction theory as the main and sole mechanism by which endocrine resistance occurs. For example, if estrogen receptor status is a marker of hormone dependence and relapse following successful endocrine treatment is caused by resistant estrogen receptor-negative cells outgrowing from suppressed receptor positive clones, the resulting hormone-independent tumor should be estrogen receptor-poor or -negative. Although this may occur,[20] most

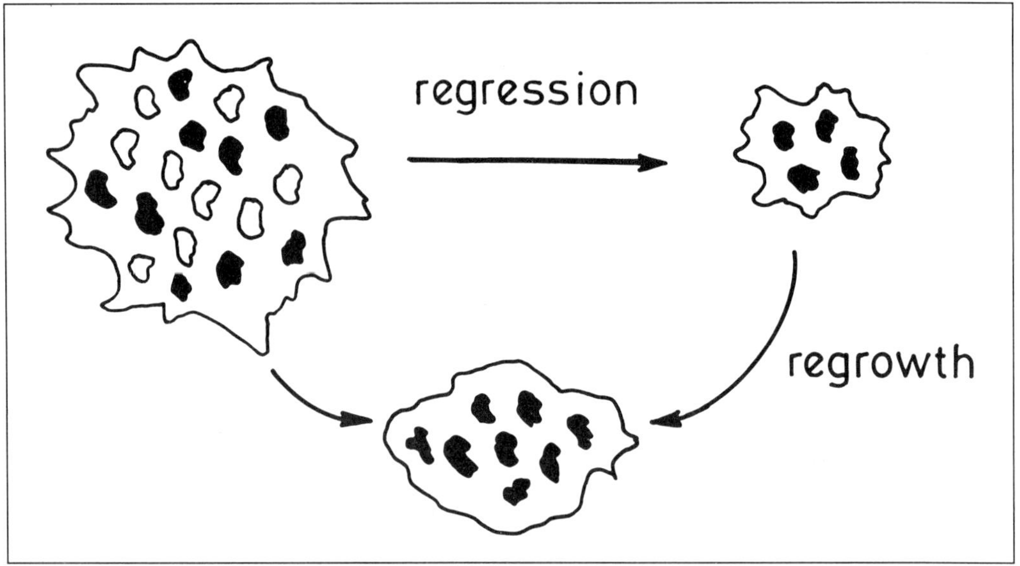

Fig. 10.2. Clonal selection as a mechanism of endocrine resistance.

often relapsing tumors are still estrogen receptor-positive.[21-23] They also may continue to express markers of estrogen function, such as progesterone receptor or pS2.[24] Results from model systems are consistent with this clinical observation, estrogen receptor positive cell lines being able to adapt to grow in culture in the absence of estrogen while maintaining their receptor status.[25] Therefore, resistance, at least in the majority of breast cancers, is not due to loss of estrogen receptors.[26]

PHENOTYPIC CHANGES

Estrogen deprivation appears to accelerate phenotypic/epigenetic adaptation which causes alterations in gene expression. Thus, long-term growth in breast cancer cell lines in culture without estrogen can result in an ordered series of phenotypic changes culminating in estrogen resistance.[27] While initial changes may be reversible on addition of steroids, later changes are irreversible.[28] As indicated above such loss of responsiveness to estrogens may occur without the loss of estrogen receptors and indeed certain inducible molecular markers. Several types of phenotypic changes could potentially lead to autonomy. These include (a) the ability of breast cancers to synthesize estrogen from alternative sources, (b) mutation/variations in the estrogen receptor and (c) constitutive production of mitogens.

Synthesis from alternative sources

Some breast cancers have the ability to synthesize estrogens[29,30] and the acquisition of such steroidogenic potential might allow tumors to become independent of external sources of estrogen. However there is little evidence that progression to autonomy is associated with enhanced capacity for estrogen biosynthesis or that hormone-independent cancers are more likely to synthesize estrogen than hormone-dependent tumors.[23,30,31]

Mutation/variants of the estrogen receptor

Variants and mutations of the estrogen receptor gene can lead to differences in the regulation of the protein and/or influence the structural function of the estrogen receptor[32,33] (Fig. 10.3). However, the incidence of "true" mutations of the estrogen receptor in breast cancer may be rare. In one study of metastatic tumors from patients, the estrogen receptor was normal in 18 out of 20 cases.[34] However, the estrogen receptor in some breast cancers appears unusual by either failing to show binding to DNA, being truncated on binding or being otherwise transcriptionally deficient. Garcia et al[35,36] identified a polymorphic variant in a region of the estrogen receptor messenger-RNA which influences the transcriptional function of the protein. In some breast cancer specimens this variant has since been correlated with lower than normal levels of hormone binding activity and preliminary data suggest that women who are heterozygous for this variance have a higher proportion of spontaneous abortions than those who are homozygous of the same mutation.[37] Forms of estrogen receptor-like messenger-RNAs truncated after exons 2 or 3 have also been identified in breast cancer biopsies by Northern blotting.[38] These messages lack substantial

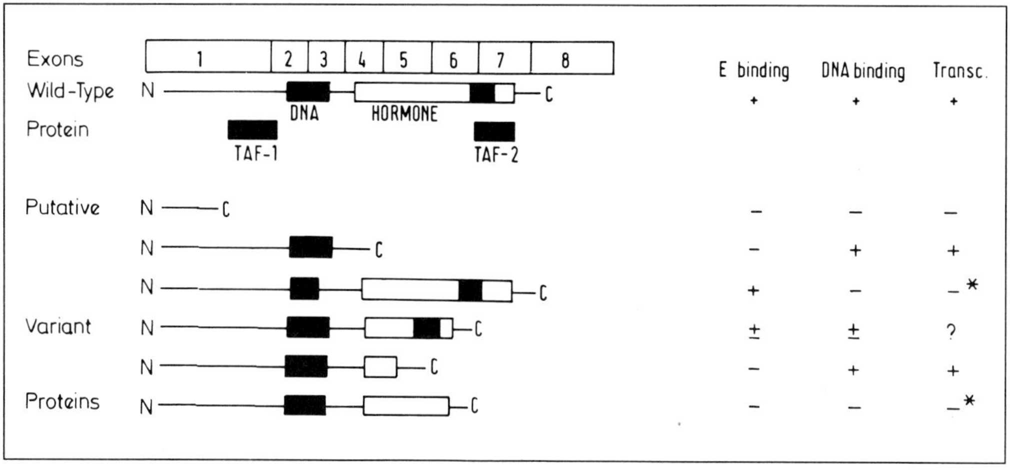

Fig. 10.3. Variants and mutations of estrogen receptors.

portions of the coding region of the gene, including that for the hormone binding domain. In addition a variant estrogen receptor message has been detected that can program an in vitro transcription system to produce a truncated estrogen receptor from an alternative transcription start site.[38,39] No function for these receptors has been demonstrated although the proteins may interfere with the function of normal estrogen receptor in vivo. Fuqua et al[40] have also identified mutant forms of the estrogen receptor missing parts of the hormone-binding domain because of deletion of exon 5. These receptors still bind DNA, are transcriptionally active whether or not estrogen is present and constitutively activate normally estrogen-dependent genes. Constitutively active estrogen receptors would be expected to confer estrogen independence. Indeed, molecular studies have shown that transfection of the exon 5 variant into MCF-7 cells (which have wild-type receptors) results in proliferation unaffected by the antiestrogen,[41] tamoxifen, which usually inhibits the growth of the MCF-7 cells. While a permanently activated estrogen receptor might therefore explain hormone independence, the exon 5 deletion variant has been found in estrogen receptor-positive and estrogen receptor-negative progestogen receptor-positive cancers which frequently respond to estrogen deprivation therapy.[42] The data have also yet to be expanded to the level of protein. This is important as the variants of messenger-RNA do not guarantee the presence of protein variants. Fuqua et al[39,43] also identified an estrogen receptor variant lacking exon-7 which, although transcriptionally inactive itself, inhibited the function of wild type estrogen receptor. Dominantly negatively active mutants of this type were able to confer resistance to tamoxifen in cell systems and by-pass the requirement for estrogen-occupied estrogen receptor for growth. The selection of tamoxifen-resistant estrogen receptor variants could therefore be clinically significant with the drug actually providing selective pressure for the eventual outgrowth of cells containing these variants.

Constitutive production of mitogens

Because estrogens may exert their growth promoting effects through induced mitogenic growth factors, it has been hypothesized that the transition from an estrogen-dependent to an estrogen-autonomous growth state is associated with a change in which estrogen-mediated growth factor loops are supplemented or supplanted by constitutive growth factor production (Fig. 10.4).

The known mitogenic and angiogenic properties of transforming growth factors make them good candidates in this respect. Experiments using exogenous TGFα or antibodies/antisense mRNA against TGFα demonstrate that this growth factor has growth promoting autocrine activities in breast cancer cell lines.[44-46] Furthermore levels of mRNA for TGFα have been found to be elevated in estrogen-independent as compared with estrogen-dependent breast cancer cell lines.[47] Recent

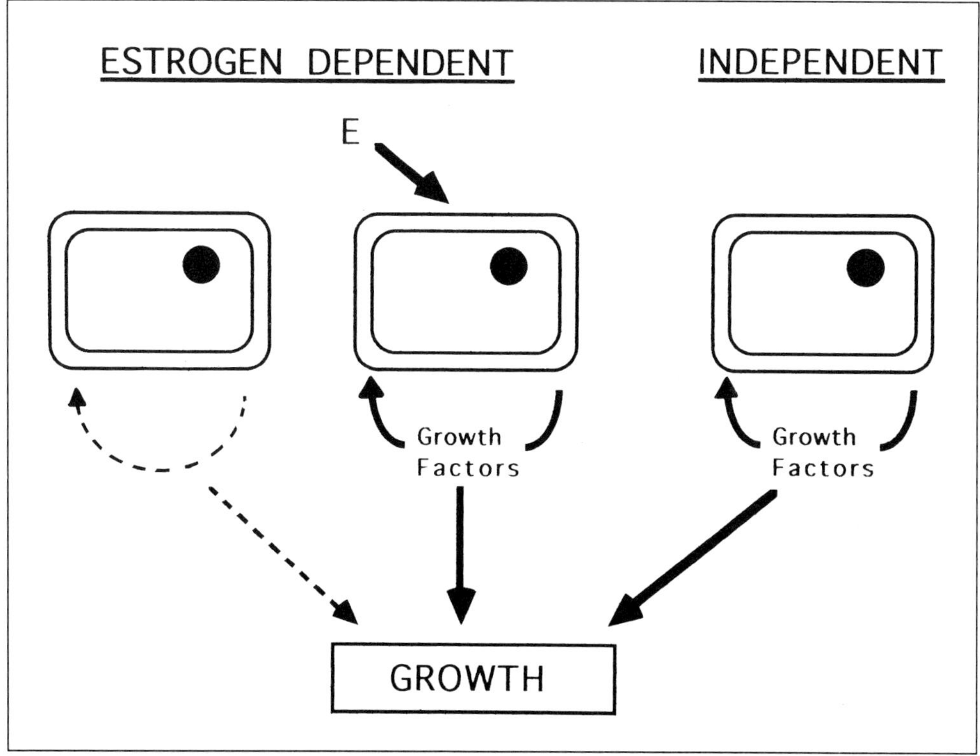

Fig. 10.4. Constitutive growth factor production as a mechanism of endocrine resistance.

studies also indicate that changes in growth rates of breast cancer cells in response to steroid deprivation are associated with a transient decrease in TGFα and an increase in TGFβs but there is a return to parental levels in those cells which begin to proliferate in a steroid-deprived state.[48] It may be therefore that insensitivity to TGFαs and TGFβs occurs with long-term steroid depletion and this is reflected in altered production of growth factors. In clinical specimens the lack of response to antiestrogen in estrogen receptor-positive advanced breast cancer has been reported to correlate with elevated TGFα levels[49] and elevated cell proliferation rates.[50,51] This evidence linking increased production of TGFα to estrogen resistance needs to be balanced against the observation that transfection of the TGFα gene with an inducible promoter into estrogen-dependent cells does not by-pass the requirement for estrogen even when induced fully (see Fig. 10.5). It should be emphasized, however, that while in cell lines hormone independent cells may secrete greater amounts of TGFα than hormone dependent cells,[48,53] work in primary breast cancers has not produced consistant results.[49,54-56]

Model systems support the notion that insulin-like growth factors are important mediators of breast tumor growth. IGF-II expression

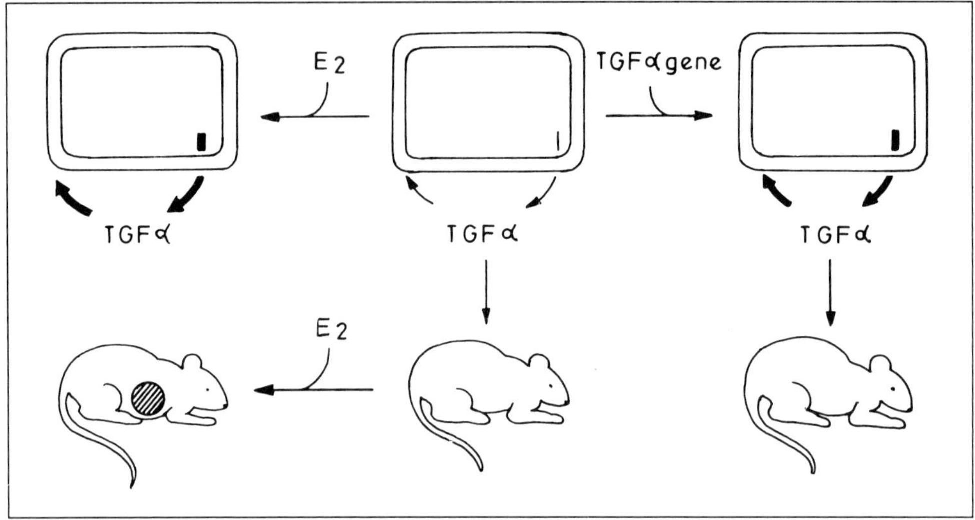

Fig. 10.5. Overexpression of TGFα does not by-pass requirement for estrogen.

appears to be closely linked to hormone responsiveness[57] and, in certain estrogen independent cell lines and xenografts, IGF-II is constitutively expressed.[51,58] Estrogen increases the sensitivity of breast cancer cells to the proliferative effects of IGFs,[59,60] at least in part by increasing the number of IGF-I receptor sites.[59] Breast tumors also express variable levels of IGF-I receptors that are positively correlated with those of estrogen receptors.[61,62]

Interestingly, although the transforming growth factor beta (TGFβ) family has been most frequently identified as negative autocrine regulators in the breast,[63] the TGFβs appear to be elevated in more aggressive cancers.[64,65] Arteaga et al[66] have also reported that the introduction of TGFβ1 cDNA into a breast cancer cell line results in the formation of estrogen-independent tumors in nude mice.

Involvement of growth factors in the transition from endocrine-responsive to unresponsive breast cancer might also entail changes in growth factor receptor levels. It is thus pertinent that the epidermal growth factor receptor may be overexpressed in tumors unresponsive to estrogen deprivation therapy.[51,67-69] However, this need not be a functional relationship as evidenced by the observation that an antibody to EGF receptor, while being able to block the proliferative effect of TGFα, failed to have similar effects on estradiol-mediated growth.[70] The *erb*B-2 oncogene encodes for a growth factor receptor which has extensive homology to the EGF receptor.[71] Studies of *erb*B-2 in breast cancer have shown that over-expression is associated with aggressive tumor phenotype and poor prognosis.[72-75] There are also data which suggest that *erb*B-2 amplification is associated with poor disease-free survival in steroid receptor-positive breast cancers and it has been

Receive a FREE BOOK of your choice

Please help us out—Just answer the questions below, then select the book of your choice from the list on the back and return this card.

R.G. Landes Company publishes five book series: *Medical Intelligence Unit, Molecular Biology Intelligence Unit, Neuroscience Intelligence Unit, Tissue Engineering Intelligence Unit* and *Biotechnology Intelligence Unit*. We also publish comprehensive, shorter than book-length reports on well-circumscribed topics in molecular biology and medicine. The authors of our books and reports are acknowledged leaders in their fields and the topics are unique. Almost without exception, there are no other comprehensive publications on these topics.

Our goal is to publish material in important and rapidly changing areas of bioscience for sophisticated scientists. To achieve this goal, we have accelerated our publishing program to conform to the fast pace in which information grows in bioscience. Most of our books and reports are published within 90 to 120 days of receipt of the manuscript.

Please circle your response to the questions below.

1. We would like to sell our *books* to scientists and students at a deep discount. But we can only do this as part of a prepaid subscription program. The retail price range for our books is $59-$99. Would you pay $196 to select four *books* per year from any of our Intelligence Units–$49 per book–as part of a prepaid program?

    Yes   No

2. We would like to sell our *reports* to scientists and students at a deep discount. But we can only do this as part of a prepaid subscription program. The retail price range for our reports is $39-$59. Would you pay $145 to select five *reports* per year–$29 per report–as part of a prepaid program?

    Yes   No

3. Would you pay $39–the retail price range of our books is $59-$99–to receive any single book in our Intelligence Units if it is spiral bound, but in every other way identical to the more expensive hardcover version?

    Yes   No

To receive your free book, please fill out the shipping information below, select your free book choice from the list on the back of this survey and mail this card to:

R.G. Landes Company, 909 S. Pine Street, Georgetown, Texas 78626   U.S.A.

Your Name ____

Address ____

City_____________________________   State/Province:_______________________

Country: _________________________   Postal Code:_______________________

My computer type is Macintosh________ ; IBM-compatible _______ ; Other _______

Do you own _____ or plan to purchase ____ a CD-ROM drive?

Available Free Titles

*Please check three titles in order of preference.
Your request will be filled based on availability. Thank you.*

☐ Water Channels
*Alan Verkman,
University of California-San Francisco*

☐ The Na,K-ATPase:
Structure-Function Relationship
J.-D. Horisberger, University of Lausanne

☐ Intrathymic Development of T Cells
*J. Nikolic-Zugic,
Memorial Sloan-Kettering Cancer Center*

☐ Cyclic GMP
Thomas Lincoln, University of Alabama

☐ Primordial VRM System and the Evolution
of Vertebrate Immunity
John Stewart, Institut Pasteur-Paris

☐ Thyroid Hormone Regulation
of Gene Expression
Graham R. Williams, University of Birmingham

☐ Mechanisms of Immunological Self Tolerance
*Guido Kroemer, CNRS Génétique Moléculaire et
Biologie du Développement-Villejuif*

☐ The Costimulatory Pathway
for T Cell Responses
Yang Liu, New York University

☐ Molecular Genetics of Drosophila Oogenesis
Paul F. Lasko, McGill University

☐ Mechanism of Steroid Hormone Regulation
of Gene Transcription
M.-J. Tsai & Bert W. O'Malley, Baylor University

☐ Liver Gene Expression
*François Tronche & Moshe Yaniv,
Institut Pasteur-Paris*

☐ RNA Polymerase III Transcription
R.J. White, University of Cambridge

☐ src Family of Tyrosine Kinases in Leukocytes
Tomas Mustelin, La Jolla Institute

☐ MHC Antigens and NK Cells
*Rafael Solana & Jose Peña,
University of Córdoba*

☐ Kinetic Modeling of Gene Expression
James L. Hargrove, University of Georgia

☐ PCR and the Analysis of the T Cell Receptor
Repertoire
*Jorge Oksenberg, Michael Panzara & Lawrence
Steinman, Stanford University*

☐ Myointimal Hyperplasia
Philip Dobrin, Loyola University

☐ Transgenic Mice as an In Vivo Model
of Self-Reactivity
*David Ferrick & Lisa DiMolfetto-Landon,
University of California-Davis and Pamela Ohashi,
Ontario Cancer Institute*

☐ Cytogenetics of Bone and Soft Tissue Tumors
*Avery A. Sandberg, Genetrix & Julia A. Bridge ,
University of Nebraska*

☐ The Th1-Th2 Paradigm and Transplantation
Robin Lowry, Emory University

☐ Phagocyte Production and Function Following
Thermal Injury
*Verlyn Peterson & Daniel R. Ambruso,
University of Colorado*

☐ Human T Lymphocyte Activation Deficiencies
*José Regueiro, Carlos Rodríguez-Gallego
and Antonio Arnaiz-Villena,
Hospital 12 de Octubre-Madrid*

☐ Monoclonal Antibody in Detection and
Treatment of Colon Cancer
Edward W. Martin, Jr., Ohio State University

☐ Enteric Physiology of the Transplanted Intestine
Michael Sarr & Nadey S. Hakim, Mayo Clinic

☐ Artificial Chordae in Mitral Valve Surgery
Claudio Zussa, S. Maria dei Battuti Hospital-Treviso

☐ Injury and Tumor Implantation
*Satya Murthy & Edward Scanlon,
Northwestern University*

☐ Support of the Acutely Failing Liver
A.A. Demetriou, Cedars-Sinai

☐ Reactive Metabolites of Oxygen and Nitrogen
in Biology and Medicine
Matthew Grisham, Louisiana State-Shreveport

☐ Biology of Lung Cancer
*Adi Gazdar & Paul Carbone,
Southwestern Medical Center*

☐ Quantitative Measurement
of Venous Incompetence
*Paul S. van Bemmelen, Southern Illinois University
and John J. Bergan, Scripps Memorial Hospital*

☐ Adhesion Molecules in Organ Transplants
Gustav Steinhoff, University of Kiel

☐ Purging in Bone Marrow Transplantation
*Subhash C. Gulati,
Memorial Sloan-Kettering Cancer Center*

☐ Trauma 2000: Strategies for the New Millennium
*David J. Dries & Richard L. Gamelli,
Loyola University*

suggested that this effect may be related to the non-responsiveness of these tumors to adjuvant tamoxifen therapy.[76,77] Indeed, tamoxifen may enhance the aggressiveness of these tumors.[77] Experimental evidence showing an estrogen receptor-dependent up-regulation of *erb*B-2 expression upon tamoxifen administration[78] and transfection of hormone-sensitive breast cancer cells with c-*erb*B-2 confers resistance to tamoxifen[79] would support this.

RESISTANCE ASSOCIATED WITH INDIVIDUAL TYPES OF ESTROGEN DEPRIVATION

Since the estrogen stimulus for hormone-dependent tumors may be potentially derived from three different sources, glandular synthesis of estrogen by the ovary, extraglandular synthesis of estrogen in peripheral tissues and (ixogenous supplies, individual types of estrogen deprivation might be more or less effective depending on their mode of action. For example, measures which act by blocking at the level of tumor estrogen receptors would be expected to be effective irrespective of the source of estrogen. Other therapies which are specific for particular sources may ineffectively blockade estrogen action. For example, ovariectomy will effectively reduce the trophic effects of estrogen in premenopausal women but is likely to be ineffective in postmenopausal women in whom the major source of tumor estrogen is extra-glandular. Similarly aromatase inhibitors, which are effective in reducing extraglandular synthesis, may be ineffective in premenopausal women because of their inability to inhibit estrogen biosynthesis in the ovary; they may also be ineffective in those postmenopausal women in whom exogenous estrogens are primarily responsible for maintaining tumor growth. The corollary of this is that alternative forms of endocrine manipulation may induce regression of evidently estrogen-resistant tumors. It is therefore an interesting exercise, as is shown in Table 10.2, to plot the pattern of theoretical responses to endocrine therapies according to dependence for individual hormone classes. Thus,

Table 10.2. Theoretically expected response to major forms of endocrine therapies subdivided according to dependence on different hormonal sources

Response to	Dependence upon			
	Endogenous estrogens	Δ 5 androgens	Exogenous estrogens	No hormones
Aromatase Inhibitor	√	x	x	x
Adrenalectomy	√	√	x	x
Hypophysectomy	√	√	x	x
Antiestrogens	√	√	√	x

if a tumor is dependent upon adrenal androgens, it should be insensitive to aromatase inhibitors but responsive to hypophysectomy, adrenalectomy and antiestrogens. Similarly, if a tumor is dependent upon exogenous sources of estrogen, it would appear resistant to aromatase inhibitors and endocrine ablation but not antiestrogens. This scheme suggests that all types of estrogen deprivation are not equivalent and, this being the case, certain forms of resistance may be specific to individual methods of treatment. The following sections therefore review aspects of resistance that might be specific to antiestrogens and aromatase inhibitors.

ANTIESTROGENS

Almost all tumors which are initially responsive to tamoxifen acquire resistance to the drug.[80] This represents a major restriction in the current use of tamoxifen. Thus, while patients with advanced breast cancer may experience responses to tamoxifen which vary from several weeks to several years, virtually all patients can expect to encounter disease progression while taking tamoxifen.[81] Similarly when tamoxifen is used as an adjuvant treatment nearly 60% of node-positive patients (compared to almost 70% of untreated controls) suffer disease recurrence within ten years.[82] However, between 35-60% of women who develop disease that is refractory to tamoxifen, will respond favorably to second-line endocrine treatment;[81] some may experience disease response attributable only to the withdrawal of tamoxifen treatment[83,84] and others apparently are resistant to any hormone manipulation.[80]

Models have been developed in vitro and in vivo to study the progression of breast cancer growth from tamoxifen sensitive to tamoxifen resistant states. Both long-term estrogen deprivation and/or long-term tamoxifen exposure result in cell lines and tumors capable of growth in the presence of tamoxifen.[85-89]

Because breast cancer is a highly heterogenous disease, it is likely that the mechanisms which cause tamoxifen-resistant growth are equally heterogenous. These are summarized in Table 10.3 and potentially include:

Endocrine compensation

Because tamoxifen is a competitive inhibitor of estrogen action at the estrogen receptor,[90] increases in circulating or local estrogen may reduce the antitumor effectiveness in patients. For example, tamoxifen can be an effective agent in premenopausal patients[91,92] but it does cause a major increase of circulating estradiol in women with functioning ovaries.[93] Furthermore, in premenopausal women with advanced breast cancer who respond and then fail on tamoxifen therapy, there is a 50% chance of a second response to oophorectomy.[91] These observations would be consistent with ovarian estrogens reversing the

Table 10.3. Potential causes of resistance to antiestrogens

Cause	Observation
Endocrine compensation	Increased levels of estrogens following treatment with tamoxifen in premenopausal women
Antiestrogen binding proteins	Increase in tumors during treatment with antiestrogens act as sink for tamoxifen
Drug metabolism	Increased metabolism of tamoxifen in resistant tumors Increased expression of p-glycoprotein in a subset of resistant tumors
ER expression	Lack of ER expression associated with antiestrogen failure Deletion of hormone-binding domain leads to constitutive ER activation
ER mutants/variants	Altered characteristics cause antiestrogen bound receptor to behave as if occupied by estrogen
Gen transcription and activation	Accessory proteins produce abnormal ER transcription
Second messenger cross-talk	Increased levels of cyclic-AMP alter cellular response to antiestrogens Anti-estrogens influence protein kinase C and calmodulin-mediated signal transduction
Growth factor enhancement	Increased production of mitogenic growth factors reverse effects of antiestrogens

antitumor actions of tamoxifen, an effect which can be countered by the removal of the source of elevated estrogen, viz. the ovaries.

Antiestrogen binding proteins

An interesting observation is that antiestrogen binding sites in tumors appear to increase during treatment with antiestrogen therapy.[94] Since these sites can sequester and soak up tamoxifen they may prevent the drug binding to estrogen receptors and allow estrogen to regain access to the estrogen receptor so stimulating tumor growth.[95]

Drug metabolism

Tamoxifen undergoes extensive metabolism in patients[96] and alterations in metabolism can produce less active or even estrogenic metabolites thereby reducing therapeutic efficiency (Fig. 10.6).[80,97] Changes in uptake or the induction of an active excretion system can also lower intracellular concentrations of tamoxifen and its metabolites to a point when they no longer act efficiently as competitive blockers of the estrogen receptor.[98] It is thus interesting that breast tumors which are resistant to tamoxifen appear to have reduced levels of the drug compared with responsive cancers (Table 10.4).[99,100] Long-term administration of tamoxifen to athymic mice bearing MCF-7 breast cancer cells may also be associated with tamoxifen-stimulated growth,[101,102] a phenomenon which has been used to explain the tumor regressions following tamoxifen withdrawal.[98] More recently Osborne and colleagues found that tamoxifen-stimulated tumors have lower intratumoral concentrations of the parent drug itself than do tamoxifen-inhibited cancers.[103] Under these circumstances tamoxifen metabolism may account for continued growth of these tumors in that, as tumors become refractory to tamoxifen, they may also be stimulated by the estrogenic properties of some triphenylethylene metabolites. However doubts surround this possibility as levels of estrogenic metabolites are also reduced in stimulated tumors and non-isomerizable tamoxifen analogues which do not undergo metabolism to the common estrogenic products[103,104] are still associated with the phenomenon of tamoxifen resistance and dependence.[105,106]

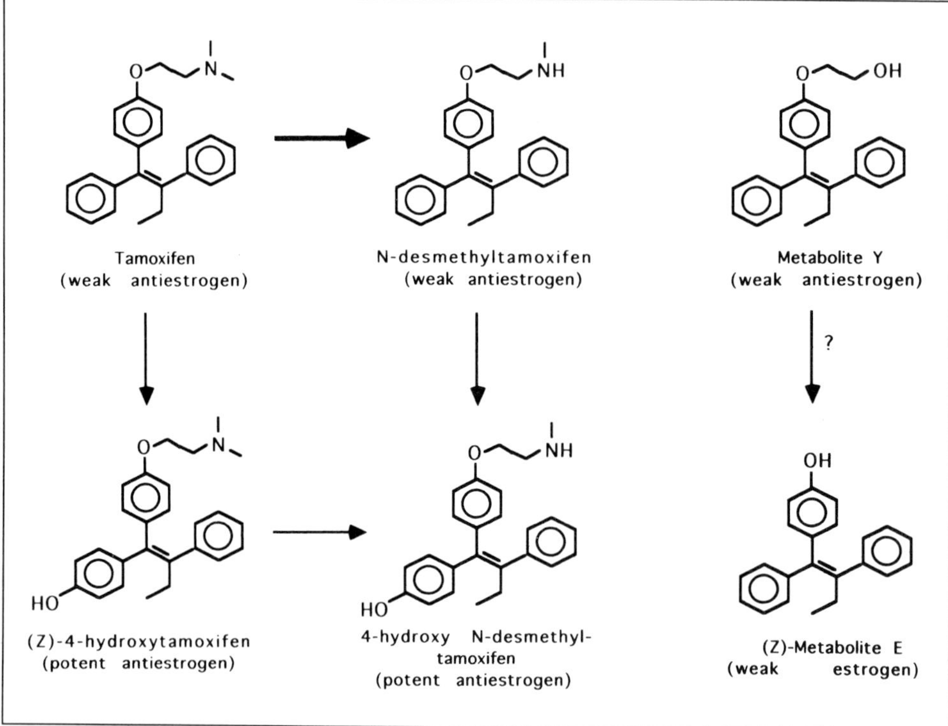

Fig. 10.6. *Metabolites of tamoxifen.*

Table 10.4. Levels of tamoxifen and metastasis in sensitive and resistant breast cancer

	Tamoxifen Sensitive	Tamoxifen Resistant
Tamoxifen	36.0 mg/g	4.4 mg/g
4-OH (cis) (V anti-oestrogenic)	104.1 ng/g	58.4 ng/g
4-OH (trans) (oestrogenic)	162.6 ng/g	49.9 ng/g

Data derived from Osborne et al. JNCI 1991; 83:1477-1482.

Estrogen receptor variants and mutants

The possibility that estrogen receptor mutants and variants might be associated with resistance has been reviewed earlier. However, this has additional relevance to resistance to antiestrogens if a mutated receptor could convert the pharmacology of an antiestrogen to an estrogen such that an antiestrogen occupied receptor behaves as though it were occupied by an estrogen. Interestingly, studies in which mutant receptors have been transfected in hormone sensitive cells have demonstrated a phenotype in which both estradiol and 4-hydroxy-tamoxifen act as estrogen receptor agonists but a pure antiestrogen does not.[107]

Gene transcription and activation

It is also possible that while the estrogen receptor mechanism itself may be normal in resistant cells, abnormalities exist in other aspects of gene transcription and activation. Altered expression of accessory proteins could modify the transcriptional signal generated by ligands binding to the estrogen receptor. As a result cells may become estrogen independent by developing a mechanism to bypass the requirement whereby an estrogen-occupied estrogen receptor induces transcription; in contrast, tamoxifen-occupied estrogen receptor may still be capable of interfering with transcriptional activity. Persuasive evidence for this has been derived from some model systems and is reviewed by Wolf and Jordan.[80] It is also possible to speculate that changes in accessory proteins affecting transcriptional activity through the estrogen receptor might contribute to tamoxifen-stimulated growth.

Cross-talk

Cross-talk between polypeptide growth factor pathways and estrogen receptor mediated events could also theoretically result in tamoxifen resistance. For instance, it has been shown that increasing the level of cellular cyclic AMP pharmacologically alters the cellular response to

tamoxifen converting it from an antiestrogen to a weak estrogen agonist.[108] These effects may also account for the observation that tamoxifen
has estrogen agonist properties in some tissues while antagonistic effects predominate in others.

Cell cycle interactions

Antiestrogen treatment of breast cancer cells in vitro leads to growth
arrest with the accumulation of cells in the GI phase[109,110] (see Fig. 10.7).
Indeed, it can be shown that sensitivity of cells to antiestrogens is
restricted to the GI phase of the cell cycle; elsewhere in the cycle,
cells are essentially insensitive and proceed through S-phase of mitosis
at the same rate as untreated cells.[111,112] This suggests that antiestrogens
may control the expression of key cell cycle regulatory genes, the products
of which determine rates of GI progression. The important molecules
involved in this process are cell cycle regulatory cyclins, cyclin-inde-
pendent kinases and inhibitors of these kinases.[113,114] Of the various
cyclins, cyclin D1 seems to be particularly important and is rate limiting for progress through the GI phase.[115] Alterations in cell cycle control may be involved in endocrine resistance. Thus, steroids and their
antagonists can determine the rate of breast cancer cell proliferation
by direct effects on genes controlling the cell cycle.[116] If, therefore,

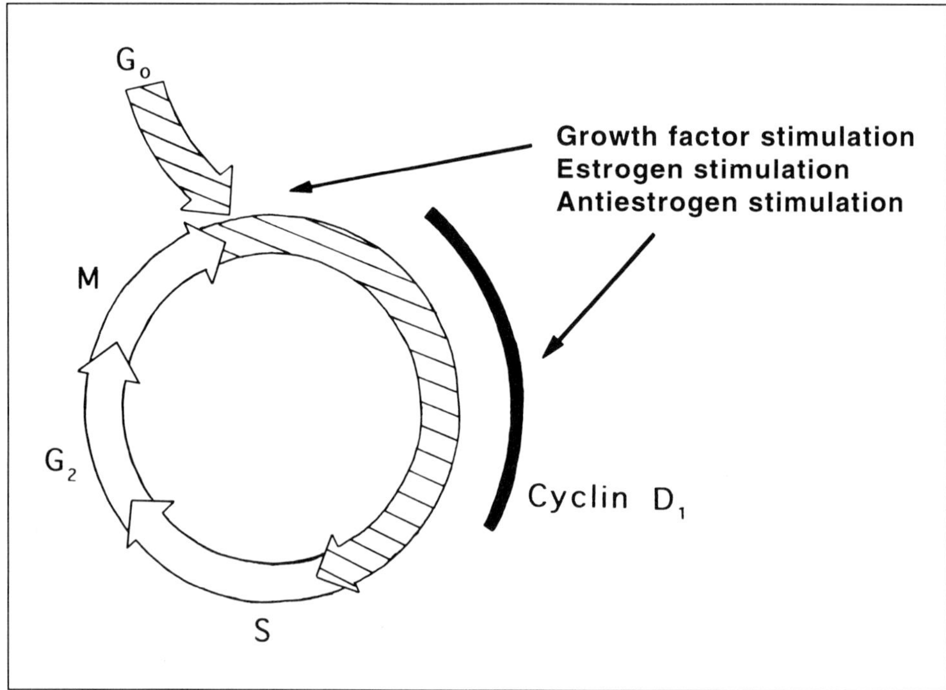

Fig. 10.7. Antiestrogens and cell-cycle control.

normal function of these genes was disrupted, for example by their underexpression or overexpression or by mutation, this could contribute to autonomous growth or loss of hormone sensitivity. Because aberrant expression of oncogenes, (for example c-*myc* and *cyclin* D1) and tumor suppressor genes (such as p53) which may be downstream targets for steroids is relatively common in breast cancer,[117-119] such genes potentially contribute to the acquisition of steroid insensitivity and resistance to endocrine agents. In particular, the central role for *cyclin* D1 in control of breast cancer cell progression[115] and the rapid decline in *cyclin* D1 messenger RNA levels after antiestrogen treatment of breast cancer cells[120,121] suggest that it may be involved in mediating antiestrogen inhibition of growth and the development of antiestrogen resistance. Failure of antiestrogens to inhibit *cyclin* D1 expression because of constitutive overexpression or upregulation/amplification of other signaling pathways[122,123] may result in continuous *cyclin* D1/CDK activation and cell cycle progression even in the presence of the growth inhibitor. Although such mechanisms are speculative at this time, several studies have described overexpression of *cyclin* D1 in breast cancer cell lines.[124]

Changed phenotype

Comparative studies of parental and tamoxifen-resistant cell lines have detected informative differences in patterns of secreted proteins. In particular, tamoxifen resistance may be associated by the lack of tamoxifen up-regulation of the synthesis of a 42 kD protein with presumed growth inhibitory functions.[128] Interestingly, pure antiestrogens which exert normal up-regulation of the protein also inhibit growth in the tamoxifen-resistant cells. Another candidate protein which appears to be selectively altered in tamoxifen resistant cells is the type 1 IGF receptor[129] which may be relevant because of the potential involvement of insulin-like growth factors in endocrine resistance.[60-63]

"Pure" antiestrogens and cross-resistance

Antiestrogens devoid of estrogenic activity such as ICI 182780[130] are currently being investigated as potential second-line endocrine treatments for tamoxifen-resistant patients. These drugs cause a decrease in cellular content of estrogen receptor protein by markedly reducing its half-life[131] and blocking nuclear-cytoplasmic shuttling so that the receptor is predominantly nuclear under equilibrium conditions.[132] In the presence of ICI 182780, nuclear re-entry does not occur and degradation takes place probably through lysozymes.

Recently, cross-resistance between the different types of antiestrogens using cell lines of breast cancer has been examined.[87,88] This has shown that tamoxifen-resistant cells generally retain responsiveness to 'pure' steroidal antiestrogens (Table 10.5). However, cells selected for resistance against the steroidal antiestrogens are usually cross-resistant to

Table 10.5. Cross-resistance to antiestrogens

Cell line	Selection Anti-estrogens	Test Antiestrogen	Cross-Resistance
LY2	LY 117018	Tamoxifen	Yes
LCC2	4-OH-Tamoxifen	ICI 164,384	No
MCF7-Tam^R-1	Tamoxifen	ICI 164,384	No
RL-3	Tamoxifen	4-OH Tamoxifen	Yes

tamoxifen.[88] Similar resistance patterns are apparent in patients. The logical sequence of treatment therefore is likely to be tamoxifen as first-line and steroidal antiestrogens as second-line therapies.[8,88,133]

AROMATASE INHIBITORS

Clinical experience suggests that as with other forms of endocrine therapy, cross-resistance to aromatase inhibitors is a major restraint on their use.[23,134] Given that their mechanism of action is to inhibit the enzyme activity associated with the aromatization of androgen to estrogen, consideration needs to be given to circumstances in which resistance may occur through differences in the aromatase enzyme.

Mutant aromatase

With the characterization of the molecular structure of the aromatase gene,[135] structure-function analyses have been performed.[136,137] Studies in which introduction of site mutations into the cDNA encoding for the enzyme have been informative. One particular point mutation has been shown to decrease sensitivity to the aromatase inhibitor 4-hydroxy-androstenedione without either changing that to aminoglutethimide or aromatase activity itself.[138] This phenotype has some relevance to breast tumors as a subset of cancers appears to have aromatase activity which is relatively insensitive to the inhibitory effects of 4-hydroxy-androstenedione while maintaining sensitivity to other aromatase inhibitors such as aminoglutethimide and fadrazole.[139,140]

High or induced aromatase

Resistance to aromatase inhibitors may also occur when levels of aromatase activity are so high that they cannot be blocked by the doses of inhibitors which are employed clinically. This seems to be the situation in premenopausal women in whom aromatase inhibitors have produced few successful results.[141] The high levels of aromatase in the ovary are difficult to block and, even when this is achieved, the resultant fall in circulating estrogens produces decreased feedback inhibition at the hypothalamus and pituitary; as a consequence, levels of gonadotrophins rise. This produces secondary increases in both androgen substrate and aromatase in the ovary.[134]

Drug treatment may also induce aromatase activity in peripheral tissues. Paradoxically, breast cancers derived from patients treated with aminoglutethimide display elevated levels.[142] This treatment regime also induces the aromatase system in model systems of fibroblast cell lines derived from breast adipose tissue which display a pronounced increase in aromatase activity when incubated with aminoglutethimide.[23,143] If these results are reproduced in vivo this may represent a mechanism by which tumors escape from the inhibitory effects of aminoglutethimide. However more potent inhibitors would offer the promise of second-line responses in such tumors.

ASSOCIATION WITH OTHER FEATURES OF AGGRESSIVE BEHAVIOR

The transformation from estrogen-dependent growth to that of an independent phenotype is frequently associated with other features of increased tumor aggressiveness, such as enhanced potential for metastasis and angiogenesis and decreased patient survival.[144-146] These characteristics can be mimicked in model systems in which hormone-dependent breast cancer cell lines are deprived of steroids on a long-term basis. Such cells have the ability to form estrogen-independent tumors in nude mice while displaying increased invasive capacity both in vitro and in vivo.[146]

SUMMARY

Breast cancer models have been developed with varying degrees of endocrine responsiveness and antiestrogen sensitivity which may represent different steps in the development of a fully endocrine non-responsive cell type. The fact that these do not conform to a single model suggests that multiple pathways lead to therapeutic failure and endocrine resistance. The cause of resistance may therefore differ in individual patients and consequently it may be necessary to use a variety of methods by which to overcome such resistance. The definition of the optimal route in individual patients may require specific information such as hormone status, tumor phenotype and the pharmokinetics of drug systems used to achieve endocrine deprivation.

REFERENCES

1. Anderson TJ, Miller WR. Morphological and biological observations relating to the development and progression of breast cancer. In: Dickson R, Lippman M, eds. Mammary tumorigenesis and malignant progression. Kluwer Academic Publishers 1994:3-27.
2. Hamm JT, Allegra JC. Loss of hormonal responsiveness in cancer. In: Stoll BA, ed. Endocrine management of cancer—biological bases. Basel, Karger Press 1988:61-71.
3. Hawkins RA, Roberts MM, Forrest APM. Oestrogen receptors and breast cancer: current status. Br J Surg 1980; 67:153-169.
4. Jordan VC, Wolf MF, Mirecki DM et al. Hormone receptor assays: clinical usefulness in the management of carcinoma of the breast. CRC Crt Rev Clin Lab Sciences 1988; 26:97-151.

5. Dowsett M, Johnston SRD, Newby J et al. Mechanisms of hormone response: a role for apoptosis. Endocrine Related Cancer 1995; 2:3-11.

6. Moore JW, Thomas BS, Wang DY. Endocrine status and the epidemiology and clinical course of breast cancer. Cancer Surveys 1986; 5:537-559.

7. Dowsett M, Harris AL, Smith IE et al. Endocrine changes associated with relapse in advanced breast cancer patients on aminoglutethimide therapy. J Clin Endocrinol Metab 1984; 58:99-104.

8. Howell A, Defriend D, Anderson E. Clues to the mechanism of endocrine resistance from clinical studies in advanced breast cancer. Endocrine Related Cancer 1995; 2:131-139.

9. Harris AL, Dowsett M, Jeffcoate SL et al. Endocrine and therapeutic effects of aminoglutethimide in premenopausal patients with breast cancer. J Clin Endocrinol Metab 1982; 55:718-720.

10. Santen RJ. Overall experience with aminoglutethimide in the management of advanced breast carcinoma. In: Elsdon-Dew RW, Jackson IM, Birdwood GFB, eds. Aminoglutethimide: an alternative endocrine therapy for breast carcinoma. London: Academic Press 1982:3.

11. Juranka PF, Zastawny RL, Ling V. P-glycoprotein multidrug resistance and a super family of membrane-associated transport proteins. FASEB 1989; 3:2583-2592.

12. Keen JC, Miller EP, Bellamy C et al. P-glycoprotein and resistance to tamoxifen. (Letter) Lancet 1994; 343:1047.

13. Santen RJ, Samojlik E, Worgul TJ. Aminoglutethimide product profile. In: Santen RJ, Henderson IC, eds. Pharmanual: a comprehensive guide to the therapeutic use of aminoglutethimide. Basel: S Karger 1981:101-160.

14. Murray FT, Santner S, Samojlik EA et al. Serum aminoglutethimide levels: studies of serum half-life, clearance and patient compliance. J Clin Pharmacol 1979; 19:704-711.

15. Greene GL, Sobel NB, King WJ et al. Immunochemical studies of estrogen receptors. J Steroid Biochem 1984; 20:51-56.

16. Isaacs JT. Clonal heterogeneity in relation to response. In: Stoll BA, ed. Endocrine management of cancer: biological bases. Basel: Karger, 1988:125-140.

17. Gross GE, Clark GM, Chamness GC. Multiple progesterone receptor assays in human breast cancer. Cancer Res 1984; 44:836-840.

18. Baildam AD, Zalrudik J, Howell A et al. Effects of tamoxifen upon cell DNA analysis by flow cytometry in primary carcinoma of the breast. Br J Cancer 1987; 55:561-566.

19. Stoll BA. Second endocrine response in breast, prostatic and endometrial cancers. Rev Endocr Related Cancers 1988; 30:19-25.

20. Taylor RE, Powles TJ, Humphreys J et al. Effects of endocrine therapy on steroid receptor content of breast cancer. Br J Cancer 1982; 45:80-85.

21. Allegra JC, Barlock A, Huff KK et al. Changes in multiple or sequential estrogen receptors in breast cancer. Cancer 1980; 45:792-794.

22. Hawkins RA, Tesdale AL, Anderson EDC et al. Does the oestrogen receptor concentration of a breast cancer change during systemic therapy? Br J Cancer 1990; 6:877-880.
23. Miller WR, Hawkins RA, Mullen P et al. Aromatase inhibition: determinants of response and resistance. Endocrine Related Cancer 1995; 2:73-85.
24. Johnston SRD, Saccani-Jotti G, Smith IE et al. Change in oestrogen receptor expression and function in tamoxifen-resistant breast cancer. Endocrine Related Cancer 1995; 2:105-110.
25. Darbre PD, Daly RJ. Effects of estrogen on human breast cancer cells in culture. Proc Roy Soc Edin 1989; 95B:119-132.
26. Hull DF III, Clark GM, Odborne CK et al. Multiple estrogen receptor assays in human breast cancer. Cancer Res 1983; 43:413-416.
27. Darbre PD, King RJB. Progression to steroid autonomy in S115 mouse mammary tumor cells: role of DNA methylation. J Cell Biol 1984; 99:1410-1415.
28. King RJB, Darbre PD. Progression from steroid responsive to unresponsive state in breast cancer. In: F Cavalli, ed. Endocrine therapy of breast cancer III. Berlin, Springer Verlag 1989:1-15.
29. Miller WR, Forrest APM. Oestradio synthesis from C19 steroids by human breast cancer. Br J Cancer 1974; 33:16-18.
30. Miller WR, Anderson TJ, Jack WJ. Relationship between tumour aromatase activity, tumour characteristics and response to therapy. J Steroid Biochem Molec Biol 1990; 37:1055-1059.
31. Miller WR. Endocrine treatment for breast cancers: biological rationale and current progress. J Steroid Biochem Molec Biol 1990; 37:467-480.
32. Katzenellenbogen BS. Antiestrogen resistance: mechanisms by which breast cancer cells undermine the effectiveness of endocrine therapy. JNCI 1991; 83:1434-1435.
33. Fuqua SAW. Abnormalities of the estrogen receptor in breast cancer—introduction. Breast Cancer Res Treat 1993; 26:117-118.
34. Karnik PS, Kulkarni S, Liu XP et al. Estrogen-receptor mutations in tamoxifen-resistant breast cancer. Cancer Res 1994; 54:349-353.
35. Garcia T, Lehrer S, Bloomer WD et al. A variant estrogen receptor messenger ribonucleic acid is associated with reduced levels of estrogen binding in human mammary tumors. Mol Endocrinol 1988; 2:785-789.
36. Garcia T, Sanchez M, Cox JL. Identification of a variant form of the human estrogen receptor with an amino acid replacement. Nucleic Acids Research 1989; 17:8364.
37. Lehrer S, Sanchez M, Song HK. Oestrogen receptor B-region polymorphism and spontaneous abortion in women with breast cancer. Lancet 1990; 335:622-624.
38. Murphy LC. At the cutting edge: Estrogen receptor variants in human breast cancer. Mol Cell Endocrinol 1990; 74:C83-C86.
39. McGuire WL, Chamnes GC, Fuqua SAW. The importance of normal and abnormal oestrogen receptor in breast cancer. Cancer Surveys 1992; 14:31-40.

40. Fuqua SA, Fitzgerald SD, Chamness GC et al. Variant human breast tumor estrogen receptor with constitutive transcriptional activity. Cancer Res 1991; 51:105-109.

41. Fuqua SAW, Wiltschke C, Castles C et al. A role for estrogen-receptor variants in endocrine resistance. Endocrine Related Cancer 1995; 2:19-25.

42. Zhang QX, Borg A, Fuqua SAW. An exon 5 deletion variant of the estrogen receptor frequently coexpressed with wild-type estrogen receptor in human breast cancer. Cancer Res 1993; 53:5882-5884.

43. Fuqua SAW, Falette NF, McGuire WL. Sensitive detection of estrogen receptor RNA by polymerase chain reaction assay JNCI 1990; 82:858-861.

44. Arteaga CL, Osborne CK. Growth factors as mediators of estrogen-antiestrogen action in human breast cancer cells. In: Lippman ME, Dickson RB, eds; Regulatory mechanisms in breast cancer. Boston: Kluwer Academic Press 1991:289.

45. Morishige K, Kuriche H, Amemiya K et al. Evidence for the involvement of transforming growth factor α and epidermal growth factor receptor in autocrine growth mechanism in primary human ovarian cancer in vitro. Cancer Res 1991; 51:5322-5328.

46. Reddy KB. Yee D, Hilsenbeck SG et al. Inhibition of estrogen-induced breast cancer cell proliferation by reduction in autocrine transforming growth factor a expression. Cell Growth & Differentiation 1994; 5:1275-1282.

47. Murphy LC, Dotzlaw H. Endogenous growth factor expression in T-47D, human breast cancer cells, associated with reduced sensitivity to antiproliferative effects of progestins and antiestrogens. Cancer Res 1989; 49:599-604.

48. Herman ME, Katzenellenbogen. Alterations in transforming growth factor-α and -β production and cell responsiveness during the progression of MCF-7 human breast cancer cells to estrogen-autonomous growth. Cancer Res 1994; 54:5867-5874.

49. Nicholson RI, McClelland RA, Gee JMW et al. Transforming growth factor-α and endocrine sensitivity in breast cancer. Cancer Res 1995; 54:1684-1689.

50. Nicholson RI, Bouzubar N, Walker KJ et al. Hormone sensitivity in breast cancer: influence of heterogeneity of oestrogen receptor expression and cell proliferation. Eur J Cancer 1991; 27:908-913.

51. Nicholson RI, McClelland RA, Finlay P et al. Relationship between EGF-R, c-erbB-2 protein expression and Ki67 immunostaining in breast cancer and hormone sensitivity. Eur J Cancer 1993; 39A:1018-1023.

52. Clarke R, Brunner N, Katz D. The effects of a constitutive expression of transforming growth factor-α on the growth of MCF-7 human breast cancer cells in vitro snf in vivo. Mol Endocrinol 1989; 3:372-380.

53. King RJB, Wang DY, Daly RJ et al. Approaches to studying the role of growth factors in the progression of breast tumours from the steroid sensitive to insensitive state. J Steroid Biochem 1989; 34:133-138.

54. Lundy J, Schuss A, Stanick D et al. Expression of neu protein, epidermal growth factor receptor and transforming growth factor a in breast cancer. Am J Pathol 1991; 138:1527-1534.

55. Umekita Y, Enokitono N, Sagara Y et al. Immunohistochemical studies on oncogene products (EGF-R, c-erbB-2) and growth factors (EGF, TGFα) in human breast cancer: their relationship to oestrogen receptor status, histological grade, mitotic index and nodal status. Virchows Arch A Pathol Anat 1992; 420:345-351.

56. Dublin EA, Barnes DM, Wang DY et al. TGFα and TGFβ in mammary carcinoma. J Pathol 1993; 170:15-22.

57. Brünner N, Moser C, Clarke R et al. IGF-I and IGF-II expression in human breast cancer xenografts: relationship to hormone independence. Breast Cancer Res Treat 1992; 22:39-45.

58. Brünner N, Yee D, Kern FG et al. Effect of endocrine therapy on growth of T61 human breast cancer xenografts is directly correlated to a specific down-regulation of insulin-like growth factor II (IGF-II). Eur J Cancer 1993; 29A:562-569.

59. Stewart AJ, Johnson MD, Mays FEB et al. Role of insulin-like growth factors and the type I insulin-like growth factor receptor in the estrogen-stimulated proliferation of human breast cancer cells. J Biol Chem 1990; 265:21172-21178.

60. Van der Burg B, Rutteman GR, Blankenstein A et al. Mitogenic stimulation of human breast cancer cells in a growth factor-defined medium: synergistic action of insulin and estrogen. J Cell Physiol 1988; 134:101-108.

61. Pekonen F, Partenen S, Makinen T et al. Receptors for epidermal growth factor and insulin-like growth factor 1 and their relation to steroid receptors in human breast cancer. Cancer Res 1988; 48:3716-3719.

62. Foekens JA, Portengen H, Janssen M et al. Insulin-like growth factor-1 receptors and insulin-like growth factor-1-like activity in human primary breast cancer. Cancer 1989; 63:2139-2147.

63. Knabbe C, Lippman ME, Wakefield LM et al. Evidence that transforming growth factor-beta is a hormonally regulated negative growth factor in human breast cancer cells. Cell 1987; 48:417-428.

64. MacCallum J, Bartlett JMS, Thompson AM et al. Expression of transforming growth factor beta mRNA isoforms in human breast cancer. Br J Cancer 1994; 69:1006-1009.

65. Walker RA, Dearing SJ, Gallacher B. Relationship of transforming growth factor beta 1 to extracellular matrix and stromal infiltrates in invasive breast carcinoma. Br J Cancer 1994; 69:1160-1165.

66. Arteaga CL, Carty-Dugger T, Moses HL et al. Transforming growth factor beta 1 can induce estrogen-independent tumorigenicity of human breast cancer cells in athymic mice. Cell Growth Differ 1993; 4:193-201.

67. McClelland RA, Finlay P, Dixon AR et al. Epidermal growth factor receptor and oestrogen receptor expression in breast cancer: relationship to endocrine sensitivity. Oncol (Life Sci Adv) 1993; 12:143-155.

68. Nicholson S, Halcrow P, Farndon JR et al. Expression of epidermal growth receptors associated with lack of response to endocrine therapy in recurrent breast cancer. Lancet 1989; 1:182-185.

69. Nicholson S, Wright C, Sainsbury JRC et al. Epidermal growth factor receptor as a marker of poor prognosis in node negative patients: neu and tamoxifen failure. J Steroid Biochem 1990; 37:811-814.

70. Arteaga CL, Coronado E, Osborne CK. Blockade of the epidermal growth factor receptor inhibits transforming growth factor alpha-induced but not estrogen-induced growth of hormone-dependent human breast cancer. Mol Endocrinol 1988; 2:1064-1069.

71. Yamamoto T, Ikawa S, Akiyama T et al. Similarity of protein encoded by the human c-erb-B-2 gene to epidermal growth factor receptor. Nature 1986; 319:230-234.

72. McGuire WL, Tandon AK, Allred DC et al. How to use prognostic factors in axillary node-negative breast cancer patients. JNCI 1990; 82:1006-1015.

73. Muss HB, Thor AD, Berry DA et al. c-erbB-2 expression and response to adjuvant therapy in women with node-positive early breast cancer. New Eng J Med 1993; 330:1260-1266.

74. Gullick WJ, Love SB, Wright C et al. c-erbB-2 protein overexpression in breast cancer is a risk factor in patients with involved and uninvolved lymph nodes. Br J Cancer 1991; 63:434-438.

75. Schonborn I, Zschiesche W, Spitzer E et al. C-*erb*B-2 overexpression in primary breast cancer—independent prognostic factor in patients at high risk. Breast Cancer Res Treat 1994; 29:287-295.

76. Wright C, Nicholson S, Angus B et al. Relationship between c-*erb*B-2 protein product expression and response to endocrine therapy in advanced breast cancer. Br J Cancer 1992; 65:118-121.

77. Borg A, Baldetorp B, Fernö M et al. ErbB2 amplification is associated with tamoxifen resistance in steroid-receptor positive breast cancer. Cancer Letts 1994; 81:137-144.

78. Antoniotti S, Maggiora P, Dati C et al. Tamoxifen up-regulates c-erbB-2 expression in oestrogen-responsive breast cancer cells in vitro. Eur J Cancer 1992; 28:318-321.

79. Benz CC, Scott GK, Sarup JC et al. Estrogen-dependent tamoxifen-resistant tumorigenic growth of MCF-7 cells transfected with HER2/*neu*. Breast Cancer Res Treat 1992; 24:85-95.

80. Wolf DM, Jordan VC. Drug resistance to tamoxifen during breast cancer therapy. Breast Cancer Res Treat 1993; 27:27-40.

81. Muss HB, Endocrine therapy for advanced breast cancer: a review. Breast Cancer Res Treat 1992; 21:15-26.

82. Early Breast Cancer Trialists Collaborative Group: Systemic treatment of early breast cancer by hormonal, cytotoxic or immune therapy: 133 ran-

domized trials involving 31000 recurrences and 24000 deaths among 75000 women. Lancet 1992; 339:1-15, 71-85.

83. Legault-Poisson S, Jolivet J, Poisson R et al. Tamoxifen-induced tumor stimulation and withdrawal response. Cancer Treat Rep 1979; 63:1839-1841.

84. Canney PA, Griffiths T, Latief TN et al. Clinical significance of tamoxifen withdrawal response. Lancet 1987; i:36.

85. Katzenellenbogen BS, Kendra KL, Norman MJ et al. Proliferation, hormone responsiveness and estrogen receptor content of MCF-7 human breast cancer cells grown in the short-term and long-term absence of estrogens. Cancer Res 1987; 47:4355-4360.

86. Welshons WV, Jordan VC. Adaption of oestrogen-dependent MCF-7 cells to low oestrogen (phenol red-free) culture. Eur J Cancer Clin Oncol 1987; 45:118-128.

87. Westley BR, May FEB. In vitro development of tamoxifen resistance. Endocrine Related Cancer 1995; 2:37-44.

88. Clarke R, Brünner N. Cross-resistance and molecular mechanisms in antiestrogen resistance. Endocrine Related Cancer 1995; 2:59-72.

89. Paik S, Hartmann DP, Dickson RB et al. Antiestrogen resistance in ER positive breast cancer cells. Breast Cancer Res Treat 1994; 31:301-307.

90. Jordan VC, Murphy CS. Endocrine pharmacology of antiestrogens as antitumor agents. Endocr Rev 1991; 11:578-610.

91. Sawaka CA, Pritchard KI, Paterson DJA et al. Role and mechanism of action of tamoxifen in premenopausal women with metastatic breast cancer. Cancer Res 1986; 46:3152-3156.

92. Stewart HJ. Clinical experience in the use of the antioestrogen tamoxifen in the treatment of breast cancer. Proc Roy Soc Edin 1989; 95B:231-237.

93. Jordan VC, Fritz NF, Langan-Fahey S et al. Alteration of endocrine parameters in premenopausal women with breast cancer during long-term tamoxifen monotherapy. JNCI 1991; 83:1488-1491.

94. Sutherland RL, Murphy LC, Foo MS et al. High affinity antioestrogen binding site distinct from the oestrogen receptor. Nature 1980; 288:273-275.

95. Pavlik EJ, Nelson K, Srinivasan S et al. Resistance to tamoxifen with persisting sensitivity to estrogen: possible mediation by excessive antiestrogen binding site activity. Cancer Res 1992; 52:4106-4112.

96. Adam HK, Douglas EJ, Kemp JV. The metabolism of tamoxifen in humans. Biochem Pharmacol 1979; 27:145-152.

97. Wiebe VJ, Osborne CK, McGuire WL et al. Identification of estrogenic tamoxifen metabolite(s) in tamoxifen-resistant human breast tumors. J Clin Oncol 1992; 10:990-994.

98. Osborne CK, Coronado E, Allred DC et al. Acquired tamoxifen resistance: correlation with reduced breast tumor levels of tamoxifen and isomerization of trans-4-hydroxytamoxifen. JNCI 1991; 83:1477-1482.

99. Osborne CK, Wiebe V, McGuire W et al. Tamoxifen and the isomers of 4-hydroxy-tamoxifen in tamoxifen-resistant tumors from breast cancer patients. J Clin Oncol 1992; 10:304-310.

100. Johnston SRD, Haynes BP, Smith IE et al. Acquired tamoxifen resistance in human breast cancer and reduced intra-tumoral drug concentration. Lancet 1993; 342:1521-1522.
101. Osborne CK, Coronado EB, Robinson JP. Human breast cancer in the athymic nude mouse: cytostatic effects of long-term antiestrogen therapy. Eur J Cancer Clin Oncol 1987; 23:1189-1196.
102. Gottardis MM, Jordan VC. Development of tamoxifen-stimulated growth of MCF-7 tumors in athymic mice after long-term antiestrogen administration. Cancer Res 1988; 48:5183-5187.
103. Osborne CK, Jarman M, McCague R et al. The importance of tamoxifen metabolism in tamoxifen-stimulated breast tumor growth. Cancer Cehm Pharmacol 1994; 34:89-95.
104. Murphy CS, Langan-Fahey SM, McCague R et al. Structure function relationships of hydroxylated metabolites of tamoxifen that control the proliferation of estrogen responsive T47D breast cancer cells in vitro. Mol Pharm 1990; 38:737-743.
105. Wolf DM, Langan-Fahey SM, Parker CJ et al. Investigation of the mechanism of tamoxifen-stimulated breast tumor growth with non-isomerizable analogues of tamoxifen and metabolites. JNCI 1993; 85:806-812.
106. Osborne CK. Tamoxifen metabolism as a mechanism for resistance. Endocrine Related Cancer 1995; 2:53-58.
107. Jordan VC, Catherino WL, Wolf DM. Drug resistance to tamoxifen: mutant estrogen receptors as a potential mechanism of tamoxifen-stimulated tumor growth. Endocrine Related Cancer 1995; 2:45-51.
108. Fujimoto N, Katzenellenbogen BS. Alteration in the agonist/antagonist balance of antiestrogens by activation of protein kinase A signalling pathways in breast cancer cells: antiestrogen-selectivity and promoter-dependence. Mol Endocrinol 1994; 8:296-304.
109. Sutherland RL, Green MD, Hall RE et al. Tamoxifen induces accumulation of MCF-7 human mammary carcinoma cells in the G_o/G_1 phase of the cell cycle. J Cancer Clin Oncol 1983; 19:615-621.
110. Sutherland RL, Hall RE, Tayalor IW. Cell proliferation kinetics of MCF-7 human mammary carcinoma cells in culture and effects of tamoxifen on exponentially growing and plateau-phase cells. Cancer Res 1983; 43:3998-4006.
111. Taylor IW, Hodson PJ, Green MD et al. Effects of tamoxifen on cell cycle progression of synchronous MCF-7 human mammary carcinoma cells. Cancer Res 1983; 43:4007-4010.
112. Musgrove EA, Wakeling AE, Sutherland RL. Points of action of estrogen antagonists and a calmodulin antagonist within the MCF-7 human breast cancer cell cycle. Cancer Res 1989; 49:2398-2404.
113. Motokura T, Arnold A. Cyclins and oncogenesis. Biochem Biophys 1993; 1155:63-78.
114. Pines J. Cyclins and cyclin-dependent kinases: take your partners. Trends Biol Sci 1993; 18:195-197.

115. Musgrove EA, Lee CSL, Buckley MF et al. Cyclin D1 induction in breast cancer cells shortens G_1 and is sufficient for cells arrested in G_1 to complete the cell cycle. Proc Nat Acad Sci USA 1994; 91:8022-8026.
116. Sutherland RL, Watts CKW, Musgrove EA. Cell cycle control by steroid hormones in breast cancer: implications for endocrine resistance. Endocrine Related Cancer 1995; 2:87-96.
117. Callahan R, Cropp CS, Merlo GR et al. Somatic mutations of human breast cancer—a status-report. Cancer 1992; 69:1582-1588.
118. Deng G, Chen-LC, Schott DR et al. Loss of heterozygosity and p53 gene mutations in breast cancer. Cancer Res 1994; 54:499-505.
119. Shiu RPC, Watson PH, Dubik D. c-myc oncogene expression in estrogen-dependent and -independent breast cancer. Clin Chem 1993; 39:353-355.
120. Musgrove EA, Hamilton JA, Lee CSL et al. Growth factor steroid and steroid antagonist regulation of cyclin gene expression associated with chantes in T-47D human breast cancer cell cycle progression. Mol Cell Biol 1993; 13:3577-3587.
121. Watts CKW, Sweeney KJE, Warlters A et al. Antiestrogen regulation of cell cycle progression and cyclin D1 gene expression in MCF-7 human breast cancer cells. Breast Cancer Res Treat 1994; 31:95-105.
122. Daly RJ, Binder MD, Sutherland RL. Overexpression of the Grb2 gene in human breast cancer cell lines. Oncogene 1994; 9:2723-2727.
123. Janes PW, Daly RJ, deFazio A et al. Activation of the Ras signalling pathway in human breast cancer cells overexpressing erbB-2. Oncogene 1994; 19:3601-3608.
124. Fantl V, Smith R, Brookes S et al. Chromosome 11q13 abnormalities in human breast cancer. Cancer Surveys 1993; 18:77-93.
125. Buckley MF, Sweeney KJE, Hamilton JA et al. Expression and amplification of cyclin genes in human breast cancer. Oncogene 1993; 8:2127-2133.
126. Barktova J, Lukas J, Müller H et al. Cyclin D1 protein expression and function in human breast cancer. Int J Cancer 1994; 57:353-361.
127. Gillett C, Fantl V, Smith R. Amplification and overexpression of cyclin D1 in breast cancer detected by immunohistochemical staining 1994; Cancer Res 1994; 54:1812-1817.
128. Lykkesfeldt AE, Madsen MW, Briand P. Altered expression of estrogen-regulated genes in a tamoxifen-resistant and ICI 164,383 and ICI 182,780 sensitive human breast cancer cell line MCF-7/TAM[R]-1[1]. Cancer Res 1994; 54:1587-1595.
129. Wiseman LR, Johnson MD, Wakeling AE et al. Type I IGF receptor and acquired tamoxifen resistance in oestrogen-responsive human breast cancer cells. Eur J Cancer 1993; 29A:2256-2264.
130. Wakeling AE, Dukes M, Bowler J. A potent specific pure antiestrogen with clinical potential. Cancer Res 1991; 51:3867-3873.
131. Dauvois S, Danielian PS, White R et al. Antiestrogen ICI 164,384 reduces cellular estrogen receptor content by increasing its turnover. Proc Nat Acad Sci USA 1992; 89:4037-4041.

132. Dauvois S, White R, Parker MG. The antiestrogen ICI 182780 disrupts estrogen receptor nucleocytoplasmic shuttling. J Cell Sci 1993; 106: 1377-1388.

133. De Friend DJ, Howell A, Nicholson RI et al. Investigation of a new pure antiestrogen (ICI 182780) in women with primary breast cancer. Cancer Res 1994; 54:1-7.

134. Miller WR. Aromatase inhibitors in the treatment of advanced cancer. Canter Treat Revs 1989; 16:83-93.

135. Corbin CJ, Graham-Lorence S, McPhaul M et al. Isolation of a full-length cDNA insert encoding human aromatase system cytochrome P-450 and its expression in nonsteroidogenic cells. Proc Nat Acad Sci USA 1988; 85:8948-8952.

136. Graham-Lorence S, Khaili MW, Lorence MC et al. Structure-function relationships of human aromatase cytochrome P-450 using molecular modeling and site-directed mutagenesis. J Biol Chem 1991; 266: 11939-11946.

137. Chen S, Zhou D. Functional domains of aromatase cytochrome P450 inferred from comparative analyses of amino acid sequences and substantiated by site-directed mutagenesis experiments. J Biol Chem 1992; 267:22587-22594.

138. Kadohama N, Yarborough C, Zhou D et al. Kinetic properties of aromatase mutants Pro308Phe, Asp309Asn and Asp309Ala and their interactions with aromatase inhibitors. J Steroid Biochem Mol Biol 1992; 43:693-701.

139. James VHT, Reed MJ, Adams EF et al. Oestrogen uptake and metabolism in vivo. Proc Roy Soc Edin 1989; 95B:185-193.

140. Miller WR. In vitro and in vivo effects of 4-hydroxyandrostenedione on steroid and tumour metabolism. In: Coombes RC, Dowsett M (eds), 4-Hydroxyandrostenedione—a new approach to hormone-dependent Cancer. Roy Soc Med Services Ltd Int Congress & Symposium Series 1992:45-50.

141. Harris AL, Dowsett M, Jeffcoate SL et al. Endocrine and therapeutic effects of aminoglutethimide in premenopausal patients with breast cancer. J Clin Endocrinol Metab 1982; 55:718-720.

142. Miller WR, O'Neill JS. The importance of local synthesis of estrogen within the breast. Steroids 1988, 50:537-548.

143. Miller WR, Mullen P. Factors influencing aromatase activity in the breast. J Steroid Biochem Molec Biol 1993; 44:597-604.

144. Howell A, Barnes DM, Harland RN et al. Steroid hormone receptors and survival after first relapse in breast cancer. Lancet 1984; 1:588-591.

145. Macaulay VM, Fox SB, Zhang H et al. Breast cancer angiogenesis and tamoxifen resistance. Endocrine Related Cancer 1995; 2:97-103.

146. Brünner N, Johnson MD, Holst-Hansen C et al. Acquisition of estrogen independence and antiestrogen resistance in breast cancer: association with the invasive and metastatic phenotype. Endocrine Related Cancer 1995; 2:27-35.

FUTURE PERSPECTIVES

To put the future into context it is useful to reflect on the past. There is no doubt that we have come a long way since the initial observations by Sir Percival Potts and Sir George Beatson in the 18th and 19th centuries, that ovarian function can influence both the development of the normal breast and the natural history of breast cancer. Since then the natural principles responsible for these effects have been identified as steroid hormones, in particular estrogens. Their chemical structures have been characterized and their pathways of biosynthesis elucidated. It is also clear that biosynthesis occurs not only in endocrine glands such as the ovary but also in peripheral sites which include breast adipose tissue and cancer. The factors controlling biosynthesis within the ovary have been identified but those in peripheral tissues remain largely undefined. Despite the comparatively low levels of estrogen which circulate and are needed for trophic effects, assays have been established for the measurement of estrogens in blood and other biological fluids.

The diverse nature of estrogenic influences is recognized and their mechanism of action is defined as involving specific protein receptors which act as nuclear transcription factors. Key molecules which mediate and modulate estrogenic effects have been identified. These include mitogenic growth factors and cell cycle regulators, providing an explanation for the influences that estrogens have on key developmental processes, such as proliferation and differentiation.

In parallel with these discoveries, corresponding advances have been made in relation to the risk, development, progression and prognosis of breast cancer. Many established risk factors for breast cancer implicate estrogens, at least in a permissive role. Molecules involved in carcinogenesis have been recognized and cellular factors have been uncovered which determine the behavior of established tumors and thereby influence prognosis. In terms of treatment, endocrinology and tumor biology have come together so that drug therapy based on inhibition of hormone release, synthesis and action can be applied in a rational management strategy. While at this stage the effects on mortality are limited, there has been a major improvement in terms of sparing patients the unnecessary side-effects of ineffective treatment.

Despite these advances, the causes of breast cancer are still largely unknown, the incidence of the disease has not been markedly diminished (and indeed may be increasing in underdeveloped countries), and survival rates have not been substantially reduced. Therefore we need to look to the promise of the future.

ESTROGEN AND THE NORMAL BREAST

While estrogens are critical to the development and function of the normal breast, there are many questions to be answered. Does estrogen play a primary or permissive role on proliferation within resting TDLU? Physiological levels of estrogen are evidently stimulatory—the breast shows little activity before puberty and after the menopause; in contrast, estrogen levels and proliferative activity are less closely linked during the menstrual cycle when proliferation is highest in the luteal phase, many days after the peak level of estrogen. Is estrogen simply a primer inducing other agents which are true mitogens. There are also other unanswered questions such as (i) what are the target cells for estrogen within the breast? (can stromal cells be ignored?), (ii) what is the significance of the heterogeneous staining for ER within and between lobules? (iii) what causes the apparent up-regulation of ER which can occur during the transition to malignancy in the breast?

There are practical difficulties in addressing such questions in terms of limited access to relevant clinical material (which has recently been exacerbated by the more conservative surgical management of benign breast disease) and the paucity of good model systems for the human breast. The future offers hope in both these areas. We can look forward to non-invasive monitoring of the breast by imaging techniques. For example, although still in its infancy NMR may crudely assess phosphorylation status within the breast.[1] Additionally, the use of natural and artificial basement membranes has allowed reconstruction of the three-dimensional lobular structure[2] and the establishment of xenografts of human breast in immunosuppressed animals.[3] These model systems will be complimented by transgenic and knock-out animals in which specific gene products such as estrogen receptors and inducible products can be switched on and off so that their role in mammary development may be assessed under controlled experimental conditions.

ESTROGENS AND RISK OF BREAST CANCER

While established risk factors for breast cancer point to hazards of cumulative life-time exposure to bio-available estrogen, the data are not totally conclusive and it is important to collect more supportive evidence. In this respect, more definitive data will shortly be available on the use of exogenous estrogens. Thus, clinical investigations of estrogen replacement therapy and oral contraception are maturing and the latency period which might be expected between estrogen exposure and appearance of breast cancers will be exceeded in substantive numbers of women.

Whether increased exposure to environmental estrogens augments risk also needs to be evaluated. Initially it will be necessary to screen industrial pollutants for their inherent estrogenicity/carcinogenicity. Test-systems are being developed based on breast cells transfected with estrogen receptors and reporter genes and experimental animals genetically engineered to be deficient to estrogen receptor protein (indeed the latter model will answer the fundamental question of whether estrogen receptors are required for the development of breast cancer[4]).

If these studies confirm the association between increased risk and cumulative exposure to diverse estrogenic stimuli, there remain the further problems of how to assess this risk accurately and how to develop preventative strategies. In terms of the latter, both tamoxifen and LHRH agonists are now the subject of clinical studies[5] but the feeling remains that while such interventions may be feasible in committed high-risk individuals, they will not be acceptable to the general population. The search must therefore continue for less artificial methods of reducing risk. The concept of identifying natural antiestrogens and adopting dietary approaches may yet prove to be fruitful. Current social trends are not necessarily in the correct direction. The pattern of oral contraceptive use has changed—teenagers are taking oral contraceptives earlier and the average age at first pregnancy is later. Consequently, the duration of uninterrupted use before pregnancy is becoming extended. The possibility of inducing an "artificial" pregnancy needs to be explored.

ESTROGENS AND TUMOR BEHAVIOR

There are practical questions which have to be considered for patients who have been diagnosed with breast cancer and wish either to continue the use of contraceptive steroids, start hormone replacement therapy for menopausal symptoms or become pregnant. The particular concern is whether estrogen supplementation or excess will stimulate occult metastatic disease and adversely affect prognosis. Definitive results are expected from ongoing clinical studies designed to address these issues.

SOURCES OF ESTROGEN

That the ovary is the major site of estrogen biosynthesis in premenopausal women is undeniable; yet the suggestion persists that other estrogenic stimuli may be influential. Phytoestrogens in the diet may have a direct action on the breast or modify the menstrual cycle. Effects on the development and growth of breast cancer are controversial and it still remains to be determined whether industrial pollutants such as plasticizers and pesticides have sufficient estrogenicity to be effective against a background of more potent natural estrogens, especially in premenopausal women. Nevertheless, as was indicated earlier, the systems by which to test this are being developed. Effects of exogenous estrogens are much more feasible in postmenopausal women in whom the sources of estrogen are less well defined. While the capacity of estrogen biosynthesis has been demonstrated in many peripheral tissues, most notably adipose tissue, muscle and breast tumors, it still has to be resolved whether distant aromatase activity (via endocrine supply) or local biosynthesis (functioning in an autocrine/paracrine manner) maintains the growth of estrogen-dependent breast cancers. In vitro studies whereby androgen and estrogen are simultaneously administered to patients before and after treatment with antiestrogens and aromatase inhibitors will be informative. Research into the aromatase enzyme and its molecular controls is also ongoing. Recent work suggests that the promoters for transcription of the aromatase gene may be tissue-specific,[7] opening up the possibility of differential controls by which to switch estrogen biosynthesis on and off selectively at particular sites.

The future development of non-invasive non-radioactive technology will also allow a more accurate assessment of in situ metabolism such that it will become possible to assess the relevance of alternative pathways of estrogen biosynthesis and metabolism.

LEVELS AND PATTERNS OF ESTROGEN IN THE BREAST

The monitoring of estrogen dynamics in situ within the breast will undoubtedly shed light on the origin of the unusual patterns of estrogen within breast fluids and tissues. Parallel advances in histochemistry and molecular pathology should also confirm the tissue and cellular distribution of such estrogens. Microdissection of the breast for estrogen analyses and molecular painting for estrogen inducible genes and products will also indicate whether the estrogens are in a biologically active form.

MECHANISM OF ESTROGEN ACTION

This is an area in which the future offers the prospect of rapid progress. Technical advances in molecular biology mean that in the next few years promoters for the estrogen receptor gene will have been characterized, the significance of variants of the estrogen receptor molecules will be clarified and the factors which influence estrogen-induced transcription identified.[8] Genetically engineered systems in which estrogen receptors and estrogen-induced products are selectively switched on or suppressed will distinguish between effects directly attributable to estrogen and those involving other signaling pathways.[4] The opportunity will arise to target specific estrogen-related products differentially and to direct effects to particular target sites.

ESTROGEN DEPRIVATION THERAPY

Drugs which have the characteristics of "pure" antiestrogens and "pure" aromatase inhibitors are now entering the clinic.[9,10] These agents have high specificity and potency and can provide a complete blockage of estrogen action and synthesis. Within a few years it will be known whether treatment is associated with increased response rates and, if so, whether this translates into an improved cure rate.[3] Results from clinical trials will determine the place of such therapies in the context of other forms of treatment modalities. While the drugs will be initially used in advanced breast cancer, there will be pressure for use in earlier stages of the disease, particularly in an adjuvant situation. As this will probably entail long-term therapy, acceptability will depend upon the side-effects of prolonged estrogen deprivation and the possibility of reversing such effects in non-malignant tissues, in particular protecting bone and the vasculature. Combining drugs with targeting vectors could be the answer whereby site-directed therapies control breast cancer without having detrimental effects on coronary heart disease and osteoporosis.

Gene therapy targeting the overexpression of estrogen receptors in tumors has yet to be fully exploited. Similarly, other molecules on the downstream pathway of estrogen action such as cyclins, growth factors and their receptors could be usefully disabled to produce anti-tumor effects.

PREDICTION OF ESTROGEN SENSITIVITY/DEPENDENCY

Molecular technology can be expected to identify important markers which predict for estrogen sensitivity. Methods by which to assess ER functionality have already been developed such as RT-PCR for variant molecules, gel shift assays to assess DNA binding activity and antibodies to measure ER functional domains.[11] Accurate prediction of both degree and type of estrogen sensitivity and the molecules to target as therapy can be envisaged. This should lead to a fully rational management strategy for estrogen deprivation.

RESISTANCE TO ENDOCRINE THERAPY

The most important challenge facing estrogen deprivation therapy is acquired resistance. Hopefully, a greater understanding of the mechanism involved will lead to strategies by which to circumvent the process. Such knowledge may also help to by-pass de novo resistance and that of other treatment modalities. Progress is being facilitated by the development of appropriate model cell lines and xenograft systems.[12] Even at this stage it is clear that no single model reflects the spectrum of clinically resistant tumors. Just as multiple pathways lead to therapeutic failure, circumvention is likely to be multifactorial. Nevertheless, measurements in these model systems and clinical material from resistant patterns are informative. To date, most attention has focused on the estrogen receptor and the possibility that ER variants may be either dominant-positive (transcriptionally active in the absence of estrogen) or dominant-negative (inactivate wild-type function).[13] In the next few years the role of truncated and alternative estrogen receptors in estrogen-resistant disease will be fully evaluated. Experiments are already underway in which mutant and variant estrogen receptors are being introduced into animals whose wild type expression has been deleted.[4] Similar models will determine the role of genes normally induced as a result of estrogen action.

It is also clear that the mechanism by which estrogens and antiestrogens regulate cellular proliferation may be underpinned by interacting with growth factor signaling; a greater knowledge of the process may therefore lead to a better understanding of how such controls are by-passed.

Finally, the introduction of the ER gene into receptor-negative breast cancer cells might theoretically confer hormone sensitivity and produce a more differentiated and less aggressive phenotype. Current experimentation suggests that the effect of transfecting ER genes depends upon the cell into which ER is being introduced, the levels of ER expressed and the ER responsive genes induced.[14] Interestingly the growth of transfected cells may be inhibited (rather than stimulated) by physiological levels of estrogen.[14,15]

SUMMARY

The links coupling estrogens to the breast were forged many years ago and, if the future reflects the past, it may be some time before answers are available to fundamental questions. However, these are exciting times and the potential is almost unlimited. Furthermore, the twin prizes of prevention and cure of breast cancer will yield immense rewards. A prevention strategy with even a modest success rate of 1 in 5 is calculated to reduce worldwide incidence by 250,000 cases per year. Similarly an effective estrogen deprivation therapy combined with efficient measures to circumvent acquired resistance will offer personal cures to the majority of women with a diagnosis of breast cancer.

REFERENCES

1. Twelves CJ, Lowry M, Porter DA et al. Phosphorus-31 metabolism of human breast—an in vivo magnetic resonance spectroscopic study at 1.5 Tesla. Br J Radiol 1994; 67:36-45.
2. Yang J, Guzman RC, Popnikolov N et al. Phenotypic characterization of collagen gel embedded primary human breast epithelial cells in athymic nude mice. Cancer-Lett 1994; 81:117-27.
3. Miller FR, Soule HD, Tait L et al. Xenograft model of progressive human proliferative breast disease. J Natl Cancer Inst 1993; 85:1725-1732.
4. Korach KS. Insights from the study of animals lacking functional estrogen receptor. Science 1994; 266:1524-1527.
5. Fentiman IS. Prevention of Breast Cancer. Austin: RG Landes Co. 1993.

6. Russo J, Russo IH. The etiopathogenesis of breast cancer prevention. Cancer Letters 1994; 90:81-89.
7. Simpson ER, Mahendroo MS, Nichols JE et al. Aromatase gene expression in adipose tissue: relationship to breast cancer. Int J Fertil Menopausal Stud 1994; 39:75-83.
8. Halachmi S, Marden E, Martin G et al. Estrogen receptor-associated proteins—possible mediators of hormone-induced transcription. Science 1994; 264:1455-1458.
9. De Friend DJ, Howell A, Nicholson RI et al. Investigations of a new pure antiestrogen (ICI-182780) in women with primary breast cancer. Cancer Res 1994; 54:408-414.
10. Lipton A, Demers LM, Harvey HA et al. Letrozole (CGS 20267)—a phase I study of a new potent oral aromatase inhibitor of breast cancer. Cancer 1995; 75:2132-2138.
11. Traish AN, Al-Fadhli S, Klinge C et al. Identification of structurally altered estrogen receptors in human breast cancer by site-directed monoclonal antibodies. Steroids 1995; 60:467-474.
12. Clarke R, Brünner N. Cross-resistance and molecular mechanisms in antiestrogen resistance. Endocrine-Related Cancer 1995; 2:59-72.
13. Wiltschke C, Fuqua SAW. Clinical relevance of estrogen receptor variants in breast cancer. Trends Endocrinol Metab 1995; 6:77-82.
14. Catherino WH, Jordan VC. The biological action of cDNAs from mutated estrogen receptors transfected into breast cancer cells. Cancer Lett 1995; 90:35-42.
15. Levenson AS, Jordan VC. Transfection of human estrogen receptor (ER) cDNA into ER-negative mammalian cell lines. J Steroid Biochem Mol Biol 1994; 51:229-239.

═══ INDEX ═══

Page numbers in italics denote figures (f) or tables (t).

A

Abe R, 63
ACTH, 82, 139
adrenalectomy, 20, 65, 76, 125, 127-128, 139-140,
　　153, *179t*, 180
adriamycin, 20
albumin, 7, 48
amenorrhea, 129, 136
aminoglutethimide (CGS16949), 84-85, 139-141,
　　173, 186-187
androgens
　　Δ5-, 81
　　adrenal, 27, 38, 81, 142, 180
androstenedione, 6-7, 81
　　Δ4-, 3, 81, 86
　　4-hydroxy-, *140t*, 141, 186
anovulation, 37
antiestrogen(s), 20, *65t*, 114-116, 125, 132-137,
　　176-177, *179t*, 180-187, 199. *See also*
　　　tamoxifen
　　pure, 143, 183, 185-186, 200
aromatase, 78, 80-86, 107
　　inhibitor(s), 20, 65, 76, 81, 126, 137-143, 153,
　　　173, *179t*, 180, 186-187, 200
Arteaga CL, 178

B

Banders-van Halewun EA, 46
Beatson GT, 125, 197
benign breast disease, 16, *47t*, 97
Bergkvist L, 41
Bradlow, HL, 51, 99
breast fluid(s), 95-98, 107
Bulbrook RD, 45, 49, 67

C

C18 steroids, 1, 10
c-*erb*B-2, 20, 117, 162, 179
c-*fos*, 52
c-*myc*, 20, 52, 117, 185
cancer, endometrial, 39
castration, 20, 35, 39, 125, 128, 131, 137
cathepsin D, *9t*, 101, 116
CGS20267, 141
contraceptive(s), oral, 11, 29, 42-43, 198-199
cross-talk, 183-184
cyclin D1, 184-185
cyst fluid(s), 98-101
cytochrome p450, 3, 137, 139, 141

D

daidzein, 11, 76-78
Dao TL, 65
De Waard F, 46
dehydroepiandrosterone (DHA), 81, 97, 99, 100,
　　101f
detergents, 11, 75, 78
DHEA sulfate, 86
diethylstilbestrol, 11, 39, 41, 52, 65, 132
dysgenesis, gonadal, 25

E

efflux pump, 172-173
ELISA, 156
endometrium, 9, 20, 29, 68, 103
enterodiol, 11
enterolactone, 77
equol, 11, 77, *78t*
erbA oncogene protein, 10
*erb*B-2, 178
ERICA, 156-157
estradiol, 1, 3-7, 9-10, 37, 45-49, 66-67, 76,
　　80-81, 85-86, 88, 96-99, 101-107, 113-115,
　　117, 131, 135, 180, 183. *See also*
　　　phytoestrogen(s).
　　-17β, 1, 42, 88
　　ethinyl, 11
　　glucoronide, 45
　　sulfate, 86, 99
estriol, 45, 96, 99-100
estrogen(s)
　　catechol, 8, 52
　　17β dehydrogenase, 4, 7
　　endogenous, 11, 45, 50, 53, 102, 107, 132,
　　　135, 142
　　environmental, 11, 75, 199
　　exogenous, 38-44, 53, 64, 75-78, 135, 179,
　　　198-199
　　lipoidal (E_2-L), 88
　　receptor(s)(ER), 29, 68-69, 103, 111-112, 127,
　　　133, 151-157, 162, 175-176, 179-180,
　　　181t, 183, 198, 201-202
　　　-negative cells, 69, 87-88, 115, 134-135,
　　　　140, 153-160, 162, 171-173, 176
　　　-positive cells, 69, 86-87, 113, 115, 126,
　　　　129, 132-134, 140, 151-161, 174, 176
　　replacement therapy (ERT), 39-42, 64
　　sulfatase, 86

estrone, 1, 3, 5-7, 9, 45, 48, 67, 76, 86, 96-99,
        102-103, 105-107
    glucosiduronate, 96
    sulfate, 6-7, 45, 85, 86, 99-100, 102-103, 105,
        143
ethinyl estradiol, 132
exon 5, 159, 176

F
fadrazole, *140t*, 186
fibroblast growth factors, 113, 115
Fishman J, 51
follicle stimulating hormone (FSH), 4, 131
Fuqua SA, 176

G
Garcia T, 175
genistein, 76-78
glucocorticoids, 32, 82, 125
GnRH, 78
gonadotrophin(s), 5, 32, 77, 80, 82, 128-129, 136,
        186
    FSH, 78, 80
    LH, 78, 80
Guernsey, Island of, 45-46, 49, 67

H
H-*ras*, 20
Harris AL, 67
heat shock protein(s), 111
    HSP27, 68, 161-162
Henderson BE, 48
hormone replacement therapy, 69
Howell A, 155
Husbey RA, 30
hydroxyestrone
    2-, 51-52
    4-, 52
    16a-, 51-52
17-hydroxylase C17-20 lyase, 78, 80
hydroxylation
    2-, 8, 50-51
    16a-, 8, 50-51, 68
17β-hydroxysteroid dehydrogenase (EDH), 86-87,
        107
hyperestrogenaemia, 48
hyperestrogenization, 44
hyperplasia, 17, *18f*, 44, 68
hypophysectomy, 20, 65, 125, 127, 140, 153, *179t*,
        180

I
ICI164383, 135
ICI182780, 135, 185
inhibin, 80

insulin-like growth factor(s) (IGF), 27, 80, 113, 177,
        185
    -I, 27, 82, 113-116, 178
    -II, 114-116, 177-178
ionizing radiation, 16-17
isoflavones, 76-78

J
Jensen, 151
Jordan VC, 183

K
ketoconazole, 142
Klinefelter's syndrome, 44

L
Lachelin GCL, 96
LHRH agonists, 20, 65, 125, 128-132, 143, 154,
        199
luteinizing hormone (LH), 5

M
mastectomy, 20, 66, 105
MCF-7, 114-117, 135, *136f*, 160, 176, 182
McGarrigle HHG, 96
menarche, *36t*, 37, *47t*
menopause, 29-32, *36t*, *37t*, 132
menstrual cycle(s), 25, *28f*, 36-37, 96, 152
mestranol, 11
methoxyestrone
    -2, 66
milk, 95-97
mitogens, 176-179

N
[Na⁺]:[K⁺] ratio, 99-101
NADPH, 3
nipple aspirates, 95-98, 107
Northern blotting, 175

O
O-quinone, 52
obesity, 16, 40, *47t*, 48, *49t*, 63, 75
oophorectomy, 39, 126-127, 136-137, 180
Osborne CK, 182
osteoporosis, 39, 201
Ottman R, 63
ovariectomy, 20, 54, 65, 125-126, 153
    medical, 129, 132

P
p53, 20, 117, 185
pesticides, 11, 78, 199
Petrakis NL, 96

phytoestrogen(s), 11, 77*t*, 78*t*, 199
    coumestrol, 77
    daidzein, 11, 76-78
    equol, 77, 78*t*
    estradiol. *See* estradiol
    genistein, 76-78
Pike MC, 38
plasticizers, 199
platelet-derived growth factor (PDGF), 115
pLIVI, 161
Potts P, 197
pregnancy, 25, 32, 64
premarin, 39
progesterone, 37, 87-88, 152
    receptor(s), 158-160, 162, 174
        -negative cells, 158-159
        -positive cells, 87, 159, 176
progestins, 20, 28
progestogen(s), 37*t*, 38, 42, 142
prolactin, 113
pS2, 101, 160, 174
puberty, 25-27, 32, 198

R

Rochefort H, 116

S

Schinzengier, 125
Schon HJ, 99
sex hormone-binding globulin (SHBG), 7, 9*t*, 37,
    46, 48-51, 67
soya, 76-78
Symmers WS, 44
synthesis
    extraglandular, 75-76, 81-88, 179
    glandular, 75, 78-81

T

T47D, 114-115
tamoxifen, 77, 116, 131-137, 140, *153t*, 154, 160,
    173, 176, 179-186, 199. *See also* antiestrogen(s)
terminal-duct lobular units (TDLU), 17, 51, 198
    epithelium, 28
Terrenius, 151
Thomas LB, 30
tissue:plasma gradient, 103, 105
toiletries, 11, 78
transforming growth factor (TGF)
    α, 82, 113-116, 176-178
    β, 82, 113-116, 135, 177-178
tumor:plasma gradient, 104

V

vorazole

W

Wang DY, 67
Wolf DM, 183

Z

zinc, 111

Molecular Biology Intelligence Unit

Available and Upcoming Titles

- **Organellar Proton-ATPases**
  Nathan Nelson, Roche Institute of Molecular Biology

- **Interleukin-10**
  Jan DeVries and René de Waal Malefyt, DNAX

- **Collagen Gene Regulation in the Myocardium**
  M. Eghbali-Webb, Yale University

- **DNA and Nucleoprotein Structure In Vivo**
  Hanspeter Saluz and Karin Wiebauer, HK Institut-Jena and GenZentrum-Martinsried/Munich

- **G Protein-Coupled Receptors**
  Tiina Iismaa, Trevor Biden, John Shine, Garvan Institute-Sydney

- **Viroceptors, Virokines and Related Immune Modulators Encoded by DNA Viruses**
  Grant McFadden, University of Alberta

- **Bispecific Antibodies**
  Michael W. Fanger, Dartmouth Medical School

- **Drosophila Retrotransposons**
  Irina Arkhipova, Harvard University and Nataliya V. Lyubomirskaya, Engelhardt Institute of Molecular Biology-Moscow

- **The Molecular Clock in Mammals**
  Simon Easteal, Chris Collet, David Betty, Australian National University and CSIRO Division of Wildlife and Ecology

- **Wound Repair, Regeneration and Artificial Tissues**
  David L. Stocum, Indiana University-Purdue University

- **Pre-mRNA Processing**
  Angus I. Lamond, European Molecular Biology Laboratory

- **Intermediate Filament Structure**
  David A.D. Parry and Peter M. Steinert, Massey University-New Zealand and National Institutes of Health

- **Fetuin**
  K.M. Dziegielewska and W.M. Brown, University of Tasmania

- **Drosophila Genome Map: A Practical Guide**
  Daniel Hartl and Elena R. Lozovskaya, Harvard University

- **Mammalian Sex Chromosomes and Sex-Determining Genes**
  Jennifer A. Marshall-Graves and Andrew Sinclair, La Trobe University-Melbourne and Royal Children's Hospital-Melbourne

- **Regulation of Gene Expression in *E. coli***
  E.C.C. Lin, Harvard University

- **Muscarinic Acetylcholine Receptors**
  Jürgen Wess, National Institutes of Health

- **Regulation of Glucokinase in Liver Metabolism**
  Maria Luz Cardenas, CNRS-Laboratoire de Chimie Bactérienne-Marseille

- **Transcriptional Regulation of Interferon-γ**
  Ganes C. Sen and Richard Ransohoff, Cleveland Clinic

- **Fourier Transform Infrared Spectroscopy and Protein Structure**
  P.I. Haris and D. Chapman, Royal Free Hospital-London

- **Bone Formation and Repair: Cellular and Molecular Basis**
  Vicki Rosen and R. Scott Thies, Genetics Institute, Inc.-Cambridge

- **Mechanisms of DNA Repair**
  Jean-Michel Vos, University of North Carolina

- **Short Interspersed Elements: Complex Potential and Impact on the Host Genome**
  Richard J. Maraia, National Institutes of Health

- **Artificial Intelligence for Predicting Secondary Structure of Proteins**
  Xiru Zhang, Thinking Machines Corp-Cambridge

- **Growth Hormone, Prolactin and IGF-I as Lymphohemopoietic Cytokines**
  Elisabeth Hooghe-Peters and Robert Hooghe, Free University-Brussels

- **Human Hematopoiesis in SCID Mice**
  Maria-Grazia Roncarolo, Reiko Namikawa and Bruno Péault, DNA Research Institute

- **Membrane Proteases in Tissue Remodeling**
  Wen-Tien Chen, Georgetown University

- **Annexins**
  Barbara Seaton, Boston University

- **Retrotransposon Gene Therapy**
  Clague P. Hodgson, Creighton University

- **Polyamine Metabolism**
  Robert Casero Jr, Johns Hopkins University

- **Phosphatases in Cell Metabolism and Signal Transduction**
  Michael W. Crowder and John Vincent, Pennsylvania State University

- **Antifreeze Proteins: Properties and Functions**
  Boris Rubinsky, University of California-Berkeley

- **Intramolecular Chaperones and Protein Folding**
  Ujwal Shinde, UMDNJ

- **Thrombospondin**
  Jack Lawler and Jo Adams, Harvard University

- **Structure of Actin and Actin-Binding Proteins**
  Andreas Bremer, Duke University

- **Glucocorticoid Receptors in Leukemia Cells**
  Bahiru Gametchu, Medical College of Wisconsin

- **Signal Transduction Mechanisms in Cancer**
  Hans Grunicke, University of Innsbruck

- **Intracellular Protein Trafficking Defects in Human Disease**
  Nelson Yew, Genzyme Corporation

- **apoJ/Clusterin**
  Judith A.K. Harmony, University of Cincinnati

- **Phospholipid Transfer Proteins**
  Vytas Bankaitis, University of Alabama

- **Localized RNAs**
  Howard Lipschitz, California Institute of Technology

- **Modular Exchange Principles in Proteins**
  Laszlo Patthy, Institute of Enzymology-Budapest

- **Molecular Biology of Cardiac Development**
  Paul Barton, National Heart and Lung Institute-London

- **RANTES,** *Alan M. Krensky, Stanford University*

- **New Aspects of V(D)J Recombination**
  Stacy Ferguson and Craig Thompson, University of Chicago

Neuroscience Intelligence Unit

Available and Upcoming Titles

❐ Neurodegenerative Diseases and Mitochondrial Metabolism
M. Flint Beal, Harvard University

❐ Molecular and Cellular Mechanisms of Neostriatum
Marjorie A. Ariano and D. James Surmeier, Chicago Medical School

❐ Ca²⁺ Regulation By Ca²⁺-Binding Proteins in Neurodegenerative Disorders
Claus W. Heizmann and Katharina Braun, University of Zurich, Federal Institute for Neurobiology, Magdeburg

❐ Measuring Movement and Locomotion: From Invertebrates to Humans
Klaus-Peter Ossenkopp, Martin Kavaliers and Paul Sanberg, University of Western Ontario and University of South Florida

❐ Triple Repeats in Inherited Neurologic Disease
Henry Epstein, University of Texas-Houston

❐ Cholecystokinin and Anxiety
Jacques Bradwejn, McGill University

❐ Neurofilament Structure and Function
Gerry Shaw, University of Florida

❐ Molecular and Functional Biology of Neurotropic Factors
Karoly Nikolics, Genentech

❐ Prion-related Encephalopathies: Molecular Mechanisms
Gianluigi Forloni, Istituto di Ricerche Farmacologiche "Mario Negri"-Milan

❐ Neurotoxins and Ion Channels
Alan Harvey, A.J. Anderson and E.G. Rowan, University of Strathclyde

❐ Analysis and Modeling of the Mammalian Cortex
Malcolm P. Young, University of Oxford

❐ Free Radical Metabolism and Brain Dysfunction
Irène Ceballos-Picot, Hôpital Necker-Paris

❐ Molecular Mechanisms of the Action of Benzodiazepines
Adam Doble and Ian L. Martin, Rhône-Poulenc Rorer and University of Alberta

❐ Neurodevelopmental Hypothesis of Schizophrenia
John L. Waddington and Peter Buckley, Royal College of Surgeons-Ireland

❐ Synaptic Plasticity in the Retina
H.J. Wagner, Mustafa Djamgoz and Reto Weiler, University of Tübingen

❐ Non-classical Properties of Acetylcholine
Margaret Appleyard, Royal Free Hospital-London

❐ Molecular Mechanisms of Segmental Patterning in the Vertebrate Nervous System
David G. Wilkinson, National Institute of Medical Research-UK

❐ Molecular Character of Memory in the Prefrontal Cortex
Fraser Wilson, Yale University